Single-Cell Mutation Monitoring Systems

Methodologies and Applications

TOPICS IN CHEMICAL MUTAGENESIS

Series Editor: Frederick J. de Serres

National Institute of Environmental Health Sciences
Research Triangle Park, North Carolina

A Continuation Order Plan is available for this series. A continuation order will bring delivery of each new volume immediately upon publication. Volumes are billed only upon actual shipment. For further information please contact the publisher.

Single-Cell Mutation Monitoring Systems

Methodologies and Applications

Edited by

AFTAB A. ANSARI

Northrop Services, Inc.
Research Triangle Park, North Carolina

and

FREDERICK J. DE SERRES

National Institute of Environmental Health Sciences
Research Triangle Park, North Carolina

PLENUM PRESS • NEW YORK AND LONDON

Library of Congress Cataloging in Publication Data

Main entry under title:

Single-cell mutation monitoring sytems.

(Topics in chemical mutagenesis; v. 2)
Includes bibliographical references and index.
1. Mutagenicity testing. I. Ansari, Aftab A. II. de Serres, Frederick J. III. Title:
Mutation monitoring systems: methodologies and applications. IV. Series.
QH465.C5S56   1984   574.87′322   84-3368

ISBN 978-1-4684-4666-1   ISBN 978-1-4684-4664-7 (eBook)
DOI 10.1007/978-1-4684-4664-7

© 1984 Plenum Press, New York
Softcover reprint of the hardcover 1st edition 1984

A Division of Plenum Publishing Corporation
233 Spring Street, New York, N.Y. 10013

Contributors

RICHARD J. ALBERTINI, Department of Medicine, University of Vermont College of Medicine, Burlington, Vermont 05405

JAMES W. ALLEN, Genetic Toxicology Division, Health Effects Research Laboratory, U. S. Environmental Protection Agency, Research Triangle Park, North Carolina 27711

AFTAB A. ANSARI, Northrop Services, Inc., Research Triangle Park, North Carolina 27709

MASROOR A. BAIG, Laboratory of Genetics, National Institute of Environmental Health Sciences, Research Triangle Park, North Carolina 27709; *present address:* Department of Biochemistry, University of Kashmir, Hazratbal, Srinagar 190006, India

WILLIAM L. BIGBEE, Lawrence Livermore National Laboratory, Biomedical Sciences Division, University of California, Livermore, California 94550

ELBERT W. BRANSCOMB, Lawrence Livermore National Laboratory, Biomedical Sciences Division, University of California, Livermore, California 94550

MARTHA BRICE, Division of Medical Genetics, University of Medicine, University of Washington, Seattle, Washington 98195

KAREN BROCK, Northrop Services, Inc., Research Triangle Park, North Carolina 27709

JAMES CAMPBELL, Northrop Services, Inc., Research Triangle Park, North Carolina 27709

MARGARET FARQUHAR, Division of Medical Genetics, Department of Medicine, University of Washington, Seattle, Washington 98195

HOWARD G. GRATZNER, Institute for Cell Analysis, Department of Medicine, University of Miami School of Medicine, Miami, Florida 33124

ROBERT W. KAPP, Jr., East Laboratory, Bio/dynamics, Inc., East Millstone, New Jersey 08873

PHILIP C. KELLEHER, Department of Medicine, University of Vermont College of Medicine, Burlington, Vermont 05405

MARVIN S. LEGATOR, Division of Environmental Toxicology, Department of Preventive Medicine and Community Health, The University of Texas Medical Branch, Galveston, Texas 77550

DALE LINDSLEY, Division of Medical Genetics, Department of Medicine, University of Washington, Seattle, Washington 98195

BERNHARD E. MATTER, Sandoz Ltd., Preclinical Research, Toxicology, CH-4002 Basle, Switzerland

JON C. MIRSALIS, Cellular and Genetic Toxicology Department, SRI International, Menlo Park, California 94025

ANN D. MITCHELL, Cellular and Genetic Toxicology Department, SRI International, Menlo Park, California 94025

BETTY NAKAMOTO, Division of Medical Genetics, Department of Medicine, University of Washington, Seattle, Washington 98195

PETER NUTE, Department of Anthropology, University of Washington, Seattle, Washington 98195

THALIA PAPAYANNOPOULOU, Division of Hematology, Department of Medicine, University of Washington, Seattle, Washington 98195

R. JULIAN PRESTON, Biology Division, Oak Ridge National Laboratory, Oak Ridge, Tennessee 37830

ROBERT R. RACINE, Sandoz Ltd., Preclinical Research, Toxicology, CH-4002 Basle, Switzerland

MATTHEW D. SCHARFF, Department of Cell Biology, Albert Einstein College of Medicine, Bronx, New York 10461

YOUSUF SHARIEF, Northrop Services, Inc., Research Triangle Park, North Carolina 27709

GEORGE STAMATOYANNOPOULOS, Division of Medical Genetics, Department of Medicine, University of Washington, Seattle, Washington 98195

D. L. SYLWESTER, Biometry Facility, University of Vermont College of Medicine, Burlington, Vermont 05405

DONALD J. ZACK, Department of Cell Biology, Albert Einstein College of Medicine, Bronx, New York 10461

Preface

There is general agreement that increased environmental pollution poses a potential health hazard to humans and that effective control of such genetic injury requires monitoring the exposed individuals for genetic damage and identifying chemicals that may cause mutation or cancer. Tests available for identifying mutagens or carcinogens range from relatively simple, rapid assays in prokaryotes and test systems utilizing mammalian cells in tissue culture to highly elaborate tests in intact animals. No single test can provide data for an unequivocal assessment of the mutagenicity of a given chemical and the risk it might pose to human health. A tier approach, therefore, was suggested for mutagenicity testing in which the suspected agents would be initially evaluated with simple, inexpensive tests that would give qualitative results. Chemicals found to be positive in the first-tier testing would then be evaluated with more complex tests, including those based on mammalian cells in culture. Testing in the final tier requires whole-animal studies, and is expensive and time-consuming, and even the results from these studies need to be extrapolated for human risk assessment.

The mutation systems based on whole animals require scoring large numbers of animals, and therefore are not practical for the routine testing of mutagens. As an alternative to monitoring the pedigree, cells from exposed individuals may be considered for screening for point mutations through the use of an appropriate marker protein. The advantage of such a single-cell screening system (cell specific-locus test) would be that each cell, rather than each individual, could be examined for mutational events.

Single-cell mutation monitoring systems are the ones that detect mutational events in individual cells rather than whole animals. A few single-cell mammalian mutation systems have been developed and are in use in various laboratories. Several others are in various stages of development. The purpose of this book is to bring together such mutation detection methods. Special attention has been paid to include enough experimental details to allow easy adaptation of the techniques by different investigators. Each chapter is divided into sections comprised of experimental details and sample results.

Each chapter in this book describes a mutation monitoring system that uses one of the easily available cell samples from animals or humans, e.g., red blood cells, lymphocytes, and spermatozoa. The Chapters 1–3 and 9 describe methods based on the use of red blood cells. Six chapters describe methods that use lymphocytes. The last chapter is based on the use of spermatozoa.

Aftab A. Ansari
Frederick J. de Serres

Research Triangle Park, North Carolina

Contents

Chapter 2. Use of Fluorescence-Activated Cell Sorter for Screening Mutant Cells   37

WILLIAM L. BIGBEE AND ELBERT W. BRANSCOMB

Chapter 5. Application of Antibodies to 5-Bromodeoxyuridine for the Detection of Cells of Rare Genotype

HOWARD G. GRATZNER

Chapter 9. The Micronucleus Test as an Indicator of Mutagenic Exposure 217

ROBERT R. RACINE AND BERNHARD E. MATTER

Chapter 10. The Identification of Somatic Mutations in Immunoglobulin Expression and Structure 233

DONALD J. ZACK AND MATTHEW D. SCHARFF

**Chapter 11. Detection of Chemically Induced Y-Chromosomal
Nondisjunction in Human Spermatozoa**

MARVIN S. LEGATOR AND ROBERT W. KAPP, JR.

Single-Cell Mutation Monitoring Systems

Methodologies and Applications

Somatic-Cell Mutation Monitoring System Based on Human Hemoglobin Mutants

GEORGE STAMATOYANNOPOULOS, PETER NUTE,
DALE LINDSLEY, MARGARET FARQUHAR, MARTHA BRICE,
BETTY NAKAMOTO, AND THALIA PAPAYANNOPOULOU

1. INTRODUCTION

1.1. The Approach

The system described in this chapter was developed as a means of detecting rare red cells, in genetically normal (HbA/HbA) individuals, that are heterozygous for an abnormal hemoglobin. It is assumed, first, that mutations arise spontaneously in human hemopoietic stem cells, as they do in gametal stem cells, and second, that somatic mutations of globin-chain genes do not diminish the viability of affected stem cells. The latter assumption is a reasonable one, since phenotypic expression of such mutations occurs very late in hemopoietic cell differentiation. It is expected that as a result of these stem cell mutations, lines of stem cells containing the mutant globin genes are established and produce erythrocytes heterozygous for structurally abnormal globin chains. Development of appropriate methods of screening blood samples should then permit

GEORGE STAMATOYANNOPOULOS, DALE LINDSLEY, MARGARET FARQUHAR, MARTHA BRICE, AND BETTY NAKAMOTO • Division of Medical Genetics, Department of Medicine, University of Washington, Seattle, Washington 98195. THALIA PAPAYANNOPOULOU • Division of Hematology, Department of Medicine, University of Washington, Seattle, Washington 98195. PETER NUTE • Department of Anthropology, University of Washington, Seattle, Washington 98195.

detection and enumeration of red cells that contain an abnormal hemoglobin as a result of somatic mutation in a stem cell.

In principle, an efficient and sensitive method for detecting mutant erythrocytes in genetically normal persons would be of significant value to mutation research, since the study of but a few subjects would be required to assess mutagenic effects of various environmental agents. Similarly, the monitoring of populations for the effects of known mutagens would require longitudinal studies of only a few persons. Since the effects of mutagens on human subjects could be studied directly, the relevance of such studies to human health problems would be apparent. Questions concerning age- or sex-related differences in metabolism or the possibility of polymorphic variation in systems involved in biotransformation of mutagens could be investigated in studies of both populations and families. Finally, a system for scoring somatic mutants of hemoglobin in animal models could be used to correlate frequencies of somatic and gametal mutation.

1.2. Previous Studies

Detection of red cells bearing somatic mutations was first attempted by Atwood[1] and Atwood and Scheinberg.[2,3] They noted that a small proportion (about one in 10^3) of erythrocytes from subjects of blood type AB or A failed to carry the agglutinogen A. Such cells were originally regarded as somatic mutants. On these grounds, Atwood and Scheinberg[2] calculated a somatic mutation rate of 7×10^{-6} per cell division. The mutational origin of the abnormal red cells was subsequently tested by measuring the frequencies of non-A or non-B erythrocytes in AB heterozygotes and BB homozygotes.[4] If the abnormal cells were mutants, their frequency in BB homozygotes should have equaled the square of their frequency in AB heterozygotes. Although BB homozygotes had fewer abnormal cells than did the heterozygous subjects, the frequency of these cells was 50–200 times higher than expected. These findings suggested that it is unlikely that the absence of an A or B agglutinogen from a rare red cell represents the outcome of a somatic-cell mutation.

Sutton[5,6] attempted to relate the presence of red cells with the phenotype characteristic of hereditary persistence of fetal hemoglobin (HPFH; Section 2.2) to the occurrence of somatic mutations. This condition is associated with continuation of synthesis of fetal hemoglobin in all circulating red cells of adult carriers of the abnormal gene. Rare red cells (F cells) that contain fetal hemoglobin are also found in persons who are not carriers of an HPFH determinant. It was postulated that F cells were somatic mutants.[5,6] Results of studies, using sensitive methods, render this a highly unlikely possibility, since F cells constitute from 0.5% to 5.0% of the erythrocytes in every normal adult,[7,8] and their frequencies are elevated in various states, including anemias and hemopoietic malignancies. It is clear now that F cells in the normal adult are generated by mechanisms that are unrelated to somatic mutational events[9-13] and hence they are phenocopies of the HPFH mutation.

1.3. Requirements of a Red Cell Screening System

Methods based on screening of blood samples to detect erythrocytes that carry somatic mutations do not permit direct testing, by the criterion of transmission, of the mutational origin of phenotypically abnormal cells. Since genetic criteria cannot be used to distinguish between somatic mutants and their phenocopies, red cell abnormalities that can arise epigenetically cannot be employed as indicators of somatic cell mutation. For instance, tests that allow detection of an enzyme deficiency in a single red cell are expected to be unreliable; the activities of several enzymes decline with red cell aging and cellular phenotypes that mimic heterozygosity for an enzyme deficiency can be produced epigenetically. For example, there is a drastic decrease in the activity of glucose-6-phosphate dehydrogenase in senescent erythrocytes in normal persons, and glutathione reductase deficiency can appear upon reduction of the dietary supply of riboflavin.[14] If a microenvironmental influence produces a phenotype that mimics heterozygosity for an enzyme deficiency in a small proportion of erythroblasts or erythrocytes, these cells will be mistakenly identified as "somatic mutants" upon screening single cells for this deficiency. The same considerations hold when enzyme-dependent screening methods are applied to other types of differentiated cells. On the other hand, methods for detecting the presence, in individual cells, of specific, structurally abnormal proteins (e.g., abnormal hemoglobins) are unlikely to detect abnormalities that are produced epigenetically. Somatic mutants of structurally abnormal hemoglobins are, however, expected to appear much less frequently than protein deficiency mutants, since the latter can be produced by several types of mutational events.

2. THE HEMOGLOBIN MUTANTS

2.1. Hemoglobin Loci

Human globin chains are encoded by series of α-like and β-like genes. The α-like genes are located on chromosome 16,[15] and are arranged in the order $5'\text{-}\zeta2\text{-}\psi\zeta1\text{-}\psi\alpha1\text{-}\alpha2\text{-}\alpha1\text{-}3'$.[16-18] The coding portions of the $\alpha1$ and $\alpha2$ genes differ by only two nucleotide substitutions, neither of which changes the amino acid encoded.[19] The β-like genes are located on chromosome 11,[20] in the order $5'\text{-}\psi\beta2\text{-}\epsilon\text{-}{}^G\gamma\text{-}A_\gamma\text{-}\psi\beta1\text{-}\delta\text{-}\beta\text{-}3'$.[16,21] The $\psi\zeta1$, $\psi\alpha1$, $\psi\beta1$, and $\psi\beta2$ pseudogenes are not expressed. The 5' to 3' orientation of the genes in each cluster reflects the timing of their expression during ontogeny. The ζ and ϵ genes are active during yolk-sac erythropoiesis. The α genes are expressed during the fetal stage of erythropoiesis, and remain active throughout life. Of the β-like genes, $^G\gamma$ and $^A\gamma$ participate in the formation of fetal hemoglobin ($\alpha_2\gamma_2$). They are expressed predominantly during fetal life and in a small proportion of cells (F cells) in adults. The β chains are expressed at low levels in fetuses (in which they constitute about 5% of the non-α chains); their level increases around the perinatal period, when the switch from production of fetal to adult globin occurs. Switching is completed by the sixth month of life; thereafter HbA ($\alpha_2\beta_2$) predominates in normal subjects. The δ gene, whose period of activity matches that of the β gene, contributes only about 2.5% of the non-α chains in adults (HbA$_2$: $\alpha_2\delta_2$). In addition to these genetically determined hemoglobins, secondarily modified hemoglobins, such as HbA$_{1c}$ (in which the amino termini of the β chains are glycosylated), also exist in normal red cells.[22]

2.2. Types of Mutations

Mutations affecting the globin genes fall into three broad categories.

1. There are mutations, defined as thalassemias, that produce deficiencies in synthesis of one or more hemoglobin polypeptide chains. Deficiencies in α chains (α-thalassemias) are usually consequences of deletion of one (α-thalassemia-2) or both (α-thalassemia-1) α loci.[23] The α-thalassemias are common in several populations. For example, over 20% of individuals of African descent are heterozygous for α-thalassemia-2[24]; α-thalassemias are also common in persons of Mediterranean and Asian origin.[25,26]

The β-thalassemia syndromes derive from a variety of events (reviewed in Ref. 27): termination mutations,[28,29] frameshifts,[30] mutations at mRNA splicing sites,[31-33] mutations creating alternate splicing sites,[34-38] mutations at the promoter regions of β genes,[32,39] and deletions of significant portions of β genes.[40]

In the $\delta\beta$-thalassemias, there are deficiencies of both δ and β chains. This type of anomaly can be produced by a cross-over between δ and β genes that leads to a $\delta\beta$ fusion ("Lepore") gene[41,42] by deletions that start near the 5' end of the δ gene and include the β gene,[42-46] and by inversion of a portion of the β-like cluster that includes the $^A\gamma$ and δ genes.[47] Similarly, deletion of several β-like genes underlies the $\gamma\delta\beta$-thalassemias.[48,49]

2. Hereditary persistence of fetal hemoglobin is characterized by continuation of γ-chain synthesis in adults who are otherwise hematologically normal. Globin gene mapping distinguishes two general categories of HPFH: (a) the deletion mutants, in which various lengths of the flanking sequence between the $^A\gamma$ and δ genes, together with the δ and β genes, are removed[42,44,46,50-52]; (b) the nondeletion mutants,[51,53-58] which are, presumably, consequences of changes in regulatory sequences that reside in the β-globin gene complex.

3. Structurally abnormal hemoglobins generally arise, like many β-thalassemias, through replacements of single nucleotides. When the substitution compromises mRNA processing or transcription, or when it creates a codon that signals premature termination, a thalassemic phenotype is produced. If mRNA is not adversely affected, and if the substituted nucleotide both resides in an exon and changes a codon so that a new amino acid is specified, an abnormal hemoglobin is formed. The distinction, however, is not always this clear. For instance, HbE is the product of mutation in the translated codon $\beta26$; however, this nucleotide substitution creates a new mRNA splicing site and processing of β^E mRNA is adversely affected, resulting in deficient production of β^E chain.[59]

During the past 30 years, structural analyses of abnormal hemoglobins have resulted in characterization of nearly 350 different variants.[60] Structural variants of all chains save ζ and ϵ have been observed. The types of abnormalities observed to date are summarized in Table I. Though the majority of the variants contain single amino acid substitutions in α or β subunits, abnormal chains characterized by additions or deletions of one or several amino acids, shortened chains arising through generation of premature termination codons,

Table I

Types of Structural Abnormalities Found in Human Hemoglobins[a]

Type of abnormality	Number of different variants
Single amino acid substitutions in the:	
α Chain	97
β Chain	183
$^G\gamma$ Chain	7
$^A\gamma$ Chain	6
γ chain ($^G\gamma$ or $^A\gamma$ not specified)	4
δ Chain	10
$\delta\beta$ Fusion ("Lepore") variants	3
$\beta\delta$ Fusion ("anti-Lepore") variants	3
$\gamma\beta$ Fusion variant	1
β Chains with deletions	10
α-chain frameshift	1
β-Chain frameshifts	2
Elongated α chains (stop-code mutants)	3
Elongated α chain (insertion)	1
Shortened β chain (premature termination)	1
Chains with more than one amino acid substitution:	
α Chain	1
β Chains	4
Total	337

[a]Compiled from lists in Ref. 60.

elongated chains deriving from nucleotide substitutions in termination codons, and frameshift mutants arising by deletions or insertions of nucleotides have also been observed.

From a functional point of view, the abnormal hemoglobins can be placed into two categories: the functionally normal and the functionally abnormal hemoglobins.[61] The unstable hemoglobins constitute the major proportion of the latter category. In addition to producing clinical manifestations in heterozygotes, unstable mutants are characteristically present, in red cells, in smaller amounts than are stable variants. Stable β-chain mutants usually constitute 40% and stable α-chain mutants 20% of the hemoglobin in the red cells of heterozygotes, the difference being related to the presence of single β and duplicate α loci.

3. HEMOGLOBIN IN MUTATION RESEARCH: GAMETAL MUTATION RATES

With the exception of the studies by Neel on biochemically detectable *de novo* mutants[62,63] and of the estimates based on hemoglobin mutants, information on gametal mutation rates in humans has traditionally depended upon enumeration of clinically defined, autosomal-dominant (e.g., achondroplasia, neurofibromatosis, aniridia, etc.) or X-linked (e.g., hemophilias A and B, Duchenne muscular dystrophy, etc.) phenotypes (reviewed in Ref. 64). Hemoglobin variants have been used to estimate mutation rates using indirect and direct approaches.

3.1. Indirect Estimates

Motulsky[65] indirectly estimated rates of mutation per nucleotide from the frequency of rare hemoglobin variants among northern Europeans. Given the frequency x of a variant in a population and the proportion q of carriers with unaffected parents, Motulsky derived the relationship $\mu^n = xq/2$, where μ^n is the rate at which a particular nucleotide is replaced by another to effect the amino acid substitution in question. Assuming that the frequency of replacement is uniform over all nucleotides in the exons of α and β genes, the frequency of a given abnormal nucleotide in a population is $x = (2z/2)(1/n)$ $(1/c) = z/nc$, where z is the combined frequency of all variant hemoglobins in the population (roughly 0.0005 as estimated from electrophoretic screening), n is the approximate number of amino acids in a globin chain ($\sim$ 140), and c is the potential number of amino acid substitutions that could be effected by single-nucleotide substitutions in a codon (approximately seven).

Thus, the frequency of a specific abnormal allele in a large population is $x = 0.0005(1/140)(1/7) = 5 \times 10^{-7}$.

Estimating that about 1% of all people with hemoglobinopathic methemoglobinemia (which appears as an autosomal dominant condition) were born to unaffected parents, Motulsky calculated the rate at which any one of the five known variants of Hb M arises: $\mu^n = xq/2 = (5 \times 10^{-7})(1/2)(0.01) = 2.5 \times 10^{-9}$ per nucleotide per generation. If the proportion of affected subjects born to normal parents is 10%, the estimate increases to 2.5×10^{-8} per nucleotide per generation. These figures represent estimates of the rate of substitution of any nucleotide in the coding portion of an α-globin or β-globin gene, since it is assumed that the rate is the same over all sites. If we amend these results to account for the presence of duplicate alpha loci, each estimate is reduced by one-third, to 1.7×10^{-8} and 1.7×10^{-9} substitutions per nucleotide per generation.

Vogel and Rathenberg[64] applied Motulsky's approach to data collected in Japan by Kimura and Ohta.[66] They concluded that substitutions in globin genes occur at a rate of about 5×10^{-9} per nucleotide per generation.

3.2. Direct Estimates

Direct estimates of mutation rates[67–69] were obtained using data from 55 cases of *de novo* Hb mutation, of which 40 were unstable β-chain mutants, 10 methemoglobins with abnormal β chains, and five methemoglobins with abnormal α chains, all derived from substitutions of single nucleotides. These abnormalities produce autosomal-dominant disorders, and are expressed as chronic hemolytic anemia or methemoglobinemic cyanosis. Because ascertainment is clinical, abnormal electrophoretic mobility is not requisite to detection, and mutation rates need not be corrected to compensate for failure to detect electrophoretically silent variants. The 40 cases of unstable hemoglobin were observed among 464.8×10^6 live births, and 10 cases of β^M mutants appeared among 260.9×10^6 births, and the five cases of α^M mutants appeared among 189.7×10^6 births.

Assuming that the cases of *de novo* mutation producing an unstable hemoglobin disease were the only ones that arose in the populations in question, the rate of β-gene mutation producing unstable Hb disease ($n/2n$, where n is the number of cases and N is the number of births) is 4.3×10^{-8} per β gene per generation. Knowledge of the structural abnormality in each of these mutants allows calculation of the rate of mutation per β-gene nucleotide, $(n/2N)(3/x)$. The number x of *different* nucleotides substituted in the 40 cases of unstable Hb disease is 22. Thus, $(n/2N)(3/x) = 5.9 \times 10^{-9}$ per β-gene nucleotide per generation.

Similar calculations based on the frequency of *de novo* β^M mutants yielded mutation rates of 1.9 $\times$ 10^{-8} per β gene per generation, and 19 $\times$ 10^{-9} per β-gene nucleotide per generation.

Rates calculated using the five cases of HbM disease arising from α-gene mutation were calculated as described above, with the exception that $n/2N$ was replaced by $n/4N$ to reflect the presence of four α-globin genes per subject. Mutation rates for HbM disease resulting from α-gene mutation are 7 $\times$ 10^{-9} per α gene per generation, while the mutation rates per nucleotide per generation are 10 $\times$ 10^{-9}.

The above estimates of mutation rates per nucleotide per generation range from 5.9 $\times$ 10^{-9} to 19 $\times$ 10^{-9}. When the rate is calculated using all 50 cases of β-chain mutants, the result is 7.4 $\times$ 10^{-9} per β-gene nucleotide per generation.

4. A SYSTEM FOR DETECTING SOMATIC MUTATIONS OF HEMOGLOBIN

4.1. Appropriate Mutants

A procedure for detecting products of somatic mutation at globin-chain loci must permit unambiguous identification, in a genetically normal person, of individual erythrocytes that are heterozygous for such mutations. Though tremendous mutational heterogeneity exists at the globin-chain loci, mutants in most of the categories are not appropriate targets of such a detection system.

The β- and $\delta\beta$-thalassemias are, in general, not useful, since they are expressed in red cells as quantitative deficiencies of β- or β- and δ-globin chains. The same applies to the α-thalassemias, though a comment upon these conditions is in order.

In erythroid cells, α-chain deficiency is associated with a relative excess of β chains. In a compound heterozygote for α-thalassemia-1 and α-thalassemia-2 (HbH disease), there is but one active α gene.[23,25] The excess β chains associate in tetramers (Hbβ_4 = HbH), which form, upon incubation of red cells with brilliant cresyl blue, multiple intracellular inclusion bodies of characteristic appearance.[70,71] In heterozygotes for α-thalassemia-1, who have only two active α genes, the extra β chains may be proteolytically degraded in the early stages of erythroblast maturation; only rarely do red cells (ranging in frequency from 1 $\times$ 10^{-3} to 1 $\times$ 10^{-5}) appear with phenotypes typical of the doubly heterozygous cells (i.e., those appearing in HbH disease). The origin of these rare "HbH inclusion" cells in α-thalassemia-1 heterozygotes is unclear. Perhaps they are derived from rare erythroblasts in which proteolytic degradation of the β-chain excess failed to occur. Alternatively, some cells with this phenotype could represent products of somatic mutations that converted cells heterozygous for α-thalassemia-1 into compound heterozygotes for α-thalassemia-1 and α-thalassemia-2.

Cells containing HbH are extremely rarely (if ever) seen in persons who have α-thalassemia-2 (in whom only one of the four α genes is inactivated or deleted). It is thus possible that a test for "HbH cells" in persons with α-thalassemia-2 could be used to measure the frequencies of such cells and assess their value as markers of somatic mutations. In the past, such a test was not feasible, since the existence of an individual with α-thalassemia-2 (described in the older literature as the carrier of a silent α-thalassemia gene) was inferred only from the results of family studies. Now, however, α-thalassemia-2 heterozygotes (which, as mentioned in Section 2.2, are frequent in several populations) can be readily detected by gene mapping. Since microscopic detection of HbH-containing cells is relatively easy and several million red cells can be efficiently screened after incubation with brilliant cresyl blue, the idea of using "HbH inclusion" cells are markers of somatic α-gene deletions could be resurrected.

Mutations producing the erythrocytic phenotype of HPFH are generally inappropriate, primarily because the phenotype is produced very frequently by other means (e.g., in the F cells of normal adults). Both $^G\gamma$ and $^A\gamma$ chains appear in normal F cells. Certain forms of hereditary persistence of fetal hemoglobin are associated with continuation of synthesis of either the $^G\gamma$ or $^A\gamma$ type of γ chain.[25] Hence, somatic mutants producing an $^A\gamma$- or $^G\gamma$-HPFH phenotype can, in theory, be distinguished from normal F cells by the presence of only one of the two types of γ chain in the heterozygous mutant red cell. Early in our research we attempted, without success, to develop procedures for distinguishing cells containing one type of γ chain from cells with both.

The requirements (specified in Section 1.3) for a somatic-mutation screening system are best met by mutants of the hemoglobin genes that lead to production of structurally abnormal globin chains. An ideal system for detecting single red cells containing an abnormal hemoglobin would employ electrophoresis of the contents of single cells. Although single red-cell electrophoresis has been carried out,[72,73] currently available techniques do not meet the need to screen millions of cells efficiently. Thus, we chose to test the feasibility of immunochemical screening of red cells by developing antibodies against abnormal hemoglobins and then using fluorescent conjugates of these antibodies to detect mutant hemoglobins in individual erythrocytes.

4.2. Immunochemical Detection of Abnormal Hemoglobins in Single Cells

The approach developed is, in brief, as follows. Using the methods described in Section 5, a panel of anti-mutant Hb antibodies was produced.

After conjugation with fluorochromes (usually fluorescein isothiocyanate, FITC), the antibodies were used in direct immunofluorescent assays that permitted detection of abnormal hemoglobins in single cells. Since hemoglobin is an intracellular protein, coupling of the FITC–antibody with the mutant hemoglobin required prior fixation of red cells smeared on glass slides; fixation resulted in exposure of intraerythrocytic protein to the fluorescent antibody. Results of fluorescent labeling of red cells bearing abnormal hemoglobins appear in Figures 1 and 2.

The panel of monospecific antibodies produced included antibodies that detect specific amino acid substitutions resulting from single-nucleotide replacements (transitions or transversions) in the α and β genes (Table II). In addition, we have prepared antibodies specific for the abnormal structures of two human frameshift mutants, Hb Wayne (an α-gene frameshift) and Hb Cranston (a β-gene frameshift). These mutants were included in our study for the following reasons.

The α chains of Hb Wayne contain 146 amino acid residues,[78] in contrast to the 141 residues found in α chains of normal length. This abnormality is derived from deletion of a nucleotide from the codon specifying the amino acid

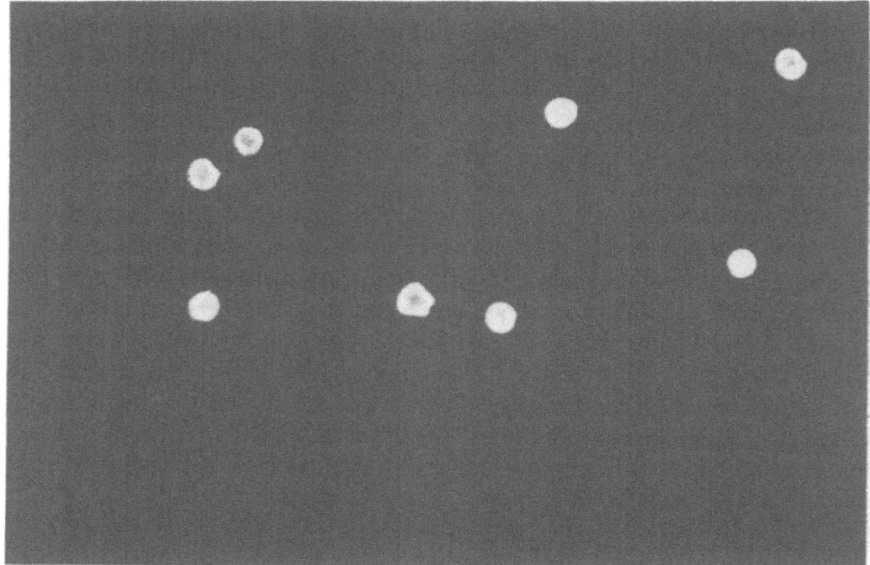

Figure 1. Microphotograph of an artificial mixture of AA and AS cells labeled with anti-HbS–FITC. The AS cells are labeled strongly, while the AA cells are barely seen over the background.

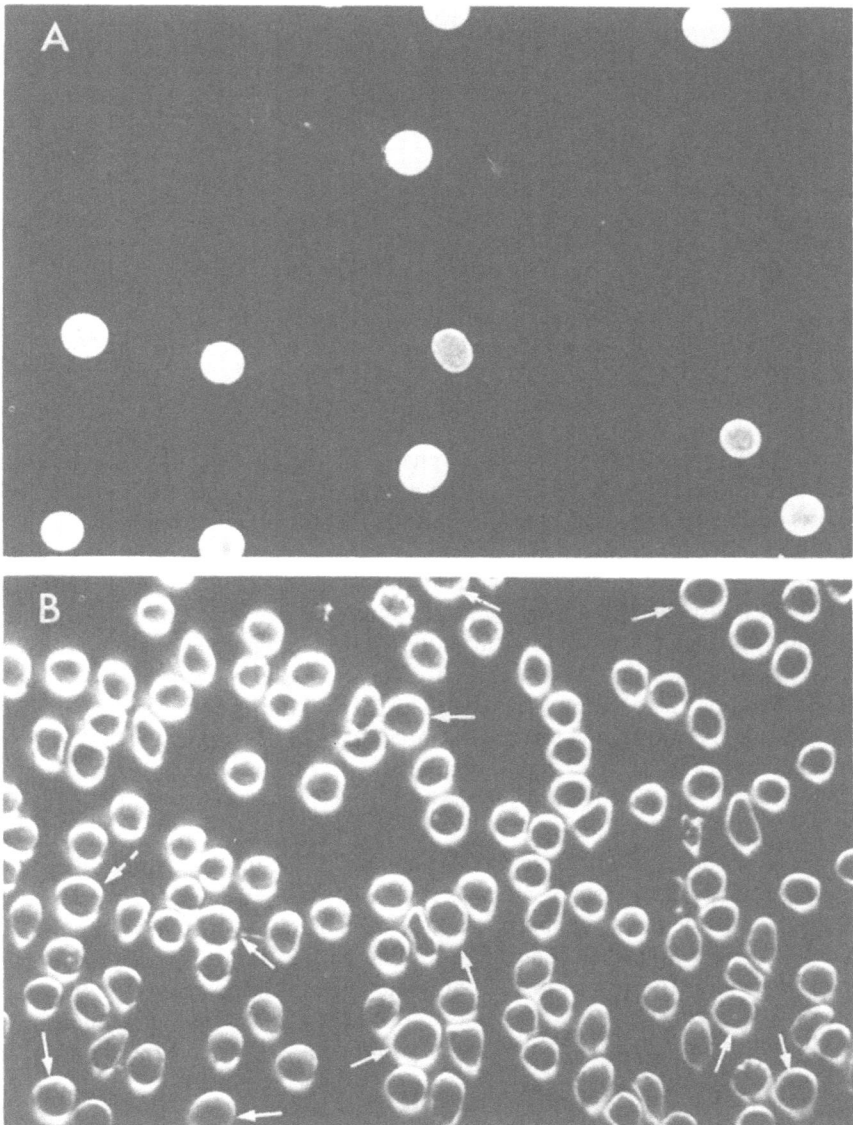

Figure 2. Microphotograph of an artificial mixture of A/Cranston and AA cells labeled with anti-Hb Cranston–FITC. (A) The preparation is viewed under the FITC-excitation beam. The Hb Cranston-containing cells fluoresce strongly. (B) The same preparation viewed under white light so that all the cells in the field are visible. Arrows point to the Hb Cranston-containing cells. (From Ref. 77, with permission.)

Table II

Abnormal Hemoglobins Recognized by Monospecific Antibodies Produced in Our Laboratory

Hemoglobin	Structural abnormality	Reference
S	$\beta 6$ Glu $\rightarrow$ Val	74
C	$\beta 6$ Glu $\rightarrow$ Lys	75
Hasharon	$\alpha 47$ Asp $\rightarrow$ His	76
Ottawa	$\alpha 15$ Gly $\rightarrow$ Arg	Unpublished
Q India	$\alpha 64$ Asp $\rightarrow$ His	Unpublished
Cranston	β Chain 157 residues long; abnormal sequence begins at $\beta 145$	77
Wayne	α Chain 146 residues long; abnormal sequence begins at $\alpha 139$	77

in position 138 or 139 of the normal chain. At the corresponding point in the coding position of the α^{Wayne} gene, the reading frame is shifted. Thus, in synthesis of α^{Wayne} chains, the normal sequence is constructed through residue 138 but new codons result in production of a novel sequence beyond that point; this sequence is terminated when, at reading frame 147, a new stop codon is reached. Antibodies that recognize the abnormal region of the α^{Wayne} chain should, in principle, also recognize the corresponding regions of α chains encoded by genes that have suffered deletion of one nucleotide or $3n + 1$ nucleotides on the 5' side of the codon specifying the residue in position 139. In each case, the carboxyl-terminal octapeptide will be identical in sequence to that found in Hb Wayne. In addition, insertions of two or $3n + 2$ nucleotides 5' to codon 139 would lead to synthesis of the same terminal sequence (Table III).

The β chains of Hb Cranston[79] contain 157 residues, 11 more than the normal β chain. The β^{Cranston} gene has sustained an insertion of two nucleotides on the 5' side of the codon specifying the amino acid residue at position 144. This leads to synthesis of a novel 13-residue carboxyl-terminal sequence that is recognized by the anti-Cranston antibodies. These antibodies should be capable of recognizing the tridecapeptide produced after deletion of one nucleotide (or $3n + 1$ nucleotides) or insertion of two (or $3n + 2$) nucleotides on the 5' side of coding site 144.

4.3. Detection of Rare Mutant Red Cells by Fluorescent Microscopy

Methods employing fluorescent labeling of cells are appropriate (as are other cytochemical procedures) for detecting relatively frequent events (i.e., those that occur at rates of from 10^{-2} to 10^{-4}). We intended to apply these methods to the detection of cells that were expected to arise much less fre-

Table III

Generation of the Novel α^Wyne Sequence by Various Insertions and Deletions Affecting an α-Globin Gene

Position in chain	135	136	137	138	139	140	141	142	143	144	145	146	147	148	149	150
α^A-Chain sequence	---Val	Leu	Thr	Ser	Lys	Tyr	Arg	Stop								
α^A-mRNA sequence	5'-GUG	CUG	ACC	UCC	AAA	UAC	CGU	UAA	CGU	GGA	GCC	UCG	GUA	GCA-3'		
α^Wyne mRNA sequence	5'-GUG	CUG	ACC	UCA	AAU	ACC	GUU	AAG	CUG	GAG	CCU	CGG	UAG	CA		
					↳ C or A deleted											
Delete 3n + 1, n = 1, bases[a]	5'-GUG	CCU	(CUG A deleted)	AAU	ACC	GUU	AAG	CUG	GAG	CCU	CGG	UAG	CA-			
		↳ CUG A deleted														
Insert 3n + 2, n = 1, bases[a]	5'-GUG	GGA	GCC	UGA	CCU	CCA	AAU	ACC	GUU	AAG	CUG	GAG	CCU	CGG	UAG	CA-
			↑ GGA GC inserted													
Underlined base sequences all encode the C-terminal octapeptide							---Asn	Thr	Val	Lys	Leu	Glu	Pro	Arg	Stop	

[a] Hypothetical example of deletion or insertion.

quently. The feasibility of detection of rare mutant red cells was tested by microscopic screening of artificial mixtures of normal and mutant erythrocytes labeled with the proper anti-mutant Hb fluorescent antibody.

For these experiments, suspensions of normal (AA) and mutant (AX, where X represents a particular abnormal hemoglobin) red cells were prepared and the number of cells per liter determined in a Coulter S electronic counter. Mixtures containing various proportions of AX and AA cells were prepared and smeared on slides, and the smears were fixed and coded. Fixed preparations that contained fairly homogeneous distributions of red cells (not too crowded, not too sparse) were selected and squares containing approximately 20,000–50,000 cells were marked. After exposing the preparations to FITC-conjugated, anti-mutant Hb antibody, all cells in the fields were viewed under white light. By using coverslips with grids that subdivided a labeled area into equal parts, and counting under white light all cells in a few subdivisions, the total number of cells contained in each field was calculated. The area was then viewed under the FITC-excitation beam and fluorescent cells were counted. The proportion of fluorescent cells observed among all cells was compared to the proportion expected from the dilution of the mutant red-cell suspension by the suspension of AA cells.

Figure 3 contains results of an experiment conducted using AS cells and anti-S labeling.[80] Results of similar tests using Hb Cranston-containing cells and anti-Hb Cranston antibodies or Hb Wayne-containing cells and anti-Hb Wayne antibodies[78] appear in Table IV. The excellent agreement between

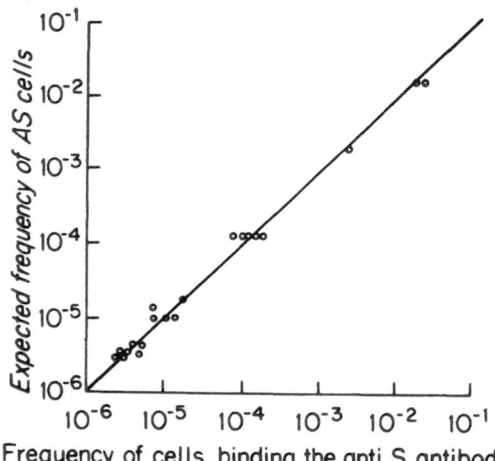

Figure 3. Correlation between observed and expected frequencies of AS cells in artificial mixtures of AA and AS cells labeled with anti-Hb S–FITC. (See text.)

Table IV

Observed and Expected Frequencies of Fluorescent Cells in Artificial Mixtures of A/A:A/Wayne Cells
Exposed to Anti-Hb Wayne–FITC and A/A:A/Cranston Cells Exposed to Anti-Hb Cranston–FITC

Antibody used		Observed fluorescent cells	Expected Hb Wayne cells	Expected Hb Cranston cells
Anti-Hb Wayne–FITC	A/A:A/Wayne cells	0.78×10^{-2}	0.81×10^{-2}	—
		0.99×10^{-2}	0.81×10^{-2}	—
		0.74×10^{-2}	0.81×10^{-2}	—
		1.21×10^{-3}	0.88×10^{-3}	—
		1.30×10^{-4}	0.88×10^{-4}	—
		0.82×10^{-5}	0.88×10^{-5}	—
		1.25×10^{-5}	0.88×10^{-5}	—
		0.75×10^{-5}	0.88×10^{-5}	—
Anti-Hb Cranston–FITC	A/A:A/Cranston cells	1.3×10^{-2}	—	1.3×10^{-2}
		1.5×10^{-3}	—	1.3×10^{-3}
		1.7×10^{-4}	—	1.2×10^{-4}
		1.3×10^{-5}	—	1.5×10^{-5}
		1.05×10^{-5}	—	1.5×10^{-5}
		1.32×10^{-5}	—	1.5×10^{-5}
		1.68×10^{-5}	—	1.5×10^{-5}
		1.26×10^{-5}	—	1.5×10^{-5}
		1.16×10^{-5}	—	1.5×10^{-5}
		1.79×10^{-5}	—	1.5×10^{-5}
		1.30×10^{-5}	—	1.5×10^{-5}
		1.46×10^{-5}	—	1.5×10^{-5}

expected and observed frequencies of fluorescent cells indicates that mutant cells can be detected even when present at frequencies as low as 1×10^{-5} to 1×10^{-6}. The typical mutant cell has a characteristically intense fluorescent labeling, as well as the morphology of an erythrocyte; thus, such cells are readily identified during the screening of artificial mixtures. Analyses of artificial mixtures also produced evidence that the frequency of a particular naturally occurring mutant cell does not exceed a value between one per 10^5 and one per 10^6 red cells. If the type of cell in question were present at a higher frequency, the proportion of labeled red cells would have exceeded that of abnormal cells originally introduced into several of the mixtures.

4.4. Screening for "S Cells" or "C Cells" in Blood of Genetically A/A Subjects

To test for the presence of cells with the immunochemical characteristics of mutant erythrocytes in normal individuals, we screened blood samples from males or females 20–35 years of age. A highly purified preparation of anti-HbS–FITC was used to label S cells. In a few instances, screening was done using a highly purified preparation of anti-HbC–FITC. Blood smears were fixed, and areas containing approximately 5×10^4 cells were exposed to the fluorescent antibody. These areas were screened under ultraviolet light using a method of overlapping fields, and labeled cells were counted. Several procedures were followed in verifying the erythrocytic nature of labeled cells, which we designate S-like and C-like erythrocytes.

Visual screening by one person of 10^8 red cells takes nearly 2 months. Blood samples from 15 healthy males and females were screened, and S-like or C-like cells were detected at frequencies ranging from 3×10^{-7} to 4×10^{-8} (mean 1.1×10^{-7}). We also conducted limited studies of persons exposed to mutagenic agents. Five subjects who received X-irradiation (dosage unknown) of the spine during treatment of ankylosing spondylitis had slightly elevated frequencies of S-like cells (mean 1.7×10^{-7}; range 3.1×10^{-7} to slightly less than 1×10^{-7}); these values were well within the range of frequencies of such cells in untreated subjects. Similarly, levels of S-like cells were measured in five patients who had received combinations of X-ray and chemotherapeutic treatment of Hodgkin's disease 2–5 years prior to screening. Levels of S-like cells in four of them fell within the upper portion of the range for untreated subjects, while the frequency of such cells in the fifth subject was the highest we have yet encountered (5×10^{-7}). Red cells from a woman who had received roughly 100 rad of total-body irradiation in the course of therapeutic treatment were also screened, as were erythrocytes from her untreated identical twin. The frequency of S-like cells in the irradiated subject (2.0×10^{-7}) fell within the range established for the controls, but it was twice the frequency (1.1×10^{-7}) found in her sister. These results suggest that red cells with the characteristics of mutant erythrocytes that contain either HbS or HbC exist at very low frequencies in genetically normal individuals.

In these studies, efforts were made to eliminate sources of artifacts that might otherwise result in mistakenly identifying cells as containing an abnormal hemoglobin. The erythrocytic identity of each labeled cell was checked cytochemically. The possibility that a fluorescent red cell nonspecifically bound the anti-mutant Hb antibody was assessed by exposing the fluorescent cell to a second antibody, of different specificity, to which was coupled a different fluorochrome. For instance, when an S-like cell was detected in a preparation labeled with anti-HbS–FITC, coordinates of the microscopic field were recorded so that the "S cell" could be found later. The preparation was then counterlabeled with an anti-HbC antibody conjugated with tetramethyl rhodamine isothiocyanate. Failure of the anti-HbC antibody to bind to the S-like cell suggested that labeling by the anti-HbS antibody was a specific phenomenon. The possibility that rare erythrocytes were nonspecifically binding FITC-conjugated antibodies were further tested as follows. Blood smears were stained with anti-IgG–FITC and from 2×10^7 to 5×10^7 cells from each of several subjects were screened. We observed no cells that fluoresced as intensely as did AS cells when labeled with anti-HbS–FITC antibodies or AC cells when labeled with anti-HbC–FITC. In addition, microcytofluorometric analysis permitted designation as mutants only those cells that were as intensely labeled as S cells or C cells from AS or AC heterozygotes. In spite of these precautions, the possibility remains that the cells we presume are mutants are, in fact, rare artifacts. Proof of mutational origin of the hemoglobin in these cells will require biochemical analysis of the globin chains from large numbers of labeled erythrocytes isolated by the cell sorter.

Detection and enumeration of these cells required tremendous expenditures of time and effort, and automated screening procedures were judged desirable. Such procedures were developed in collaboration with investigators at the Lawrence Livermore Laboratory. Methods of labeling, with fluorescent antibodies, mutant red cells in suspension permitted screening of large numbers of red cells with a cell sorter.[81] Cells that bound fluorescent anti-HbS or anti-HbC antibodies appeared at frequencies of about 1×10^{-7}.[81]

4.5. Minimum Frequencies of Somatic Mutations at Globin-Chain Loci

The observations made to date are of value in estimating the minimal frequency at which red cells containing specific abnormal hemoglobins are likely to be found in genetically HbA/HbA subjects.[82] In normal individuals, the frequencies of cells containing a particular mutant cannot exceed 1×10^{-6} because labeled cells are not found at that or higher frequencies. "Signals" appear when levels approximating 10^7 cells are approached. In spite of our current uncertainty about the origin of these signals, there is an upper limit on the frequencies of cells that contain a particular point mutation at the β-globin locus: in normal subjects, such cells do not appear at frequencies in excess of some value between 1×10^{-6} and 1×10^{-7}.

Taking 1×10^{-7} as the upper limit for the frequency of mutant cells that contain a particular abnormal globin chain, one can compute the frequency of all erythrocytes containing products of any of the 1314 different nucleotide substitutions that could arise in the β-gene exons. This overall frequency should not exceed 1.3×10^{-4}. If 12–17% of these nucleotide substitutions lead to production of electrophoretically discernible variants, the upper limit on the combined frequencies of all erythrocytes, from normal subjects, that bear electrophoretically detectable β-chain variants falls between 1.6×10^{-5} and 2.2×10^{-5}.

4.6. Relationship between Somatic Mutation Frequencies and Gametal Mutation Rates

The minimum frequency of electrophoretically detectable somatic mutants of β chains given above (between 1.6×10^{-5} and 2.2×10^{-5}) should be compared to the minimum rate of all possible electrophoretically detectable β-chain variants produced by gametal mutation. The latter can be calculated from the nucleotide mutation rate (7.4×10^{-9} given in Section 3.2), and ranges from 1.16×10^{-6} to 1.65×10^{-6}. The minimum somatic-cell frequency over all of the 1314 different nucleotide substitutions that could arise in β-gene exons is 1.3×10^{-4}, while the corresponding minimum gametal rate is 0.97×10^{-5}. According to these estimates, somatic rates exceed gametal rates by at least one order of magnitude.

The relationship between gametal and somatic mutation rates is unclear, given the several uncertainties of how frequencies of abnormal cells in a cell population are related to the rates at which the mutations themselves arise. Vogel and Rathenberg[64] reviewed the evidence for a difference in mutation rates between sexes and were inclined to attribute the disparity to differences in proliferative histories of the male and female gonadal cells. Higher gametal mutation rates in males could be related to intense proliferation of male gonadal stem cells during the years of active spermatogenesis. This rationale has also been applied to account for the well-known effect of paternal age on the occurrence of autosomal-dominant mutations in humans. If accumulation of mutations relates to proliferative behavior of a tissue, one would expect to find mutant cells at much higher frequencies among mature erythrocytes than among gametes, because continuous proliferation and self-renewal occur in the hematopoietic compartments from the time of appearance of the cells assigned to hematopoiesis in the embryo.

A more sophisticated treatment of the problem is currently unwarranted for several reasons. We do not know the actual proliferative potential of a stem cell (whether it is a hemopoietic pluripotent stem cell or a primitive spermatogonium). It may be "unlimited" (as presumed in previous hypotheses) or limited to a preprogrammed, maximum number of divisions (e.g., 20–50) inherently characteristic of normal cells (as contrasted to neoplastic cells). Hematopoiesis can be sustained throughout life given the latter of the above two assumptions, provided that, in the developing animal, the pluripotent stem-cell pool is of large size. Furthermore, in hematopoiesis a very large number of terminal cells can be produced through the expansion of the compartment of committed stem cells. The actual number of proliferative divisions a committed cell undergoes remains, however, speculative. In recent years, evidence has accumulated, through application of *in vitro* clonal methods, that committed cells may have more than one potentiality (bipotent, tripotent, or multipotent progenitors); the capacity for self-renewal of these early committed progenitors remains unknown. In view of these gaps in our knowledge, more detailed comparisons of frequency of somatic mutations in blood with rates of gametal mutation cannot be made.

4.7. Relationship between Frequencies of Somatic-Cell Mutants and Compartments in Which Mutations Occur

Mutant cells will arise in each of the hematopoietic compartments:

1. In the primitive, pluripotent stem-cell pool; mutants that do not affect proliferative capacity may persist for life; depending on the time during ontogeny that these mutations occur, they will form mutant-cell lines of various sizes.
2. In the compartment of early multipotent, but committed, stem cells; such mutants are expected to have a limited capacity for self-renewal.
3. In progenitor cells committed to erythropoiesis (erythroid stem cells).
4. In the morphologically recognizable compartment of erythropoiesis (i.e., the erythroblasts).

Mutations in compartments 2–4 are expected to produce only transient elevations in frequencies of abnormal circulating erythrocytes.

The frequency of mutant red cells in blood should represent a composite of mutations accumulated in the primitive, pluripotent stem-cell compartment and of those added in compartments 2–4. At present, it is impossible to predict how the mutant red-cell frequency will be determined. We have previously presented calculations illustrating this point.[80,82] In brief, if the number of primitive, pluripotent stem cells daily leaving the pluripotent stem-cell pool is large (e.g., in the range of 10^6–10^7, an unreasonably high number), and the rate of renewal of the cells in the pool is high (e.g., 1–10% of the cells of the pool go into cycle at a given time, again an unreasonable assumption), the frequency of mutant cells in the blood will reflect primarily those mutational events occurring among primitive, pluripotent stem cells. If, on the other hand, only a small number of pluripotent stem cells (not more than a few thousand) become committed per day, the frequency of mutant red cells in the blood will depend largely upon the number of mutational events occurring in the committed stem cells and their progeny.

The question of what the frequencies of mutant cells in the blood do represent *vis-à-vis* mutations in the hemopoietic cell pools is not a strictly theoretical one, since it bears upon the types of effects environmental mutagens produce on frequencies of abnormal erythrocytes. Given frequent stem-cell commitment and relatively frequent dividing of pluripotent stem cells, environmental mutagens will produce detectable changes in frequencies when they act either early in life, continuously throughout life, or in ways that increase mutation rates severalfold over spontaneous mutation rates. If stem cell commitment is infrequent, the main effect of environmental mutagens will be a transient increase in the frequency of mutant cells in the blood. Hence, in a person exposed to a mutagen inducing HbS or HbC mutations, there will be a rise of mutant S cells or C cells in the blood for a few weeks following exposure (i.e., until the committed stem cells present at the time of exposure are exhausted). At present, an answer to the question can be obtained only empirically with either longitudinal studies of persons acutely exposed to mutagens or, better, studies of mutagenesis in experimental animals.

5. METHODOLOGICAL ASPECTS: MONOSPECIFIC ANTI-MUTANT-HEMOGLOBIN ANTIBODIES

Antibodies specific for normal hemoglobin chains of several species have been described[7,8,83-92] and used in studies of hemoglobin switching during development. Antibodies specific for abnormal human hemoglobins have been produced by several investigators.[73-77,93-101] In these studies a variety of methods has been used for antibody production. The methods described here yield the large quantities of monospecific antibodies required for single-cell screening by immunofluorescence. Screening for mutant red cells in blood samples from normal subjects requires exposure of large numbers of fixed red-cell preparations to FITC–antibody. About 1 mg of pure anti-mutant Hb antibody is consumed during the screening of 10^7 red cells. The study of large numbers of cells from several individuals demands availability of considerable amounts of monospecific antibodies. Since hemoglobin is a poor antigen and only a small fraction of the antibody in the serum of an immunized animal is mutant-specific, large quantities of sera must be processed in order to obtain the necessary amount of an anti-mutant Hb antibody.

5.1. Immunizations

Immunizations[74-77] are carried out using abnormal hemoglobins purified by ion exchange chromatography.[102,103] The animal (a goat or a horse) is initially injected with 10 mg of the pure antigen emulsified with 4 ml of complete Freund's adjuvant, 2.5 mg of antigen being injected intramuscularly at each of four sites. After 2 and 4 weeks, the animal is given 20 mg of antigen (5 mg at each of four sites) emulsified with 4 ml of incomplete Freund's adjuvant. Sera are first collected 35–40 days following initiation of the immunization schedule. Booster injections (12 mg of antigen in 2 ml of incomplete Freund's adjuvant) are given at about 60 and 90 days. Sera are stored at $-70°C$.

5.2. Sepharose–Hb

Sepharose–mutant Hb complexes are prepared using purified abnormal Hb. Sepharose–normal Hb complexes contain HbA and the normal minor hemoglobins A_2, A_3, and F. Though the abnormal hemoglobins used as antigens are chromatographically pure, minor hemoglobins could contaminate the preparations. If antibodies against these minor hemoglobins are not removed, their presence in the final antibody preparation will result in nonspecific labeling of red cells.

Sepharose is activated[104] by the addition of a freshly prepared aqueous solution of cyanogen bromide (70 mg of CNBr per ml of packed Sepharose) and coupled with hemoglobin (7–8 mg per ml of packed activated Sepharose). After masking unoccupied sites with glycine, the Sepharose–Hb is poured into a funnel and washed extensively with 0.2 M boric acid, 0.15 M in NaCl, pH 8.0. Subsequently the Sepharose–Hb preparation is washed with cold, CO_2-saturated water. At this step, hemoglobin appears in the eluate. Washing of Sepharose–Hb with CO_2–H_2O continues until no trace of unbound hemoglobin is detected in the wash (as judged by comparing the optical density at 415 nm of the wash with that of distilled water). Hemoglobin eluted from the Sepharose–Hb column presumably derives from tetramers, not all subunits of which are attached covalently to Sepharose; treatment with CO_2-saturated water is expected to dissociate noncovalently bound subunits that are linked, through hydrophobic interactions, to the covalently bound subunits.

The Sepharose–mutant Hb complexes are subsequently washed with glycine-containing buffer and borate buffer, and, following addition of 0.02% (w/v) sodium azide, they are stored at 4°C; they can be used after several months in storage.

5.3. Purification

To remove antibodies reactive with hemoglobins A, A_2, and F, the serum is absorbed against Sepharose–normal Hb using one of two approaches. Either it is passed at 4°C through a 5.5 × 45.0 cm column of Sepharose–normal Hb at a flow rate of 15–20 ml/hr, or aliquots of serum are mixed with Sepharose–normal Hb and stirred for 48 hr at 4°C. Choice of the column or the batch method depends on the volume of serum to be processed.

Binding of the anti-mutant Hb antibody to Sepharose–mutant Hb is achieved either by passing the serum, at 4°C, through a 2.5 × 30 cm Sepharose–mutant Hb column at a flow rate of 10 ml/hr, or mixing it with Sepharose–mutant Hb and stirring for 48 hr at 4°C. The procedure is then repeated. The Sepharose–mutant Hb preparation is subsequently placed on a funnel and washed extensively with borate buffer until protein ceases to appear in the eluate (as determined optically at 280 nm).

Antibodies bound to Sepharose–mutant Hb are dissociated by developing the Sepharose–mutant Hb columns with cold CO_2–H_2O (pH 3.9–4.0) at a flow rate of 15 ml/hr. Elution profiles are monitored by measuring optical densities at 280 and 415 nm. Fractions corresponding to the protein-containing peaks are pooled, concentrated to 10–20 ml, and dialyzed against distilled water.

In spite of the pretreatment of Sepharose–mutant Hb preparations with CO_2-saturated water, small amounts of hemoglobin consistently contaminate the antibody fractions eluted from these columns. The contaminants are removed as described by Tozer *et al.*[105] A pool of protein-bearing fractions is dialyzed against cold CO_2–H_2O and applied to a 5 × 20 cm column of CM-cellulose (Whatman CM-52) equlibrated with cold CO_2–H_2O. Development at 4°C with 0.05 M $NaHCO_3$ yields a single peak of antibody; the hemoglobin

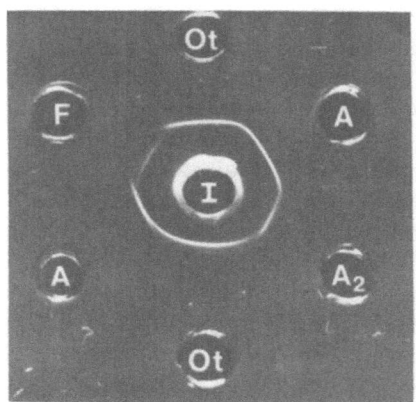
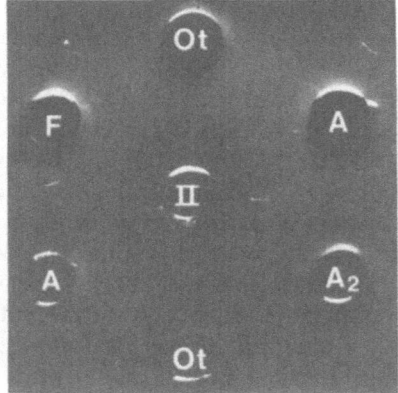
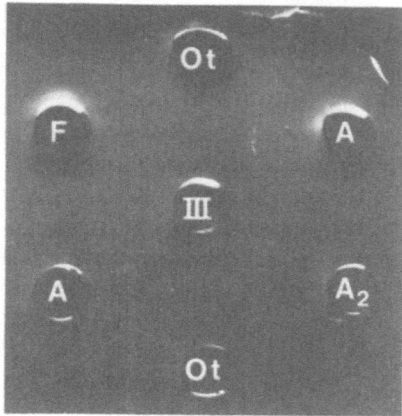

Figure 4. Double immunodiffusions using anti-Hb Ottawa antibodies. The central well contains: (I) the original serum from the horse immunized with Hb Ottawa, (II) the serum after absorption against Sepharose–normal Hb, (III) the purified antibody preparation. Note the absence of precipitation lines in II and III.

remains on the column. The antibody is recovered from solution by lyophilization after dialysis against water.

The anti-mutant Hb antibodies are nonprecipitating (Figure 4). Over 96% of the preparation recovered from the CM-cellulose colmn is IgG.[74] For conjugation with the fluorochrome,[106] 10 mg of purified antibody is reacted with FITC; unbound FITC is removed by gel filtration in a column of Sephadex G-25, and fractions showing an FITC/protein optical density ratio of 1.0 are stored at $-70°$C.

5.4. Red Cell Labeling

Smears from blood drawn in EDTA are covered with acetone–methanol (1:9, v/v) or with 100% methanol for 5–10 min, washed with phosphate-buffered saline (PBS), then with distilled water, and air-dried.[7,107] Areas with satisfactory distributions of erythrocytes are marked, covered with 5–10 μl of conjugated antibody (usually diluted 1:5 with PBS and 1% albumin) and incubated for 30–50 min in a humidified chamber at 37°C. Excess antibody is removed by washing the smears with PBS and distilled water. After air-drying, the smears are ready for examination.

Red cell labeling with FITC-conjugated antibody is used in judging if an anti-mutant Hb antibody is qualitatively adequate for mutant cell labeling and if it contains cross-reactive components. Three sets of smears are prepared: one from normal red cells, one from mutant red cells, and one from a 1:10 mixture of mutant and normal red cells. The presence of nonspecific labeling is readily apparent upon examination of the preparation of normal cells and the mixture of mutant and normal cells. To remove the cross-reacting antibodies the FITC-conjugated antibody is absorbed against Sepharose–normal Hb. After concentration by vacuum dialysis, the FITC–antibody is tested again for presence of cross-reactivities.

Highly intense labeling of mutant red cells and very faint background fluorescence of normal cells is obtained only with antibody preparations that have been absorbed repeatedly against Sepharose–normal Hb before and after FITC conjugation. The intensity of red cell labeling can be measured cytofluorometrically. The fluorescent intensity (FI) of a cell is recorded, and background fluorescence (measured in a cell-free area of the field) is subtracted from the cell's FI. Measurements of the FI of 100–200 cells allow construction of FI distribution curves. With qualitatively good antibody preparations, the FI values of mutant cells are at least 10–20 times higher than those of control cells.

The minimum amount of Hb per cell required for labeling by a fluorescent anti-Hb antibody has not been determined. That the method is very sensitive is suggested by the labeling of Hb Wayne-containing red cells with FITC-conjugated, anti-Hb Wayne antibodies. Hemoglobin Wayne constitutes 1–2% of the total Hb in red cells of heterozygotes. Given an MCH of 30 pg, the labeling of all cells from heterozygotes indicates that the anti-Hb Wayne antibodies are effective in detecting cells that contain as little as 0.15–0.3 pg of the mutant hemoglobin.

6. METHODOLOGICAL ASPECTS: MONOCLONAL ANTI-GLOBIN-CHAIN ANTIBODIES

Monoclonal anti-mutant Hb antibodies are expected to be especially useful for single-cell recognition by immunofluorescence. Production of specific anti-HbC, anti-HbS, or anti-Hb Wayne monoclonal antibodies was attempted, but no such antibodies were obtained. Several monoclonal antibodies specific for normal globin chains have been produced in this laboratory.[108] They are described here because monoclonal antibodies against normal human globin chains could be used in studies of somatic-cell mutations in animals.[109] Previously described methods[110,111] were employed in the production of these antibodies. Since the description of methods such as fusion, culture, subcloning, production of tumors in mice, and purification of antibodies from ascites fluids can be found in several texts,[112,113] only methodological aspects of relevance to the anti-globin-chain monoclonal antibodies are presented here.

6.1. Immunizations

To determine which mouse strain responds best to hemoglobin immunizations, groups of BALB/c, SJL, DBA, and AJ mice were immunized and the number of responders and antibody titers in each responder were monitored. The best responding strain was SJL, while BALB/c, the strain from which the myeloma line NS-1 is derived, showed poor response to Hb immunizations.

SJL mice are injected intraperitoneally with 200 μg of hemoglobin in complete Freund's adjuvant. Two weeks later they are injected with 100 μg of hemoglobin in incomplete Freund's adjuvant. Serum antibody titers are tested 7–10 days after the second injection. One month later, animals producing the highest immune responses are given a final intraperitoneal (IP) injection (50 μg of antigen in saline) 3–4 days before preparation of spleen-cell suspensions.

6.2. Screening

After fusion, the NS-1 × SJL hybrid cells are grown in Costar 96-well microtiter plates and the supernates are screened to detect wells containing anti-Hb antibody-producing hybrid cells. Cells from positive wells of these master plates are minicloned by plating 5–15 cells per well; positive miniclones are cloned by limiting dilution (primary clones) and positive primary clones are subcloned. Cells from stable secondary clones are injected (IP) into pristane-primed F_1 hybrids from SJL × BALB/c crosses.

An iodinated protein A (IPA) assay[108] using 96-well microtiter plates is used to screen clones. Each well is coated with a layer of Hb by adding 50 μl per well of a solution of hemoglobin (20 μg/ml in PBS) and incubating for 18 hr at 37°C. Unbound Hb is removed by aspiration. To block those sites in the wells that are not covered by hemoglobin, gelatin (1% in PBS) is added and the plates are incubated for 2 hr at 37°C. Subsequently, 50 μl of culture supernate is added and incubated at 37°C for 1 hr. At this stage, anti-Hb antibodies present in a culture supernate bind to the Hb molecules coating the wells. Following this incubation the culture supernates are aspirated, the wells are rinsed with 0.25% gelatin in PBS, and 50 μl of ^{125}I-labeled protein A [(1–2) × 10^5 counts per well] is added and the plates are incubated for 1 hr at 37°C. The wells are subsequently rinsed with PBS and air-dried, and the microtiter plates are processed for autoradiography. Wells containing Hb–Ab complexes bind IPA and on autoradiography produce black spots, while wells without Hb–Ab complexes fail to bind IPA and hence fail to produce spots on the film.

The assay described above (direct assay) detects IgG_{2a} and IgG_{2b} antibodies that bind protein A efficiently. Following the incubation with culture supernate, IgG_1 and IgG_3 antibodies are detected by incubation with the IgG fraction of rabbit anti-mouse IgG (indirect assay); this second antibody binds to the primary Ab–Hb complexes and provides the sites for binding of IPA. The other steps of the procedure remain the same. The direct or indirect method is used to monitor presence of anti-globin antibodies in sera from immunized animals, culture supernates, or ascites fluids, or in the fractions obtained from the elution of a protein A column.

Hemoglobin tetramers, solubilized globin chains, PMB-bound chains isolated after binding of p-hydroxymercuribenzoate to sulfhydryl groups, or globin-chain peptides can be used as antigen in these assays. Globin chains (1 mg/ml) are dissolved in 20% formic acid; this solution is diluted in 2% formic acid and used for coating the microwells. After incubation, the solution is aspirated and residual formic acid washed from the wells with PBS before addition of the blocking solution (1% gelatin).

6.3. Semiquantitative Assessment of Ab–Hb Binding

Characterization of the anti-globin-chain monoclonal antibodies is based on a semiquantitative assay conducted using antibodies purified by protein A column chromatography. Reactions are carried out as in the screening method,

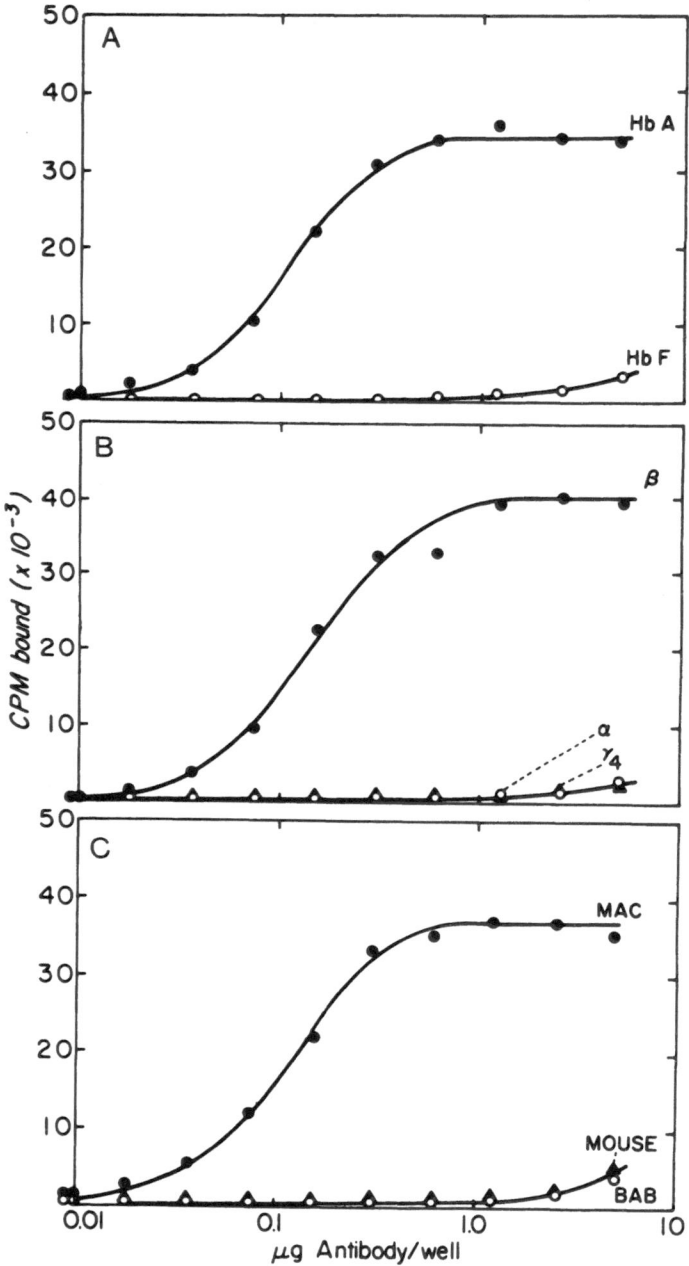

Figure 5. Binding of monoclonal antibody 16-2 (an anti-β-chain monoclonal) to various hemoglobins and globin chains. MAC, macaque Hb A; BAB, baboon Hb A.

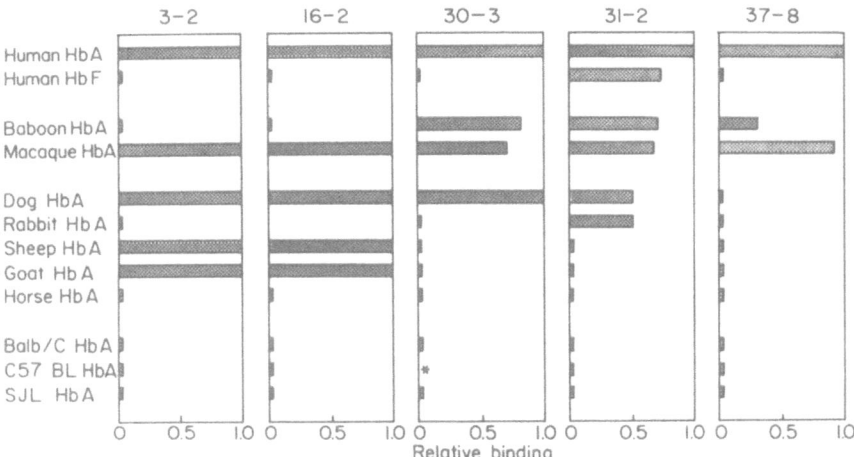

Figure 6. Binding of anti-adult human globin monoclonals to hemoglobins of various species. Relative binding is determined from the midpoints of binding curves such as those in Figure 5, using the binding of antibody to Hb A as a standard. (From Ref. 108 with permission.)

but instead of processing the microtiter plates for autoradiography, the ^{125}I bound in each well is eluted (by adding 150 μl of 2 M NaOH per well and incubating at 37°C for 2 hr) and counted in a gamma counter.[108] The Hb–Ab binding is quantitated by titrating the hemoglobin used for coating of the microwells and adding to each well identical amounts of antibody and ^{125}I-protein A counts. With some monoclonal antibodies this procedure yields high backgrounds and nonspecific binding. These problems are circumvented by applying identical amounts of antigen (1 μg/well), followed by various concentrations of antibody (antibody titration), and a constant amount of ^{125}I-protein A counts (Figure 5). For comparative purposes, findings can be expressed as percent binding (explained in the legend to Figure 6).

6.4. Mapping the Sites of Ab–Hb Binding

A summary of reactivities of anti-β-chain monoclonal antibodies with hemoglobins from various species is provided in Figure 6. The reactions with hemoglobins and globin chains of various species distinguish among antibodies that recognize different antigenic sites in a globin chain. In addition, these reactions permit deductions about the structures and positions of antigenic sites recognized by an antibody.

Each antibody is expected to bind to a structural site that is limited to about five or six amino acid residues. The globin chains of various species have diverged in structure. Divergence of structure within the antigenic sites is expected to be reflected in the extent to which monoclonal antibodies recognize these sites. Comparisons of the structures of the globins that are recognized by the antibody with the structures of those not recognized allow one to limit the number of structural sites at which the antibody might bind.

Detection of sites likely recognized by the antibody is facilitated by use of fragments of globin chains in semiquantitative Ag–Ab reactions. For instance, treatment with cyanogen bromide cleaves the globin chain at sites occupied by methionine residues, and produces fragments that can be separated by gel filtration. Monoclonal antibody 45-1, an anti-(γ + β)-chain antibody, reacts with γCB-1 but not with γCB-2 or γCB-3, suggesting that the antigenic site is contained in the 55 amino acid residues of this fragment. Comparisons of the sequence of the first 55 amino acids in globin chains that react with 45-1 with those in globin chains that fail to react with 45-1 suggest that the structural site recognized by this antibody lies between residues β12 and β20.[108]

Opportunities for testing the validity of such deductions, based on comparisons of primary structures, are provided by human Hb variants that are altered at the presumed sites of Hb–Ab binding. The usefulness of mutants is illustrated by the results of characterization of monoclonal antibody 3-2.[114]

This antibody reacts with human and macaque *(Macaca nemestrina)* β chains but not with baboon *(Papio cynocephalus)* β chains. The antigenic site must involve a portion of the β-globin sequence in which the chains from both human and macaque differ from those of the baboon.[115–117] At only two posi-

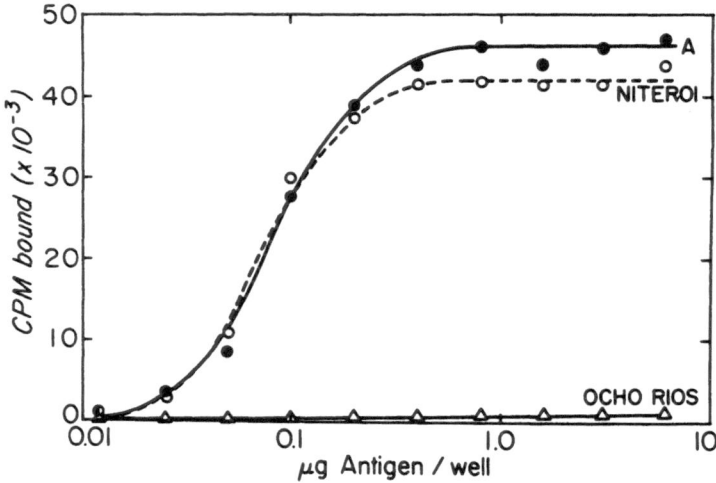

Figure 7. Reactions of antibody 3-2 (a β-chain-specific monoclonal antibody) with Hb A, Hb Niteroi, and Hb Ocho Rios. Note the absence of binding with Ocho Rios, a hemoglobin that contains a single amino acid substitution (Asp replaced by Ala) at position β52.

tions, $\beta 43$ and $\beta 52$, are these conditions satisfied. In the human and macaque β chains position $\beta 43$ is occupied by glutamic acid, while in the baboon chain, aspartic acid occupies this site. Position $\beta 52$ is occupied by aspartic acid in human and macaque and by alanine in the baboon.

Hemoglobin Niteroi[118] is a human variant whose β chains have sustained deletion of a sequence of three amino acid residues, one of which is the glutamyl residue that normally occupies position $\beta 43$. In Hb Ocho Rios,[119] the aspartyl residue that normally occupies position $\beta 52$ has been replaced by an alanyl residue.

As shown in Figure 7, Hb Niteroi (which lacks the glutamic acid normally found in position $\beta 43$) reacts with the antibody to the same extent as does the normal β chain. Conversely, Hb Ocho Rios fails to react, indicating that the aspartyl residue normally in position $\beta 52$ lies within the antigenic site and is requisite to the antigen–antibody reaction

6.5. Possible Recognition of Mutant Hemoglobins in Animals

Antibody 3-2 binds to neither the β chains of baboon hemoglobin nor of Hb Ocho Rios because the amino acid sequence at positions 51–56 of both chains is Pro-Ala-Ala-Val-Met-Gly. The same antibody does recognize the human β chain because the corresponding sequence therein is Pro-Asp-Ala-Val-Met-Gly. If in a baboon a mutation were to occur that resulted in the substitution of alanine by aspartic acid at position $\beta 52$, antibody 3-2 would recognize the abnormal baboon hemoglobin because the latter would then be identical in sequence, over positions $\beta 51$–56, to the normal human β chain.

Results of studies with Ab 3-2 suggest that in general a monoclonal antihuman globin-chain antibody that does not recognize the comparable portion of a nonhuman globin chain should react with the nonhuman globin chain if the latter is appropriately altered by mutation.[109] Presumably such antibodies could be employed in detection of nonhuman red cells that contain a mutant hemoglobin as a result of somatic mutation; they could hence be useful in experiments aimed at answering some of the questions discussed in Sections 4.6 and 4.7.

ACKNOWLEDGMENTS. The studies described here were supported by Grant GM-15253 and Contract NO1-ES-9-0002 from the National Institutes of Health.

REFERENCES

1. K. C. Atwood, The presence of A_2 erythrocytes in A_1 blood, *Proc. Natl. Acad. Sci. USA 44*, 1054–1057 (1958).

2. K. C. Atwood and S. L. Scheinberg, Somatic variation in human erythrocyte antigens, *J. Cell Comp. Physiol. 52 (Suppl. 1),* 97–123 (1958).

3. K. C. Atwood and S. L. Scheinberg, Isotope dilution method for assay of inagglutinable erythrocytes, *Science 129,* 963–964 (1959).

4. K. C. Atwood and F. J. Pepper, Erythrocyte automosaicism in some persons of known genotype, *Science 134,* 2100–2102 (1961).

5. H. E. Sutton, Monitoring somatic mutations in human populations, in: *Mutagenic Effects of Environmental Contaminants* (H. E. Sutton and M. I. Harris, eds.), pp. 121–128, Academic Press, New York (1972).

6. H. E. Sutton, Somatic cell mutations, in: *Birth Defects, Proceedings of the 4th International Conference* (A. G. Motulsky and W. Lenz, eds.), pp. 212–214, Exerpta Medica, Amsterdam (1974).

7. W. G. Wood, G. Stamatoyannopoulos, G. Lim, and P. E. Nute, F-Cells in the adult: Normal values and levels in individuals with hereditary and acquired elevations of Hb F, *Blood 46,* 671–682 (1975).

8. S. H. Boyer, T. K. Belding, L. Margolet, and A. N. Noyes, Fetal hemoglobin restriction to a few erythrocytes (F cells) in normal human adults, *Science 188,* 361–363 (1975).

9. G. Stamatoyannopoulos and Th. Papayannopoulou, Fetal hemoglobin and the erythroid stem cell differentiation process, in: *Cellular and Molecular Regulation of Hemoglobin Switching* (G. Stamatoyannopoulos and A. W. Nienhuis, eds.), pp. 323–341, Grune and Stratton, New York (1979).

10. Th. Papayannopoulou, P. E. Nute, G. Stamatoyannopoulos, and T. C. McGuire, Hemoglobin ontogenesis: Test of the gene excision hypothesis, *Science 196,* 1215–1216 (1977).

11. Th. Papayannopoulou and G. Stamatoyannopoulos, On the origin of F cells in the adult: Clues from studies in clonal hemopathies, in: *Cellular and Molecular Regulation of Hemoglobin Switching* (G. Stamatoyannopoulos and W. W. Nienhuis, eds.), pp. 73–84, Grune and Stratton, New York (1979).

12. S. H. Boyer, G. J. Dover, K. D. Smith, and A. Scott, Some interpretations of *in vivo* studies of globin gene switching in man and primates, in: *Hemoglobins in Development and Differentiation* (G. Stamatoyannopoulos and A. W. Nienhuis, eds.), pp. 225–241, Alan R. Liss, New York (1981).

13. Th. Papayannopoulou, B. Nakamoto, S. Kurachi, D. Kurnit, and G. Stamatoyannopoulos, Cell biology of hemoglobin switching. II. Studies on the regulation of fetal hemoglobin synthesis in human adults, in: *Hemoglobins in Development and Differentiation* (G. Stamatoyannopoulos and A. W. Nienhuis, eds.), pp. 307–320, Alan R. Liss, New York (1981).

14. E. Beutler, Red cell metabolism. A. Defects not causing hemolytic disease. B. Environmental modification, *Biochimie 54,* 759–764 (1972).

15. A. Deisseroth, A. Nienhuis, P. Turner, R. Velez, W. F. Anderson, F. Ryddle, J. Lawrence, R. Creagan, and R. Kucherlapati, Localization of the human α-globin structural gene to chromosome 16 in somatic cell hybrids by molecular hybridization assay, *Cell 12,* 205–218 (1977).

16. T. Maniatis, E. F. Fritsch, J. Lauer, R. M. Lawn, N. J. Proudfoot, M. H. M. Shander, and C.-K. J. Shen, The structure and chromosomal arrangement of human globin genes, in: *Organization and Expression of Globin Genes* (G. Stamatoyannopoulos and A. W. Nienhuis, eds.), pp. 15–31, Alan R. Liss, New York (1981).

17. J. Lauer, C.-K. J. Shen, and T. Maniatis, The chromosomal arrangement of human α-like globin genes: Sequence homology and α-globin gene deletions, *Cell 20,* 119–130 (1980).

18. P. F. R. Little, Globin pseudogenes, *Cell 28,* 683–684 (1982).

19. S. A. Liebhaber, M. Goossens, and Y. W. Kan, Homology and concerted evolution at the α1 and α2 loci of human α-globin, *Nature 290,* 26–29 (1981).

20. A. Deisseroth, A. Nienhuis, J. Lawrence, R. Giles, P. Turner, and F. H. Ruddle, Chromosomal localization of human β-globin gene on human chromosome 11 in somatic cell hybrids, *Proc. Natl. Acad. Sci. USA 75*, 1456–1460 (1978).

21. E. F. Fritsch, R. M. Lawn, and T. Maniatis, Molecular cloning and characterization of the human β-like globin gene cluster, *Cell 19*, 959–972 (1980).

22. H. F. Bunn, D. N. Haney, K. H. Gabbay, and P. M. Gallop, Further identification of the nature and linkage of the carbohydrate in hemoglobin A_{Ic}, *Biochem, Biophys. Res. Commun. 67*, 103–109 (1975).

23. Y. W. Kan, A. M. Dozy, H. E. Varmus, J. M. Taylor, J. P. Holland, L. E. Lie-Injo, J. Ganesan, and D. Todd, Deletion of α-globin genes in haemoglobin-H disease demonstrates multiple α-globin structural loci, *Nature 255*, 255–256 (1975).

24. A. M. Dozy, Y. W. Kan, S. H. Embury, W. C. Mentzer, W. C. Wang, B. Lubin, J. R. Davis, Jr., and H. M. Koenig, α-Globin gene organization in Blacks precludes the severe form of α thalassaemia, *Nature 280*, 605–607 (1979).

25. D. J. Weatherall and J. B. Clegg, *The Thalassaemia Syndromes*, 3rd ed., Blackwell Scientific Publications, Oxford (1981).

26. M. Pirastu, K. Y. Lee, A. M. Dozy, Y. W. Kan, G. Stamatoyannopoulos, M. G. Hadjiminas, Z. Zchariades, A. Angius, M. Furbetta, C. Rosatelli, and A. Cao, Alpha-thalassemia in two Mediterranean populations, *Blood 60*, 509–512 (1982).

27. R. A. Spritz and B. G. Forget, The thalassemias: Molecular mechanisms of human genetic disease, *Am. J. Hum. Genet, 35*, 333–361 (1983).

28. J. C. Chang and Y. W. Kan, β^0-Thalassemia, a nonsense mutation in man, *Proc. Natl. Acad. Sci. USA 76*, 2886–2889 (1979).

29. R. F. Trecartin, S. A. Liebhaber, J. C. Chang, K. Y. Lee, and Y. W. Kan, β^0 Thalassemia in Sardinia is caused by a nonsense mutation, *J. Clin Invest. 68*, 1012–1017 (1981).

30. S. H. Orkin and S. C. Goff, Nonsense and frameshift mutations in β^0-thalassemia detected in cloned β-globin genes, *J. Biol. Chem. 256*, 9782–9784 (1981).

31. R. Treisman, N. J. Proudfoot, M. Shander, and T. Maniatis, A single-base change at a splice site in a β^0-thalassemic gene causes abnormal RNA splicing, *Cell 29*, 903–911 (1982).

32. M. Baird, C. Driscoll, H. Schreiner, G. V. Sciarratta, G. Sansone, G. Niazi, F. Ramirez, and A. Bank, A nucleotide change at a splice junction in the human β-globin gene is associated with β^0-thalassemia, *Proc. Natl. Acad. Sci. USA 78*, 4218–4221 (1981).

33. S. H. Orkin, H. H. Kazazian, Jr., S. E. Antonarakis, S. C. Goff, C. D. Boehm, J. P. Sexton, P. G. Waber, and P. J. V. Giardina, Linkage of β-thalassaemia mutations and β-globin gene polymorphisms with DNA polymorphisms in human β-globin gene cluster, *Nature 296*, 627–631 (1982).

34. R. A. Spritz, P. Jagadeeswaran, P. V. Choudary, P. A. Biro, J. T. Elder, J. K. DeRiel, J. L. Manley, M. L. Gefter, B. G. Forget, and S. M. Weissman, Base substitution in an intervening sequence of a β^+-thalassemic human globin gene, *Proc. Natl. Acad. Sci. USA 78*, 2455–2459 (1981).

35. D. Westaway and R. Williamson, An intron nucleotide sequence variant in a cloned β^+-thalassemia globin gene, *Nucl. Acids Res. 9*, 1777–1788 (1981).

36. M. Busslinger, N. Moschonas, and R. A. Flavell, β^+-Thalassemia: Aberrant splicing results from a single point mutation in an intron, *Cell 27*, 289–298 (1981).

37. Y. Fukumaki, P. K. Ghosh, E. J. Benz, Jr., V. B. Reddy, P. Lebowitz, B. G. Forget, and S. M. Weissman, Identification of an abnormally spliced messenger RNA in erythroid cells from patients with β^+-thalassamia and monkey cells expressing a cloned β^+-thalassemia gene, *Cell 28*, 585–593 (1982).

38. T. J. Ley, N. P. Anagnou, G. Pepe, and A. W. Nienhuis, RNA processing errors in patients with β-thalassemia, *Proc. Natl. Acad. Sci. USA 79*, 4775–4779 (1982).

39. M. Poncz, M. Ballantine, D. Solowiejczyk, I. Barak, E. Schwartz, and S. Surrey, β-Thalassamia in a Kurdish Jew, *J. Biol. Chem. 257*, 5994–5996 (1982).

40. S. H. Orkin, J. M. Old, D. J. Weatherall, and D. G. Nathan, Partial deletion of β-globin gene in certain patients with β^0-thalassemia, *Proc. Natl. Acad. Sci. USA 76*, 2400–2404 (1979).

41. C. Baglioni, Abnormal human hemoglobins. X. A study of hemoglobin Lepore$_{Boston}$, *Biochim. Biophys. Acta 97*, 37–46 (1965).

42. S. Ottolenghi, B. Giglioni, P. Comi, A. M. Gianni, E. Polli, C. T. A. Acquaye, J. H. Oldham, and G. Masera, Globin gene deletion in HPFH, $\delta^0\beta^0$ thalassaemia and Hb Lepore disease, *Nature 278*, 654–657 (1979).

43. J. G. Mears, F. Ramirez, D. Liebowitz, F. Nakamura, A. Bloom, F. Konotey-Ahulu, and A. Bank, Changes in restricted human cellular DNA fragments containing globin gene sequences in thalassemia and related disorders, *Proc. Natl. Acad. Sci. USA 75*, 1222–1226 (1978).

44. E. F. Fritsch, R. M. Lawn, and T. Maniatis, Characterization of deletions which affect the expression of fetal globin genes in man, *Nature 279*, 598–603 (1979).

45. R. Bernards, J. M. Kooter, and R. A. Flavell, Physical mapping of the globin gene deletion in $(\delta\beta)^0$-thalassemia, *Gene 6*, 265–280 (1979).

46. S. Ottolenghi, B. Giglioni, R. Taramelli, J. P. Comi, U. Mazza, G. Saglio, C. Camaschella, P. Izzo, A. Cao, R. Galanello, E. Gimferrer, M. Baiget, and A. M. Gianni, Molecular comparison of $\delta\beta$-thalassemia and hereditary persistence of fetal hemoglobin DNAs: Evidence of a regulatory area? *Proc. Natl. Acad. Sci. USA 79*, 2347–2351 (1982).

47. R. W. Jones, J. M. Old, R. J. Trent, J. B. Clegg, and D. J. Weatherall, Major rearrangement in the human β-globin gene cluster, *Nature 291*, 39–44 (1980).

48. S. H. Orkin, S. C. Goff, and D. G. Nathan, Heterogeneity of DNA deletion in $\gamma\delta\beta$-thalassemia, *J. Clin. Invest. 67*, 878–884 (1981).

49. L. H. T. van der Plog, A. Donings, M. Oort, D. Roos, L. Bernini, and R. A. Flavell, γ-β-Thalassaemia studies showing that deletion of the γ- and δ-genes influences β-globin gene expression in man, *Nature 283*, 637–642 (1980).

50. R. Bernards and R. A. Flavell, Physical mapping of the globin gene deletion in hereditary persistence of foetal haemoglobin (HPFH), *Nucl. Acids Res. 8*, 1521–1534 (1980).

51. D. Tuan, M. J. Murnane, J. K. deRiel, and B. G. Forget, Heterogeneity in the molecular basis of hereditary persistence of fetal haemoglobin, *Nature 285*, 335–337 (1980).

52. P. Jagadeeswaran, D. Tuan, B. G. Forget, and S. M. Weissman, A gene deletion ending at the midpoint of a repetitive DNA sequence in one form of hereditary persistence of fetal haemoglobin, *Nature 296*, 469–470 (1982).

53. R. W. Jones, J. M. Old, W. G. Wood, J. B. Clegg, and D. J. Weatherall, Restriction endonuclease maps of the β-like globin gene cluster in the British and Greek forms of HPFH and for one example of $^G\gamma\beta^+$ HPFH, *Br. J. Haematol. 50*, 415–442 (1982).

54. Th. Papayannopoulou, R. M. Lawn, G. Stamatoyannopoulos, and T. Maniatis, Greek ($^A\gamma$) variant of hereditary persistence of fetal haemoglobin: Globin gene organization and studies of expression of fetal haemoglobins in clonal erythroid cultures, *Br. J. Haematol. 50*, 387–399 (1982).

55. J. M. Old, H. Ayyub, W. G. Wood, J. B. Clegg, and D. J. Weatherall, Linkage analysis of nondeletion hereditary persistence of fetal hemoglobin, *Science 215*, 981–982 (1982).

56. J. F. Balsley, E. Rappaport, E. Schwartz, and S. Surrey, The γ-δ-β-globin gene region in $^G\gamma$-β^+-hereditary persistence of fetal hemoglobin, *Blood 59*, 828–831 (1982).

57. R. W. Jones, J. M. Old, R. J. Trent, J. B. Clegg, and D. J. Weatherall, Restriction mapping of a new deletion responsible for $^G\gamma(\delta\beta)^0$ thalassemia, *Nucl. Acids Res. 9*, 6813–6825 (1981).

58. M. Farquhar, R. Gelinas, B. Tatsis, J. Murray, M. Yagi, R. Mueller, and G. Stamatoyan-nopoulos, Restriction endonuclease mapping of γ-δ-β globin region in $^G\gamma(\beta)^+$ HPFH and a Chinese $^A\gamma$ HPFH variant, *Am. J. Human Genet, 35*, 611–620 (1983).

59. S. H. Orkin, H. H. Kazazian, Jr., S. E. Antonarakis, H. Ostrer, S. C. Goff, and J. P. Sexton, Abnormal RNA processing due to the coding region mutation of the β^E globin gene, *Blood 60*, 56a (1982).

60. International Hemoglobin Information Center, Lists of variants, *Hemoglobin 4*, 215–228 (1980).

61. H. F. Bunn, B. G. Forget, and H. M. Ranney, *Human Hemoglobins*, W. B. Saunders, Philadelphia (1977).

62. J. V. Neel, C. Satoh, H. B. Hamilton, M. Otake, K. Goriki, T. Kageoka, M. Fujita, S. Neriishi, and J. Asakawa, Search for mutations affecting protein structure in children of atomic bomb survivors: Preliminary report, *Proc. Natl. Acad. Sci. USA 77*, 4221–4225 (1980).

63. J. V. Neel, H. W. Mohrenweiser, and M. H. Meisler, Rate of spontaneous mutation at human loci encoding protein structure, *Proc. Natl. Acad. Sci. USA 77*, 6037–6041 (1980).

64. F. Vogel and R. Rathenberg, Spontaneous mutation in man, *Adv. Hum. Genet. 5*, 223–318 (1975).

65. A. G. Motulsky, Some evolutionary implications of biochemical variants in man, in: *Proceedings VIII International Congress Anthropological Ethnological Sciences*, Vol. 1, pp. 364–365, Science Council of Japan (1969).

66. M. Kimura and T. Ohta, Mutation and evolution at the molecular level, *Genetics 73 (Suppl.)*, 19–35 (1973).

67. G. Stamatoyannopoulos, P. E. Nute, and M. Miller, *De novo* mutations producing unstable hemoglobins or hemoglobins M. I. Establishment of a depository and use of data to test for an association of *de novo* mutation with advanced parental age, *Hum. Genet. 58*, 396–404 (1981).

68. G. Stamatoyannopoulos and P. E. Nute, *De novo* mutations producing unstable Hbs or Hbs M. II. Direct estimates of minimum nucleotide mutation rates in man, *Hum. Genet. 60*, 181–188 (1982).

69. P. E. Nute and G. Stamatoyannopoulos, Estimates of mutation rates per nucleotide in man, based on observations of *de novo* hemoglobin mutants, in: *Population and Biological Aspects of Human Mutation* (E. B. Hook and I. H. Porter, eds.), pp. 337–347, Academic Press, New York (1981).

70. A. Gouttas, Ph. Fessas, H. Tsevrenis, and E. Xefteri, Description d'une nouvelle variété d'anémie hémolytique cogénitale étude (hématologique, électrophorétique et génétique) *Sang 26*, 911–919 (1955).

71. Th. Papayannopoulou and G. Stamatoyannopoulos, Stains for inclusion bodies, in: *The Detection of Hemoglobinopathies* (R. M. Schmidt, T. H. J. Huisman, and H. Lehmann, eds.), CRC Press, Cleveland (1974).

72. M. Rosenberg, Electrophoretic analysis of hemoglobin and isozymes in individual vertebrate cells, *Proc. Natl. Aca. Sci. USA 67*, 32–36 (1970).

73. S. I. O. Anyaibe and V. E. Headings, Identification of hemoglobins in single erythrocytes by electrophoresis, *Am. J. Hematol. 2*, 307–315 (1977).

74. Th. Papayannopoulou, T. C. McGuire, G. Lim, E. Garzel, P. E. Nute, and G. Stamatoyannopoulos, Identification of haemoglobin S in red cells and normoblasts, using fluorescent anti-Hb S antibodies, *Br. J. Haematol. 34*, 25–31 (1976).

75. Th. Papayannopoulou, G. Lim, T. C. McGuire, V. Ahern, P. E. Nute, and G. Stamatoyannopoulos, Use of specific fluorescent antibodies for the identification of hemoglobin C in erythrocytes, *Am. J. Hematol. 2*, 105–112 (1977).

76. P. E. Nute, Th. Papayannopoulou, B. Tatsis, and G. Stamatoyannopoulos, Toward a system for detecting somatic-cell mutations. V. Preparation of fluorescent antibodies to hemoglobin Hasharon, a human α-chain variant, *J. Immunol. Methods 42*, 35–44 (1981).

77. G. Stamatoyannopoulos, P. E. Nute, Th. Papayannopoulou, T. McGuire, G. Lim, H. F. Bunn, and D. Rucknagel, Development of a somatic mutation screening system using Hb mutants. IV. Successful detection of red cells containing the human frameshift mutants Hb Wayne and Hb Cranston using monospecific fluorescent antibodies, *Am. J. Human. Genet. 32*, 484–496 (1980).   .

78. M. Seid-Akhavan, W. P. Winter, R. K. Abramson, and D. L. Rucknagel, Hemoglobin Wayne: A frameshift mutation detected in human hemoglobin alpha chains, *Proc. Natl. Acad. Sci. USA 73*, 882–886 (1976).

79. H. F. Bunn, G. J. Schmidt, D. N. Haney, and R. G. Dluhy, Hemoglobin Cranston, an unstable variant having an elongated β chain due to nonhomologous crossover between two normal β chain genes, *Proc. Natl. Acad. Sci. USA 72*, 3609–3613 (1975).

80. G. Stamatoyannopoulos, Possibilities for demonstrating point mutations in somatic cells, as illustrated by studies of mutant hemoglobins, in: *Genetic Damage in Man Caused by Environmental Agents* (K. Berg, ed.), pp. 49–62, Academic Press, New York (1979).

81. W. L. Bigbee, E. W. Branscomb, H. B. Weintraub, Th. Papayannopoulou, and G. Stamatoyannopoulos, Cell sorter immunofluorescence detection of human erythrocytes labeled in suspension with antibodies specific for hemoglobin S and C, *J. Immunol. Methods 45*, 117–127 (1981).

82. G. Stamatoyannopoulos and P. E. Nute, Screening of human erythrocytes for products of somatic mutation: An approach and a critique, in: *Population and Biological Aspects of Human Mutation* (E. B. Hook and I. H. Porter, eds.), pp. 265–273, Academic Press, New York (1981).

83. G. M. Maniatis and V. M. Ingram. Erythropoiesis during amphibian metamorphosis. II. Immunochemical study of larval and adult hemoglobins of *Rana catesbeiana*, *J. Cell Biol. 49*, 380–389 (1971).

84. G. M. Maniatis and V. M. Ingram, Erythropoiesis during amphibian metamorphosis. III. Immunochemical detection of tadpole and frog hemoglobins *(Rana catesbeiana)* in single erythrocytes, *J. Cell Biol. 49*, 390–404 (1971).

85. M. Flavin, Y. Blouquit, A. M. Duprat, P. Deparis, H. Tonthat, and J. Rosa, Hemoglobin ontogeny in the salamander *Pleurodeles waltlii*, in: *Hemoglobins in Development and Differentiation* (G. Stamatoyannopoulos and A. W. Nienhuis, eds.), pp. 215–221, Alan R. Liss, New York (1981).

86. M. Reichlin, E. Bucci, C. Fronticelli, J. Wyman, E. Antonini, C. Ioppolo, and A. Rossi-Fanelli, The properties and interactions of the isolated α- and β-chains of human haemoglobin. IV. Immunological studies involving antibodies against the isolated chains, *J. Mol. Biol. 17*, 18–28 (1966).

87. T. Nishimura, T. Kogo, K. Yokomuro, Y. Kimura, A. Kajita, and R. Shukuya, Immunological studies in the multiple hemoglobins of tadpole and frog of *Rana catesbeiana, FEBS Lett. 36*, 1–4 (1973).

88. K. Shimizu and A. Hagiwara, Ontogeny of chicken hemoglobin. III. Immunological study of the heterogeneity of hemoglobin in development, *Dev. Growth Diff. 15*, 285–306 (1973).

89. A. J. Tobin, B. S. Chapman, D. A. Hansen, L. Lasky, and S. E. Selvig, Regulation of embryonic and adult hemoglobin synthesis in chickens, in: *Cellular and Molecular Regulation of Hemoglobin Switching* (G. Stamatoyannopoulos and A. W. Nienhuis, eds.), pp. 205–211, Grune and Stratton, New York (1979).

90. D. H. K. Chui, T. W. Brotherton, and J. Gauldie, Hemoglobin ontogeny in fetal mice: Adult hemoglobin in yolk sac derived erythrocytes, in: *Cellular and Molecular Regulation of*

Hemoglobin Switching (G. Stamatoyannopoulos and A. W. Nienhuis, eds.), pp. 213–224, Grune and Stratton, New York (1979).

91. R. D. Jurd and N. Maclean, Detection of haemoglobin in red cells of *Xenopus laevis* by immunofluorescent double labelling, *J. Microsc. 100* (Pt. 2), 213–217 (1973).

92. J. Benbassat, The transition from tadpole to frog haemoglobin during natural amphibian metamorphosis. II. Immunofluorescence studies. *J. Cell Sci. 16*, 143–156 (1974).

93. F. W. Boerma and T. H. J. Huisman, Serologic investigations of human hemoglobins. II. Antibodies produced by isolated human hemoglobin types with known structural differences, *J. Lab. Clin. Med. 63*, 264–278 (1964).

94. M. Reichlin, M. Hay, and L. Levine, Antibodies to human A_1 hemoglobin and their reaction with A_2, S, C, and H hemoglobins, *Immunochemistry 1*, 21–30 (1964).

95. M. Reichlin, Quantitative immunological studies on single amino acid substitution in human hemoglobin: Demonstration of specific antibodies to multiple sites, *Immunochemistry 11*, 21–27 (1974).

96. R. D. Schreiber and M. Reichlin, The occurrence of shared idiotypic specificity among the goat antibodies that distinguish human hemoglobin S from A_1, *J. Immunol. 113*, 359–366 (1974).

97. M. Reichlin and R. W. Noble, Immunochemistry of protein mutants, in: *Immunochemistry of Proteins* (M. Z. Atassi, ed.), vol. 2, pp. 311–251, Plenum Press, New York (1977).

98. S. H. Boyer, M. L. Boyer, A. N. Noyes, and T. K. Belding, Immunological basis for detection of sickle cell hemoglobin phenotypes in amniotic fluid erythrocytes, *Ann. N.Y. Acad. Sci. 241*, 699–713 (1974).

99. P. T. Rowley, R. A. Doherty, C. Rosecrans, and E. Cernichiari, Sickle hemoglobin: A specific radioimmunoassay, *Blood 43*, 607–611 (1974).

100. F. A. Garver, M. B. Baker, C. S. Jones, M. Gravely, G. Altay, and T. H. J. Huisman, Radioimmunoassay for abnormal hemoglobins, *Science 196*, 1334–1336 (1977).

101. J. G. Curd, N. S. Young, and A. N. Schechter, Antibodies to an NH_2-terminal fragment of β^S globin. II. Specificity and isolation of antibodies for the sickle mutation, *J. Biol. Chem. 251*, 1290–1295 (1976).

102. A. M. Dozy and T. H. J. Huisman, Studies on the heterogeneity of hemoglobin. XIV. Chromatography of normal and abnormal human hemoglobin types on CM-Sephadex, *J. Chromatogr. 40*, 62–70 (1969).

103. A. M. Dozy, E. F. Kleihauer, and T. H. J. Huisman, Studies on the heterogeneity of hemoglobin. XIII. Chromatography of various human and animal hemoglobin types on DEAE-Sephadex, *J. Chromatogr. 32*, 723–727 (1968).

104. J. Porath, R. Axén, and S. Ernback, Chemical coupling of proteins to agarose, *Nature 215*, 1491–1492 (1967).

105. B.T. Tozer, K. A. Cammack, and H. Smith, Separation of antigens by immunological specificity. 2. Release of antigen and antibody from their complexes by aqueous carbon dioxide, *Biochem J. 84*, 80–93 (1962).

106. T. B. Crawford, T. C. McGuire, and J. B. Henson, Detection of equine infectious anemia virus *in vitro* by immunofluorescence, *Arch. Ges. Virusforsch. 34*, 332–339 (1971).

107. M. Dan and A. Hagiwara, Detection of two types of hemoglobin (Hb A and Hb F) in single erythrocytes by fluorescent antibody technique, *Jpn. J. Hum. Genet. 12*, 55–61 (1967).

108. G. Stamatoyannopoulos, M. Farquhar, D. Lindsley, M. Brice, Th. Papayannopoulou, and P. E. Nute, Monoclonal antibodies specific for globin chains, *Blood 61*, 530–539 (1983).

109. G. Stamatoyannopoulos and P. E. Nute, Detection of somatic mutants of hemoglobin, in: *Utilization of Mammalian Specific Locus Studies in Hazard Evaluation and Estimation of Genetic Risk* (F. J. de Serres and W. Sheridan, eds.), pp. 29–38, Plenum Press, New York (1983).

2

Use of Fluorescence-Activated Cell Sorter for Screening Mutant Cells

WILLIAM L. BIGBEE AND ELBERT W. BRANSCOMB

1. INTRODUCTION

Until recently, virtually all measurements of cellular mutation frequencies have been based on clonogenic assays. In fact, clonogenicity has been considered essential for the legitimate identification of mutant cells because it confirms the transmissbility of the variant phenotype. However, largely because of the apparent connection between somatic mutagenesis and carcinogenesis, it has become important to measure mutational injury in samples of normal somatic cells that generally have little or no replicative capacity. As a result, a number of efforts are underway to develop nonclonogenic mutation assays applicable to cells obtained from *in vivo* tissue samples and to find alternative means for authenticating the mutant pedigree of detected cells.

It is primarily in this connection that the use of high-speed cytometric analysis in mutation frequency measurements is of interest. Detecting and counting individual mutant cells, particularly when relatively rare mutational phenotypes are involved, can become quite impractical without the high processing speeds and quantitative detection sensitivity these approaches can provide. However, efforts to develop nonclonogenic somatic-cell mutation assays have encountered several problems. The first of these concerns the use of null mutation markers. Nonclonogenic assays involving cells from normal, *in vivo* tissue samples must generally use forward mutation markers. The best studied, the most readily recognized, and in many respects the most informative class of forward mutation markers are the so-called null mutations, defined by the functional loss of a gene product. It appears, however, that most null pheno-

WILLIAM L. BIGBEE AND ELBERT W. BRANSCOMB • Lawrence Livermore National Laboratory, Biomedical Sciences Division, University of California, Livermore, California 94550.

types can also be expressed in a single cell for a large number of "artifactual," nonmutational reasons. As a result, assays based on null markers have proved extremely problematic in nonclonogenic form.

One can avoid this so-called *phenocopy* problem, as Dr. George Stama-toyannopoulos at the University of Washington and Dr. Heinrich Malling at NIEHS were the first to champion, by scoring "positive," forward mutations expressed in the form of a mutationally modified protein. While this strategy appears to ensure that the detected phenotypes can arise only through muta-tion, it has proven difficult to realize for quite different reasons. The foremost of these is due to the rarity of cells bearing the types of mutationally modified proteins that it so far appears possible to detect. All such methods so far pro-posed detect phenotypes that result from highly specific DNA alterations. The necessarily small target size of these mutations implies that cells bearing the mutant marker will be extremely rare, apparently as infrequent as one in 10^7–10^8.[1,2] Also, the problems associated with labeling, detecting, and counting rare cells at these frequencies has thus far prevented the development of a prac-tical method based on this approach. In any case, event frequencies in this range make it essential that some type of high-speed cytometry be used to count the mutant cells. Of course, nonclonogenic assays using null phenotypes or other markers with relatively high event frequencies may in some cases also benefit from high-speed cytometry.

Although both high-speed scanning microscopes and flow cytometers have promise in these applications, the latter have received the greatest attention thus far, and we will confine our discussion to them. Flow cytometers offer the ability to make quantitative measurements on single cells at high processing speeds, and perhaps more importantly, to sort individual cells based on the measurements obtained.

In what follows we will review our efforts to develop two different types of *in vivo*, nonclonogenic somatic-cell mutation assays applicable to erythro-cytes. The first is a "modified gene product" assay using amino acid-substituted forms of hemoglobin. The second is a null mutation assay using the red cell membrane protein glycophorin A. These two schemes employ flow cytofluo-rometry in quite different ways and together give some idea of the potential and the problems these machines bring to cellular mutation assays.

2. IMMUNOLOGIC IDENTIFICATION AND FLOW DETECTION OF ERYTHROCYTES CONTAINING AMINO ACID-SUBSTITUTED HEMOGLOBIN

In this section we will discuss from a general point of view the problems associated with using flow cytometry and immunofluorescent labeling in a somatic mutation assay that measures the frequency of red cells that contain certain singly amino acid-substituted forms of hemoglobin. We will discuss (1) the immunological and genetic considerations for producing the necessary antibodies, (2) how the cells can be labeled for flow processing, and (3) the operating parameters of flow cytometers that control the practicality of this approach.

2.1. Production of Antibodies

If two versions of a protein differ by only a single amino acid substitution, antibodies can often be found that will bind to one but not the other. This was implied quite generally by studies using immunological cross-reactivity to define protein phylogenies.[3] It was demonstrated directly in a number of specific cases through the study of antibodies raised to singly substituted variants of human hemoglobin.[4-6] We can conclude from these results that in typical globular proteins a majority of surface presented amino acid substitutions are immunologically detectable. In principle, this fact permits one to identify, by immunological labeling, cells that express the products of single-base-substitution mutations and to envisage a nonclonogenic somatic-cell mutation assay based on that ability.

Such assays rest on the assumption that rare, circulating red cells, containing roughly heterozygotic levels of a singly substituted protein, can arise only as the descendents of stem cells in which the corresponding structural gene mutation has occurred. For the assay to be useful, moreover, we must be confident that the frequency of cells presenting the variant phenotype can be related to the fraction of mutant progenitor cells. This requires, among other things, that the cells carrying the variant protein have normal survival *in vivo*. Lastly, we must have some means of demonstrating that antibodies specific for a substituted protein will only label cells that contain that protein, and only if the variant protein is present at the relatively high levels that would arise in "pseudoheterozygotic" mutant cells.

The first problem to be solved in realizing this promise is that of producing antibodies that will recognize the mutant proteins, and to do this we require immunogenic models of the substituted proteins we hope to detect. At least three possibilities for such models are apparent: heritable genetic variants, phylogenetic homologues, and synthesized peptides. Each of these will be discussed in turn.

Heritable genetic variants, in which only single amino acid substitutions are involved, are known for a number of proteins, either as allelic forms or as rare mutations present in isolated kindreds. Usually these variants can arise from the normal or alternative form by single-base-substitution mutations, and are thus suitable models for mutations in somatic cells.

Human hemoglobin is of course the best available candidate for this approach. Nearly 400 variant hemoglobins, the majority characterized by a single amino acid substitution, have been identified in the human population.[7] Individuals who synthesize any one of these mutant hemoglobins do so as a result of inheriting a mutated hemoglobin gene. The presence of rare individuals carrying such germinal mutations suggests that these same mutational events may also occur somatically in the hemoglobin genes of the blood-forming stem cells. In normal hemoglobin A individuals, such mutations would give rise to rare circulating red cells containing variant hemoglobin in addition to the normal form. Moreover, since the complete three-dimensional structure of hemoglobin is known, and the physiology of each of the variants is at least roughly known, it is possible to choose which variants are most likely to be immunologically detectable and which are likely to yield cells in the peripheral circulation in undiminished numbers. Finally, since DNA sequences for the human α- and β-globin genes are now known,[8,9] we can determine which base substitution would be involved in producing each variant.

By immunizing an animal with the variant protein, we should obtain polyclonal sera consisting of a collection of antibodies recognizing many determinants of the protein. Most of these binding sites would be presented by both the variant and normal forms of the protein, but at least some of the antibodies may bind only to the site containing the amino acid substitution and fail to bind to the normal form. Presumably, such antibodies are more likely to be produced if the substituted amino acid differs from that present at the same site in the animal's own hemoglobin.

As an alternative, homologous proteins from other species may be used. Many proteins have remained structurally and functionally stable over substantial evolutionary periods while at the same time integrating a number of amino acid substitutions. These substitutions are usually on the protein's surface, are apparently neutral or nearly neutral, and are generally presumed to be the result of genetic drift.[3,10,11] Most of these substitutions correspond to single base changes, and each of these is individually a model for one mutant form of the protein. An antibody that binds to one version of a protein rather than another because of the presence of just one of the amino acid substitutions that distinguish them should recognize the corresponding singly substituted form of the protein in the species to which the antibody normally fails to bind. In this sense, the protein homologue from one animal should function as an immunogenic model for an ensemble of independent mutant forms of the protein in another animal. At the same time, the animal in which we wish to detect mutations may be, in some respects, the ideal one in which to raise the necessary antibodies. The immunological distinction between self and "other" should minimize the production of irrelevant or confounding antibodies, for example, those that react to the unmutated form of the test animal's protein, and should maximize the probability that substitutions will be immunogenically active.

Finally, where the amino acid sequence of the protein in question is known, it should be possible to synthesize substituted analogues of peptide fragments of the protein and raise antibodies to them specific for the substituted, "mutant" form. Some fraction of these antibodies should recognize the corresponding mutant form of the intact protein. Work in many laboratories has shown that anti-peptide antibodies to external segments of proteins can very often be found that recognize the same sequence in the native protein.[12] For all of these approaches the need for relatively large supplies of highly specific antibodies is essential and constancy of the antibody reagent from batch to batch highly desirable. For these and other reasons, monoclonal antibodies offer powerful advantages. Presently we are attempting to produce monoclonal antibodies using the three strategies outlined above. These efforts will be detailed later in the cahpter.

2.2. Suspension Labeling of Red Cells with Hemoglobin Antibodies

The second major problem one encounters in the singly substituted hemoglobin approach is how to immunochemically label cells with an antibody against a soluble interior protein. There seems no obvious way to allow antibodies access to soluble hemoglobin inside a red cell without at the same time losing the antigen. The approaches so far applied to this problem involve binding some of the interior hemoglobin in place by chemical cross-linking before rendering the membrane permeable to antibodies. We have tried two extreme variations of this strategy, which attempt to permit either inside or outside labeling and which we call respectively the ghost and the hard cell methods. The ghost method follows the approach developed by Wang and Richards[13] for studies of the erythrocyte membrane. A monolayer of hemoglobin is attached to the interior of the cell membranes by light treatment with a membrane-permeable cross-linking reagent. The cells are then lysed and the resulting "pink" ghosts kept permeable to macromolecules. In the hard cell method the red cells are cross-linked to a degree that renders them completely resistant to lysis.[14] Depending on how this treatment is performed, it either itself exposes hemoglobin in the cell's outer layer to macromolecules in the exterior medium, or permits a subsequent delipidation step that does so.

2.3. Flow Cytometric Processing

Essentially all present fluorescence-activated flow cytometers have been designed to measure, with high sensitivity and resolution, the fluorescence and scatter signals from each cell in the processed sample. Such samples typically contain a few hundred thousand cells, and are processed at rates of approximately 10^3 cells/sec. This is a task quite different from counting the frequency of extremely rare, immunofluorescently labeled cells in a large sample of comparatively unstained cells, and for that purpose the operation of these machines, and perhaps ultimately their design, must be rethought. When counting rare events we are not generally interested in the distribution of signal intensities among all the cells in the sample, nor even of the rare labeled cells. We need only distinguish between unlabeled cells and very infrequent antibody-labeled cells, and determine the number of both types in the sample processed. Most importantly, we must process, in reasonable time, several orders of magnitude more cells than are typically analyzed.

As we discuss below, the normal background frequency of erythrocytes carrying singly substituted hemoglobins is apparently in the neighborhood of one in 10 million and may well be 10-fold less in some cases of interest. This implies that 10^9–10^{10} cells must be analyzed to achieve a standard error, due to counting statistics, of 10%. At typical flow cytometer processing rates of 10^3 cells/sec this task would take between 10 and 100 hr. Therefore, for flow cytometers to be useful for the task at hand, processing speeds must be very substantially increased.

What factors determine the speed with which cells can be processed in these machines? In a typical flow cytometer, the velocity of the sample stream containing the cells is 5–10 m/sec. The intensity of the laser beam illuminating the stream will have a Gaussian distribution perpendicular to its direction of travel with a nominal width of between 30 and 50 μm. Therefore, if the illumination of the sample stream is to be uniform to within a few percent, the sample stream's diameter must be quite small, typically about 5 μm. A stream of this diameter moving at 5 m/sec delivers about 1×10^{-4} ml/sec, which corresponds, for typical cell density of about 10^7 cells/ml, to a processing rate of 1×10^3 cells/sec. Thus for standard machines, the need for narrow sample streams together with the usual maximum practical densities of the cell suspensions being analyzed restricts the processing rate to a few thousand cells per second.

For our problem, however, both of these constraints can be substantially relaxed. Since we wish only to distinguish between labeled and unlabeled cells, we can afford 20–30% variations in the illumination of the cells in the beam; this permits the stream diameter to be increased to about 30 μm or six-fold. In addition red cell suspensions can be prepared that are 50-fold more dense, i.e., 5×10^8 cells/ml, and can be processed without difficulty. Together these two changes would provide, in principle, an increase in processing speed of about 2000-fold, thus affording a throughput rate approaching 10^7 cells/sec.

However, long before we reach these speeds other constraints appear, some of which are due to limits in signal processing rates. If, as is often done, the signals from the photomultipliers are integrated to increase detection sensitivity, conventional signal integration strategies cannot process more than a few thousand signals per second. One can, however, exploit alternative integration strategies that allow processing speeds limited only by the duration of the detected signals and the need to minimize coincidence (e.g., delay line clipping; Dan Pinkel and Don Peters, private communication). If such methods are followed, or if signal integration is eliminated, one can increase the signal processing rate to perhaps 50,000–100,000/sec, at which point typical analog-to-digital converters reach their limits. At these rates problems due to coincident cell detection may also arise. If the width of the laser beam intersecting the sample stream is 50 μm, then a 5 m/sec flow velocity implies that cells spend 10 μsec traversing the beam. At a flow rate of 50,000 cells/sec, the average time between cells is only 20 μsec, so the coincident occurrence of two or more cells in the beam will reach troublesome levels at such rates, assuming that every cell must be detected. Some reduction in this limit can be had by focusing the laser beam into an ellipse whose narrow axis is parallel to the flow stream. The minimum attainable dimension is apparently about 2.5 μm, which would decrease coincidence roughly 20-fold. For most applications of flow cytometers, however, it is desirable to determine and record the magnitude of each signal received using a pulse height analyzer. For this task the signal first must be processed through an analog-to-digital converter that generally cannot process signals at rates above about 100,000/sec. Therefore, this rate appears to be about as fast as such systems can process cells, given that the signal from each cell must be digitally analyzed. This rate would permit 10^9 cells to be processed in under 3 hr. For many applications this may be acceptable and provide the best available approach.

Here again, however, the special needs of rare-event counting allow one to change processing strategies in at least two different ways in order to achieve higher processing speeds. If it is only necessary to discriminate between signals based on whether or not they fall within a predetermined intensity range, a single-channel analyzer would suffice and analog-to-digital conversion would be unnccesssary. Processing faster by several orders of magnitude would be possible. Alternatively,we can decrease the rate at which signals must be analyzed without decreasing the overall cell processing rate by ignoring the signals from the "unlabeled" cells and process only the signals from the labeled cells. If this approach is adopted, as we have done in our work, we necessarily lose the ability to use other markers, notably light scatter, that all or most cells would present. We thus cannot use these signals to count the total number of cells processed, or, perhaps more importantly, to help discriminate against fluorescent artifacts. By increasing cell density and stream diameter, a few million red cells per second can be scanned, while only the signals from rare fluorescent cells are processed. At these rates, however, more than one cell is in the beam at any one time, so scatter or other labels shared by all or most cells cannot be meaningfully detected. In a stream flowing at 5 m/sec carrying 10^6 cells past a 50-μm-wide laser beam, 10 cells, on the average, are in the beam at any one time.

If we wish to sort as well as analyze, the sorting frequency is generally limited to a few thousand per second since in present systems the drop generation frequency is generally about 20 kHz. In machines operating at the low pressures commonly employed, this frequency cannot exceed approximately 30 kHz due to hydrodynamic factors.[15] One can in principle increase this rate severalfold by rejecting sorts that contain more than one cell at the cost of discarding many of the desired cells.

Therefore, statistically meaningful numbers of cells bearing single-amino-acid-substitution mutations can be detected in tens rather than in hundreds or thousands of minutes provided processing speeds at or about 10^6 cells/sec are achieved. Such speeds are possible in conventional flow cytometers if it is acceptable to detect only the rare labeled cells. In practice it is the frequency of fluorescent artifacts of the same brightness as the labeled cells that dominates the detection and sorting frequencies in these experiments, and it is this frequency that must be kept below one in 1000 total cells.

We may improve on this picture without building specialized machines by processing cells in serial passes using a sorting cytometer, provided the cells can survive passage through the flow nozzle and subsequent retrieval and reprocessing. For the first sorting step it is also necessary that the "unlabeled" cells be almost totally nonfluorescent. One might, for example, begin with a high-speed sort based only on the detection of rare objects with the appropriate fluorescence. Perhaps 5×10^9 cells would be processed at 5×10^6 per second in under 20 min. In our experience this step would yield a sample consisting of a few million cells, a number that reflects the frequency of fluorescent artifacts in such samples and the large number of unlabeled cells that are necessarily carried through in the sorting droplets. This sorted sample would then be reprocessed in a "slow" mode at perhaps 3×10^3 cells/sec. In this step, scatter as well as other labels might be used to help discriminate between cells and fluorescent artifacts. A total processing time well under 1 hr per sample could be achieved, and a sample nearly free of artifacts might result. In any case the final sample should consist of perhaps 100–1000 labeled cells, together with very few unlabeled cells and a few thousand contaminating fluorescent particles. As a result, a final count could be performed manually with relative ease using a fluorescence microscope should the flow machine still be unable to distinguish against false positive artifacts to a sufficient degree.

Whenever we forego detecting all cells passing through the machine we must determine by some other means the total number of cells processed. This presents no particular problem and can be done by a number of methods, depending on the desired accuracy. The volume of sample consumed during the time the critical processing is taking place can be measured to between 10 and 20% simply by noting the fluid level in the sample tube at the relevant times. One can improve on this quite significantly by using motor-driven syringes to introduce the sample into the flow stream at a controlled rate. Using this approach, one can determine processed volume greater than about 0.5 ml to better than 1% (Dan Pinkel, private communication).

In this discussion we have ignored the question of whether fluorescent cells can be detected when a large number of nonfluorescent cells are also present in the beam. We will outline in Sections 2.4.1 and 2.4.2 our evidence that this is not a concern, at least when red cells are being analyzed. We now turn from this general discussion of the issues to a summary outline of our experience with the approach based on amino acid-substituted hemoglobin.

2.4. Results Using Hemoglobin S- and C-Specific Antibodies

2.4.1. Red-Cell "Ghost" Labeling Approach

Our work with this approach was initiated in collaboration with Dr. George Stamatoyannapoulos at the University of Washington. Together we were seeking a flow cytometric version of the method he had previously developed for detecting cells that contain mutationally variant forms of hemoglobin. Using the "genetic variant" approach described above, Dr. Stamatoyannapoulos and his collaborators immunized horses with human hemoglobin variants S and C, absorbed the sera against normal hemoglobin A, positively purified it by immunoabsorption using the appropriate variant, and obtained specific sera for these variant proteins.[1,16,17] These antibodies recognize and bind tightly to hemoglobin S or C but not to normal hemoglobin A. These two variant hemoglobins differ from the normal hemoglobin A amino acid sequence by single amino acid substitutions in the sixth position of the β chain as a result of single base changes in the triplet codon corresponding to that position in the β-globin gene. Hence in normal hemoglobin A individuals, these point mutations in the β-globin genes in erythroid stem cells will give rise to circulating red cells containing hemoglobin S or C in addition to hemoglobin A. To identify such cells, the hemoglobin S antibody was labeled with fluorescein and incubated with red cells fixed on slides. The preparations were then manually examined under a fluorescence microscope for the presence of antibody-labeled cells. Long and laborious effort revealed the presence of labeled cells at a frequency of about one in 10^7 unlabeled cells. While these positive results were encouraging, this assay method was not practical since a single measurement was so time-consuming (about 1 human-month per sample) and it was not possible to demonstrate biochemically that the labeled cells did, in fact, contain the mutant protein.

To circumvent these difficulties we undertook to develop a high-speed version of this assay based on flow cytometry. As referred to above, two initial technical questions needed to be resolved: (1) Could a hemoglobin antibody staining method be developed for red cells in suspension, and (2) could the sorter process such samples rapidly enough to allow examination of a statistically significant number of cells in a reasonable time? To permit antibody labeling of hemoglobin, a method needed to be devised that would maintain the integrity of individual erythrocytes, fix intracellular hemoglobin *in situ,* and then permit access to antibody. Such a procedure was suggested by the work of Wang and Richards,[13] in which membrane-permeable cross-linking reagents were used to study the topography of red cell membrane proteins. They showed that, in intact red cells, these reagents cross-linked intracellular hemoglobin to itself and to many of the peripheral and intrinsic membrane proteins (bands 1, 2, 3, 4.1, 4.2, 5, 6, and 7). We successfully adapted this procedure to cross-link cells and produce ghosts that retain about 10^6 hemoglobin molecules covalently bound to the cell membrane, remain permeable to antibody, and retain the native antigenicity of hemoglobin A, S, and C.[2] Such antibody-labeled ghost suspensions can be analyzed on the flow sorter. Cross-linked ghosts prepared from cells taken from an individual heterozygous for hemoglobin S and labeled with FITC–anti-hemoglobin S produce a unimodal histogram with a coefficient of variation of about 15%. (Antibodies produced, immunopurified, and labeled by Dr. Stamatoyannapoulos were used in all of these experiments.) These ghosts are readily detectable even with the limited number of remaining hemoglobin molecules and direct fluorophor labeling of the primary antibody. This ease of detection is afforded by the very efficient 488-nm laser excitation of the fluorescein and by the performance of the flow sorter, which together provide a useful sensitivity of $\sim 10^4$ fluorescein molecules per cell.

Next, the issue of sorter processing speed was examined. As discussed in Section 2.3, to measure a frequency of one labeled cell per 10^7 negative cells one would like to analyze at least 10^9 total cells in no more than a few tens of minutes. This implies processing speeds of about 10^6 cells/sec. In our flow instruments these speeds can be obtained with a sample density of about 5×10^8 cells/ml using near maximum flow rates. Under these conditions about 20 cells are in the laser beam at any given time. Using cross-linked red cell ghosts, we wished to determine if rare fluorescent ghosts could be reliably detected under such conditions. Suspensions of fluorescent ghosts in the absence and presence of dense suspensions of unlabeled ghosts were analyzed. We found that rare ghosts could be quantitatively detected under flow conditions resulting in an overall ghost processing rate of greater than 10^6 cells/sec.[2]

To further test the specificity of antibody labeling, mixtures of red cells taken from a person with normal hemoglobin AA and from a hemoglobin AS heterozygote were processed together and examined. Microscopic observation revealed the approximate number of expected fluorescent ghosts, with the remainder nearly invisible. These ghost suspensions were then analyzed quantitatively on the sorter. By first running a calibration sample of hemoglobin AS ghosts, a fluorescence-scatter window for antibody-labeled ghosts could be determined. This window was usually defined as an area centered on the fluorescence-scatter peak and extending plus and minus two standard deviations along both axes. By integrating the signals falling within this window and determining the total number of ghosts processed by the sum of all the scatter signals, the frequency of antibody-labeled ghosts in a mixture could be calculated and compared to the known dilution. Artificial mixtures as dilute as one in $\sim 10^5$ could be accurately reconstructed before fluorescent background noise obscured the rare labeled ghosts.[2]

Since the presence of this fluorescence background prevented us from accurately counting more dilute mixtures, a detailed investigation into the potential sources of these signals was undertaken. Noise from sorter electronics was completely absent; no signals were detected when the flow stream was turned off. However, signals did appear with the flow stream on even when buffer alone was used as sample. These signals undoubtedly arise from fluorescent objects (cells, debris, etc.) that contaminate the sorter sample tubing. Careful washing with detergent buffers greatly reduced this source of signals, although they could not be entirely eliminated. Using new or thoroughly cleaned tubing reduced the frequency of such events, under actual high-speed flow condtions, to about one signal every 10–100 sec or a total of approximately 10–20 false positive signals for an entier sorter run. This contribution to the background noise was very small, however, compared to that caused by the fluoresceinated antibody itself. To ensure permeability of the cross-linked ghosts, ghost suspensions must be maintained in hypotonic buffer at $0°C$ and, for reproducible staining, several hours of incubation are required. Under these conditons, microaggregates of the antibody form. The measured fluorescence intensity of many of these particles falls within the defined window for antibody-labeled ghosts. In a typical analysis of 10^9 ghosts, about 10^4–10^5 signals will appear in the sorting window, with the vast majority being antibody precipitates. This result is obtained even in the absence of ghosts; antibody at the same concentration incubated under the same conditions produces the same spectrum of fluorescence artifacts. Thus, nonspecific binding of the antibody to normal ghosts does not contribute significantly to the frequency of false positive signals. The antibody-generated artifacts could be dramatically reduced by filtration and ultracentrifugation of the antibody solution just before sorter analysis. However, we have been unable to devise a procedure to then resuspend the ghosts while discarding the pelleted precipitates. One precipitate removal method was partially successful. Following antibody incubation, washed ghost suspensions were incubated with Sepharose 6MB beads coupled with rabbit anti-equine IgG. These microbeads bound antibody microaggregates and could be separated from the ghosts by low-speed centrifugation. The removal was not quantitative, however, and reliable direct counts of artificial mixtures more dilute than one in 10^5 could still not be obtained. A variety of other approaches, e.g., gradient centrifugation or ghost electrophoresis prior to sorting, double labeling of ghosts to discriminate against aggregates, addition of quenchers, etc., have been suggested, but due to additional uncertainties with the ghost method have not been pursued.

Since the unavoidable fluorescent background noise prevented a direct machine count of the rare antibody-labeled ghosts, we designed a two-step strategy in which the sorter served as powerful enrichment device. Starting with approximately 10^9 ghosts, all objects producing fluorescence signals falling in the defined window were first sorted into a small conical centrifuge tube. The sample was concentrated and the sorted objects, consisting mostly of fluorescent debris and unlabeled ghosts, immobilized on microscope slides. The labeled ghosts were then counted manually using a fluorescence microscope equipped with a computer-controlled scanning stage. Typically, a sorted sample was enriched approximately 3000-fold over the initial ghost suspension and could be quantitatively scanned under the microscope in about 6 hr. Positive ghosts were defined as objects that were clearly red cell ghosts under phase illumination and that displayed membrane-specific fluorescence comparable in intensity to the model AS ghosts. Using this two-step method, five samples were analyzed using the hemoglobin S-specific antibody. The measured frequencies ranged from 1.1×10^{-8} to 1.1×10^{-7}, in rough agreement with the values obtained by Stamatoyannopoulos using the slide-based method. Three determinations were also made using the hemoglobin C-specific antibody, with similar results. In spite of this initial success, this approach is compromised in several respects. The signals from the rare fluorescent ghosts cannot be separated from fluorescent background artifacts, and thus the slide preparations are contaminated and difficult to analyze. The ghosts themselves are very fragile structures and cannot be immobilized without significant and variable losses. Thus our results are only semiquantitative; a large part of the order-of-magnitude variation in the variant cell frequencies may be attributable to these technical problems. We believe a more quantitative procedure is required in order to detect an increase in the number of variant cells with age or with subtle environmental mutagen exposures. Lastly, the cells contain only about 1% residual hemoglobin, which makes biochemical verification difficult.

2.4.2. The "Hard Cell" Labeling Approach

Because of the technical problems discussed above, we have explored alternatives to the ghost procedure. A potentially useful strategy was suggested by the work of Aragon *et al.*,[14] in which red cells could be made permeable to substrates of intracellular enzymes without concomitant loss of the proteins themselves. This was accomplished by heavy cross-linking with the same membrane-permeable reagent, dimethyl suberimidate, used in the ghost procedure. The resulting "hard cells" are resistant to hypotonic lysis and retain a nearly normal biconcave shape. In certain versions of this procedure it is necessary to further permeablize the cells to permit efficient antibody access to the hemoglobin. This is done by exposing them to an organic solvent plus a detergent treatment. When this procedure is followed we add protease digestion in order to remove the outer surface of residual membrane proteins to minimize cell clumping. Cells prepared in this way bound FITC–anti-hemoglobin S specifically.[18]

Similar antigen specificity using this hard cell preparation has been demonstrated by labeling mixtures of rabbit and human red cells with rabbit anti-human hemoglobin antibodies. Unfortunately, however, the hard cell method has proven to be prey to a labeling artifact of its own. A minority of cells prepared in this way show variable nonspecific labeling whose frequency decreases sharply with intensity (i.e., the more intense the labeling, the rarer are the cells that show it), but perhaps one in 1000 are bright enough to be confused with the properly labeled cells. Although this labeling is nonspecific in that it is produced by rabbit IgG from nonimmunized animals, and a number of monoclonal mouse antibodies to irrelevant antigens, it has not been possible to block it by preexposing the cells to several standard blocking proteins, including the nonspecific IgG from another species. The staining has also resisted standard methods for reducing nonspecific labeling, such as using high levels and mixed types of detergents and minimizing the antibody amounts and incubation times in the cell labeling reactions. If this problem can be overcome and if accurate reconstructions of artificial mixtures can be then obtained, we plan to adopt this procedure as the one of choice for future work.

These "hard cells" possess a number of useful properties. They stain significantly more brightly than do the ghosts. They are mechanically very stable and leach negligible amounts of hemoglobin. This physical stability will permit serial sorting of samples. By re-sorting the initial sorted sample, we expect to obtain significantly increased enrichments of labeled cells. In model experiments using artificial mixtures. of fluorescent and nonfluorescent "hard cells" approximately 90% recovery efficiencies were obtained in a two-step serial sort. Like the ghost suspensions, these cells can be processed at throughput rates exceeding 10^6/sec. Unlike the ghost preparations, these cells can be quantitatively immobilized on microscope slides with no loss of their characteristic shapes. Also, since hemoglobin is now presented on the exterior of the cell, incubation time with the antibody can be shortened and buffers optimized for antibody stability. This property should significantly reduce fluorescent background contamination due to precipitated antibody. The exterior presentation of the antigen will permit more aggressive fluorescence amplification schemes to be tried, e.g., biotin–avidin complexes or fluorescent microspheres. If a cellular fluorescence intensification method can be found that does not also proportionately increase the number and/or the intensity of fluorescence artifacts, then cleaner sorts of labeled cells will be obtained. This possibility, coupled with serial sorting, could greatly simplify, but probably not eliminate, manual microscopic examination. Lastly, since essentially the full cellular hemoglobin content is retained in these "hard cells," almost 100-fold more protein can be obtained for biochemical analysis. By using a reversible cross-linking analogue of dimethyl suberimidate, 3,3'-dithiobispropionimidate,[13] and ultrathin-gel single-cell electrophoretic techniques[19,20] it appears feasible to directly characterize the hemoglobin content of the antibody-labeled cells and test the assumption that labeled cells contain variant hemoglobin.

3. FUTURE OF THE HEMOGLOBIN-BASED ASSAY

Continued progress on the development of this assay approach is dependent on (1) eliminating the nonspecific staining seen with the hard cells and (2) obtaining plentiful amounts of antibodies that can recognize mutant forms of hemoglobin. We are presently addressing the later point with the development of mouse monoclonal antibodies to a variety of "model" mutant hemoglobins. This approach has already been successfully applied as mouse monoclonal antibodies to myoglobin and to hemoglobin have been reported.[21,22] In no other context can the inherent advantages of high purity, exquisite specificity, and reliable production of hybridoma-derived antibodies be better exploited than in this system. All three approaches mentioned in the introduction are being pursued. First, we have made a comprehensive survey of the reported human hemoglobin single-amino acid-substitution, frameshift, and terminator variants and evaluated each for its applicability to this work. From this list we have obtained nine hemoglobin variants to begin this effort. Ultimately, if such an approach is successful, a library of monoclonal antibodies, each specific for a different and defined human hemoglobin variant, can be generated. A battery of such antibodies could then be used together to detect a variety of variant hemoglobin-containing cells, thus improving the technical ease of the assay and its biological generalizability. Damage at many sites, involving several mutational mechanisms, in the hemoglobin A gene could now be detected. Second, the phylogenetic approach is being pursued in two forms. Monoclonal antibodies to several monkey hemoglobins that do not cross-react to human hemoglobin are being sought for use in the human directed assay. Similarly, antibodies to human hemoglobin and to several rodent hemoglobins that do not cross-react with mouse hemoglobin are being sought for use in a mouse directed assay. Third, work has begun to produce monoclonal antibodies to mutant human hemoglobins by immunizing with synthetic polypeptides. These peptides are identical to a portion of an external segment of human hemoglobin except for having a single, mutationally obtainable amino acid substitution at the site of an externally presented residue.

4. DETECTION OF ERYTHROCYTES WITH MUTATIONALLY ALTERED GLYCOPHORIN A

4.1. Background

In parallel with the assay based on the detection of red cells containing single-amino acid-substituted hemoglobin, we are developing a second assay system, also using erythrocytes, utilizing glycophorin A as a marker. Glycophorin A is a glycosylated integral red cell membrane protein present at about $(5-10) \times 10^5$ copies per cell.[23,24] Its 131 amino acid residues span the membrane, with the N terminus exposed on the cell surface. The utility of this protein as a somatic cell mutation marker was suggested by the work of Furthmayer,[25] which showed that this protein carried the antigenic structures determining the M and N blood groups. These blood group determinants are defined by a polymorphism in the amino acid sequence of the protein coded for by a pair of codominantly expressed alleles located on chromosome 4.[26] The polymorphic amino acid sequence at the N terminus of glycophorin A is

Glycophorin A(M)   Ser-Ser(*)-Thr(*)-Thr(*)-Gly-Val-····
Glycophorin A(N)   Leu-Ser(*)-Thr(*)-Thr(*)-Glu-Val-····

The asterisks indicate amino acid residues glycosylated with the structure[27]

$$NeuNAc\alpha2-3Gal\beta1-3(NeuNAc\alpha2-6)GalNAc\alpha1-O-Ser(Thr)$$

Except for the amino acid substitutions at positions one and five of the sequence, the two proteins are identical, both in amino acid sequence and sites and structures of glycosylation. Individuals homozygous for the M or N allele synthesize only the A(M) or A(N) sequence, respectively, while heterozygotes present equal numbers of the two proteins on their erythrocytes.[25]

4.2. Gene Expression Loss Variants

In this approach, we wish to detect rare erythrocytes in the blood of glycophorin A heterozygotes that fail to express one or the other of the two allelic forms of the protein. This approach has several potential practical and biological advantages over the hemoglobin-based single-amino acid-substitution system. First, glycophorin A is presented on the surface of the red cell and is firmly anchored in the membrane; thus, cell preparation and antibody labeling procedures are simplified. Second, the genetic target size is greatly expanded since the mutant phenotype detected can potentially result from a variety of mutational mechanisms, i.e., single nucleotide changes, or deletions or insertions occurring anywhere within the glycophorin A structural gene or its control elements. This target size argument implies the frequency of glycophorin A "null" variant cells should be much higher, perhaps 100- to 1000-fold, than the frequency seen for a single amino acid substitution at a single site. The resulting greater number of "null" cells should be easier to detect and the frequency of such cells, representing the sum of all possible mutational mechanisms, may more accurately reflect the average integrated genetic damage in that individual.

To detect these functionally hemizygous cells using flow cytometry we require antibodies specific for the two allelic forms of glycophorin A. Such A(M)- and A(N)-specific antibodies, labeled with two different color fluorophors, will be incubated with red cells from MN heterozygotes. Variant cells, defined by binding of only one of the antibodies and hence displaying only one of the two colors, will be enumerated using the LLNL two-color dual beam flow sorter.[28] For this purpose, we have produced and characterized four mouse monoclonal antibodies directed against glycophorin A.[29] Two of these antibodies are specific for glycophorin A(M), one preferentially binds glycophorin A(N), while a fourth recognizes a determinant common to both allelic forms. We have obtained tens of milligrams of the antibodies by Sepharose-protein A purification of ascites fluids.

Our initial experiments using these antibodies have been directed toward developing a reliable immunochemical red cell labeling procedure and evaluating the preparations using the dual beam sorter (DBS). For cytometric analysis, red cells are washed, fixed with DMS or glutaraldehyde to minimize antibody-induced cell aggregation, then incubated with antibody. The purified monoclonal antibodies have been directly conjugated with either a green (fluorescein) or red fluorophor (Texas red, a derivative of rhodamine) or used unlabeled followed by commercially available anti-mouse IgG polyclonal antibodies conjugated to the same fluorophors. Preliminary flow cytometric measurements of immunofluorescently labeled red cells have confirmed the specificity of the antibodies and demonstrated their utility for use in the assay. Satisfactory fluorescence intensities have been obtained with the primary labeled monoclonal antibodies; these intensities can be increased approximately 10-fold using the fluorophor-conjugated anti-mouse reagents with little or no increase in nonspecific labeling. These sandwich-labeled cell populations, when analyzed on the DBS, display modal fluorescence intensities approximately equal to that of standard 1.7-μm fluorescent spheres with coefficients of variation of 10–12%. From the known number of glycophorin A molecules per red cell, we estimate the DBS to have adequate sensitivity to detect approximately 10^4 fluorescein molecules per cell. Given the 10-fold amplification afforded by the sandwich antibody method, this translates into a detection sensitivity of 10^3 antigens per cell. In practice, however, the useful sensitivity may not approach this limit, due to the inherent autofluorescence of the cells. In our case, red cells autofluoresce with an intensity equal to about 0.5% of standard microspheres, yielding an approximate 200-fold difference in brightness between homozygous M cells and homozygous N cells exposed to the glycophorin A(M)-specific antibodies.[30] This overall fluorescence intensity and dynamic range between positive and negative cells is more than adequate for the detection of variant cells.

With respect to operation of the sorter, we have determined the best configuration for the fluorescein and Texas red fluorophors is an argon laser for 488-nm excitation of fluorescein and a rhodamine dye laser, driven by another argon laser also tuned to 488 nm, for 590-nm excitation of Texas red. This arrangement allows for spatially independent excitation and fluorescence emission of red-cell-bound fluorophors as well as optimal spectral separation of the fluorescence emission from the two fluorophors, thus minimizing cross-talk between the green and red signals. In the "null" mutation assay the frequency of variant cells is expected to be as much as 1000-fold higher than the frequency of single-amino acid-substituted variant cells. Thus normal processing rates of 10^3–10^4 cells/sec should be quite adequate in efficiently analyzing samples of 10^6–10^7 cells. The higher frequency of variant cells should allow for direct sorter quantitation of the variant cell frequency by simultaneous measurement of light scatter as well as the two fluorescence signals for each cell in the sample. The variant frequency will be the number of green-only or red-only cells divided by the total number of cells processed determined by the sum of the scatter-gated fluorescent cells. Also, adequate numbers of variant cells can be obtained by sorting for later biochemical analysis.

In addition to excluding instrumental fluorescence artifacts, it is also critical in this assay to rigorously exclude biological artifacts; that is, since this assay is based on the detection of cells that fail to express a gene product it is critical to ensure that the counted variant cells are true glycophorin A structural gene mutants. This is important since a number of other mechanisms, both genetic and nongenetic, could cause the protein to fail to appear on the red cell membrane. For example, mutations outside the glycophorin A locus leading to loss of function of proteins necessary for processing, transporting, glycosylating, or inserting glycophorin A into the membrane could produce apparent glycophorin A "null" cells. Nongenetic events include loss of membrane integrity or insufficient levels of substrate sugars for glycosylating enzymes due to metabolic anomalies. This assay is strongly protected against such false positive "phenocopies" since it requires antibody binding to one of the glycophorin A forms. The proper cell surface presentation of the glycophorin A product of the unaffected allele ensures that the rest of the cell apparatus necessary for the expression of the protein is intact. Also, the frequency measurement can be checked for internal consistency by comparing the number of M-"null" cells against the number of N-"null" cells. Since we assume the probability of mutation of either of the two glycophorin A alleles to be the same, the number of "null" cells of each type should be equal. Finally, we can be assured that the measured variant cell frequency will accurately reflect the actual frequency of occurrence of these cells in the body since erythrocytes from genetically homozygous glycophorin A "null" individuals, completely lacking expression of the protein, appear to exhibit normal viability,[31] implying lack of *in vivo* selection.

4.3. Single-Amino Acid-Substitution Variants

The glycophorin A marker can also be exploited in a second assay exactly analogous to the hemoglobin-based single-amino acid-substitution scheme by taking advantage of the mutational basis underlying the glycophorin A(M), A(N) polymorphism. As shown in Table I, the amino acid sequence difference at position one can arise as a result of a single nucleotide change if the serine–leucine codons are TC(A or G) and TT(A or G), respectively. Similarly, the amino acid sequence difference at position five can also occur as a result of single nucleotide changes in the respective glycine and glutamic acid codons GGG and GAG.

Thus, in homozygous M individuals, there should be rare cells containing "N-like-" glycophorin A with Leu at position one or, independently, Glu at position five due to a C to T transversion or G to A transition. Similarly, the blood of N homozygotes should contain rare cells with "M-like" glycophorin A with amino acids Ser or Gly at positions one and five, respectively. As in the case of hemoglobin, heritable mutations resulting in single amino acid substitutions in this protein have now been reported.[32-34] To detect such single sub-

Table I
Amino Acid Differences between Glycophorines A(M) and A(N)

Position	Amino acid		Corresponding triplet codon	
	A(M)	A(N)	A(M)	A(N)
1	Ser	Leu	TC(A or G)	TT(A or G)
5	Gly	Glu	GGG	GAG

stitutions our A(M)- and A(N)-specific monoclonal antibodies must be capable of recognizing the amino acid differences at these two positions independently, i.e., the antibody must not depend on the presence of both substitutions for its binding specificity. It is most likely that our antibodies recognize the amino acid difference at position one. The N terminus of glycophorin A appears to be the immunodominant determinant recognized by animal anti-M and anti-N sera,[34] although some sera may be specific for the substitution at position five.[33]

Additional testing of the specificity of our antibodies with chemically modified glycophorin A is required to precisely define their target antigenic sites. Given the expected specificity, we can use these antibodies to measure the frequency of these single-amino acid-substituted glycophorins in the bloods of homozygous M and homozygous N individuals. Such a measurement would be particularly valuable in two respects: one, it would allow us to compare the frequency of single nucleotide changes in the glycophorin A genes to those measured in the hemoglobin genes, and two, it would allow us to compare the frequency of single nucleotide changes with the frequency of the loss of expression of the entire gene in the same glycophorin A structural locus.

If our initial results measuring the frequency of single-amino acid-substituted hemoglobin-containing cells are representative, we will be faced in this assay with enumerating variant cells expressing single amino acid substitutions in glycophorin A in the range of one cell in 10^7–10^8. Thus some of the attendant problems and solutions discussed for the hemoglobin system are relevant for this marker as well. Problems of cell preparation and antibody labeling, which currently plague the hemoglobin system, should not occur, however, as the same procedures used in the "null" assay can be applied.

5. SUMMARY AND CONCLUSIONS

In estimating the prospects for developing nonclonogenic somatic-cell mutation assays of the types described here, we do not see the capabilities of presently available flow sorters as imposing a significant limitation. They appear to offer quite acceptable detection sensitivity, processing rates, machine-generated noise levels, stability, and inherent discrimination ability. For "null" variant cell assays, it appears that direct sorter enumeration of mutant cell frequencies is practical. For the assays based on single amino acid substitutions, however, this is not presently possible. Nevertheless, flow sorters can function as very efficient enrichment devices, rapidly discriminating non-labeled cells and obvious fluorescent artifacts from the antibody-labeled cells. Although the cost and operational complexity of sorting flow cytometers, particularly dual-laser versions, may limit the general use of any assay requiring them, these instruments are powerful tools for the research, development, and genetic validation of these approaches.

ACKNOWLEDGMENTS. Work performed under the auspices of the U. S. Department of Energy by the Lawrence Livermore National Laboratory under contract number W-7405-ENG-48 with the financial support of the National Institutes of Health, Grant 1 RO1 CA 30613, and the Environmental Protection Agency, Grant R808642-01.

REFERENCES

1. G. Stamatoyannopoulos, Possibilities for demonstrating point mutations in somatic cells, as illustrated by studies of mutant hemoglobins, in: *Genetic Damage in Man Caused by Environmental Agents* (K. Berg, ed.), pp. 49–62, Academic Press, New York (1979).
2. W. L. Bigbee, E. W. Branscomb, H. B. Weintraub, Th. Papayannopoulou, and G. Stamatoyannopoulos, Cell sorter immunofluorescence detection of human erythrocytes labeled in suspension with antibodies specific for hemoglobins S and C, *J. Immunol. Methods.* 45, 117–127 (1981).
3. A. C. Wilson, S. S. Carlson, and T. J. White, Biochemical evolution, *Annu. Rev. Biochem.* 46, 573–639 (1977).
4. M. Reichlin, Amino acid substitution and the antigenicity of globular proteins, in: *Advances in Immunology* (F. J. Dixon and H. G. Kunkel, eds.), Vol. 20, pp. 71–123, Academic Press, New York (1975).
5. M. Reichlin, and R. W. Noble, Immunochemistry of protein mutants, in: *Immunochemistry of Proteins* (M. Z. Atassi, ed.), Vol. 2. pp. 311–349, Plenum Press, New York (1977).
6. F. A. Garver, M. B. Baker, C. S. Jones, M. Gravely, A. Gultekin, and T. H. J. Huisman, Radioimmunoassay for abnormal hemoglobins, *Science 196,* 1334–1336 (1977).
7. T. H. J. Huisman and J. H. P. Jonxis, *The Hemoglobinopathies: Techniques of Identification,* p. 341–413, Marcel Dekker, New York (1977).
8. J. T. Wilson, L. B. Wilson, V. B. Reddy, C. Cavellesco, P. K. Ghosh, J. K. deRiel, B. G. Forget, and S. M. Weissman, Nucleotide sequence of the coding portion of human α-globin messenger RNA, *J. Biol. Chem.* 255, 2807–2815 (1980).
9. C. A. Marotta, J. T. Wilson, B. G. Forget, and S. M. Weissman, Human β-globin messenger RNA III. Nucleotide sequences derived from complementary DNA, *J. Biol. Chem.* 252, 5040–5053 (1977).
10. M. Kimura, The neutral theory of molecular evolution, *Sci. Am.* Nov, 98–126 (1979).
11. M. Goodman, Decoding the pattern of protein evolution, *Prog. Biophys. Mol. Biol., 37,* 105–164 (1981).
12. R. A. Lerner, Tapping the immunological repertoire to produce antibodies of predetermined specificity, *Nature 299,* 592–596 (1982).
13. K. Wang and F. M. Richards, Reaction of dimethyl-3,3-dithiobispropionimidate with intact human erythrocytes, *J. Biol. Chem. 250,* 6622–6626 (1975).
14. J. J. Aragon, J. E. Feliu, R. A. Frenkel, and A. Sols, Permeabilization of animal cells for kinetic studies of intracellular enzymes: *In situ* behavior of the glycolytic enzymes of erythrocytes, *Proc. Natl. Aca. Sci. USA 77,* 6324–6328 (1980).

15. V. Kachel and E. Menke, Hydrodynamic properties of flow cytometric instruments, in: *Flow Cytometry and Sorting* (M. R. Melamed, P. F. Mullaney, and M. L. Mendelsohn, eds.), pp. 41–59, Wiley, New York (1979).

16. Th. Papayannopoulou, T. C. McGuire, G. Lim, E. Garzel, P. E. Nute, and G. Stamatoyannopoulos, Identification of haemoglobin S in red cells and normoblasts, using fluorescent anti-Hb S antibodies, *Br. J. Haematol. 34*, 25–31 (1976).

17. Th. Papayannopoulou, G. Lim, T. C. McGuire, V. Ahern, P. E. Nute, and G. Stamatoyannopoulos, Use of specific fluorescent antibodies for the identification of hemoglobin C in erythrocytes, *Am. J. Hematol. 2*, 105–112 (1977).

18. W. L. Bigbee, E. W. Branscomb, and R. H. Jensen, Detection of mutated erythrocytes in man, Presented at the American–Swedish Workshop on Individual Susceptibility to Genotoxic Agents in the Human Population (F. J. deSerres, ed.), held at the National Institutes of Environmental Health Sciences, Research Triangle Park, North Carolina, May 10–12, 1982 (in press).

19. H. W. Goedde, H.-G. Benkmann, and L. Hirth, Ultrathin-layer isoelectric-focusing for rapid diagnosis of protein variants, *Hum. Genet. 57*, 434–436 (1981).

20. S. I. O. Anyaibe and V. E. Headings, Identification of inherited protein variants in individual erythrocytes, *Biochem. Genet. 18*, 455–463 (1980).

21. J. A. Berzofsky, G. Hicks, J. Fedorko, and J. Minna, Properties of monoclonal antibodies specific for determinants of a protein antigen, myoglobin, *J. Biol. Chem. 255*, 11188–11191 (1980).

22. G. Stamatoyannopoulos, D. Lindsley, Th. Papayannopoulos, M. Farquhar, M. Brice, P. E. Nute, G. R. Serjeant, and H. Lehmann, Mapping of antigenic sites on human haemoblogin by means of monoclonal antibodies and haemoglobin variants, *Lancet ii*, 952–954 (1981).

23. H. Furthmayer, Structural analysis of a membrane glycoprotein: glycophorin A, *J. Supramol. Struc. 7*, 121–134 (1977).

24. C. G. Gahmberg, M. Jokinen, and L. C. Andersson, Expression of the major red cell sialoglycoprotein, glycophorin A, in the human leukemic cell line K562, *J. Biol. Chem. 254*, 7442–7448 (1979).

25. H. Furthmayer, Structural comparison of glycophorins and immunochemical analysis of genetic variants, *Nature 271*, 519–524 (1978).

26. P. J. L. Cook, J. E. Noades, C. G. Lomas, K. E. Buckton, and E. B. Robson, Exclusion mapping illustrated by the MNSs blood group, *Ann. Hum. Genet. Lond. 44*, 61–73 (1980).

27. R. Prohaska, T. A. W. Koerner Jr., I. M. Armitage, and H. Furthmayer, Chemical and carbon-13 nuclear magnetic resonance studies of the blood group M and N active sialoglycopeptides from human glycophorin A, *J. Biol. Chem. 256*, 5781–5791 (1981).

28. P. N. Dean and D. Pinkel, High resolution dual laser flow cytometry, *J. Histochem. Cytochem. 26*, 622–627 (1978).

29. W. L. Bigbee, M. Vanderlaan, S. S. N. Fong, and R. H. Jensen, Monoclonal antibodies specific for the M and N forms of human glycophorin A, *Mol. Immunol.* (in press) (1984).

30. R. H. Jensen, W. L. Bigbee, and E. W. Branscomb, Somatic mutations detected by immunofluorescence and flow cytometry, presented at Proceedings of the International Symposium on Biological Dosimetry, Approaches to Mammalian Systems (Neuherberg, West Germany, October 14–16, 1982) (in press).

31. M. J. A. Tanner and D. J. Anstee, The membrane change in En(a−) human erythrocytes, *Biochem. J. 153*, 271–277 (1976).

32. W. Dahr, K. Beyreuther, E. Gallasch, J. Kruger, and P. Morel, Amino acid sequence of the blood group M(g)-specific major human erythrocyte membrane sialoglycoprotein, *Hoppe-Seyler's Z. Physiol. Chem. 362*, 81–85 (1981a).

33. W. Dahr, M. Kordowicz, K. Beyreuther, and J. Kruger, The amino-acid sequence of the M(c)-specific major red cell membrane sialoglycoprotein—An intermediate of the blood group M- and N-active molecules, *Hoppe-Seyler's Z. Physiol. Chem. 362*, 363–366 (1981b).

34. H. Furthmayer, M. N. Metaxas and M. Metaxas-Bühler, M(g) and M(c): Mutations within the amino-terminal region of glycophorin A, *Proc. Natl. Acad. Sci. USA 78*, 631–635 (1981).

3

Development of a Plaque Assay for the Detection of Red Blood Cells Carrying Abnormal or Mutant Hemoglobins

MASROOR A. BAIG AND AFTAB A. ANSARI

1. INTRODUCTION

The potential of immunological methods for the detection of single mammalian cells carrying an altered (mutant) form of marker protein molecule (antigen) has been recently reviewed.[1] The use of immunological methods for detection of mutations has been possible by using antibodies that can specifically recognize the amino acid difference(s) between the molecule normally present in a given cell and its variant form. Techniques like immunofluorescence[2,3] have been employed to distinguish cells carrying mutant forms of a protein against which antibody is available from the normal cells. In this chapter we describe the development of a simple method that could be used for detection and quantitation of red blood cells (RBC) carrying a specific variant of hemoglobin (Hb).

2. PRINCIPLE OF THE METHOD

The RBC–antibody plaque assay is an adaptation of the hemolytic plaque assay originally developed to enumerate immunoglobulin-secreting lympho-

MASROOR A. BAIG • Laboratory of Genetics, National Institute of Environmental Health Sciences, Research Triangle Park, North Carolina 27709; *present address:* Department of Biochemistry, University of Kashmir, Hazratbal, Srinagar 190006, India. AFTAB A. ANSARI • Northrop Services, Inc., Research Triangle Park, North Carolina 27709.

cytes.[4] The lymphocyte plaque assay involves the lysis of indicator cells (sheep RBC—sRBC—coated with an antibody against the immunoglobulin) when they are plated with immunoglobulin-secreting lymphocytes, complement, and a complement-fixing anti-immunoglobulin antibody called developer. Unlike lymphocytes, RBC do not secrete the molecules to be detected. Therefore, for the RBC plaque assay to work, Hb in the test RBC should be released into the surrounding medium after all the components of the assay have been mixed and plated. To achieve the lysis of the test RBC, an antibody against the membrane of the test RBC is also incorporated in the assay mixture. For the assay, known numbers of test RBC are plated with indicator cells (sRBC coated with antibody against the Hb present in the test RBC), anti-RBC ghost antibody, a polyspecific anti-Hb antibody, and guinea pig complement. All the test RBC are lysed by the binding of anti-RBC ghost to the surface of the test RBC and subsequent activation of the complement. The Hb thus released binds to the specific anti-Hb antibody on the indicator cells and the developer, complement gets activated, and all the indicator sRBC surrounding the test RBC are lysed, resulting in the formation of a clear zone or plaque. One such plaque would correspond to one test RBC containing the type of Hb against which the antibody is coupled to the indicator sRBC. The possible sequence of events occurring in the RBC antibody plaque assay is shown in Figure 1.

    Let us now consider two kinds of RBC, one containing Hb variant H1 and the other containing the variant H2. If H1 and H2 have some structural and

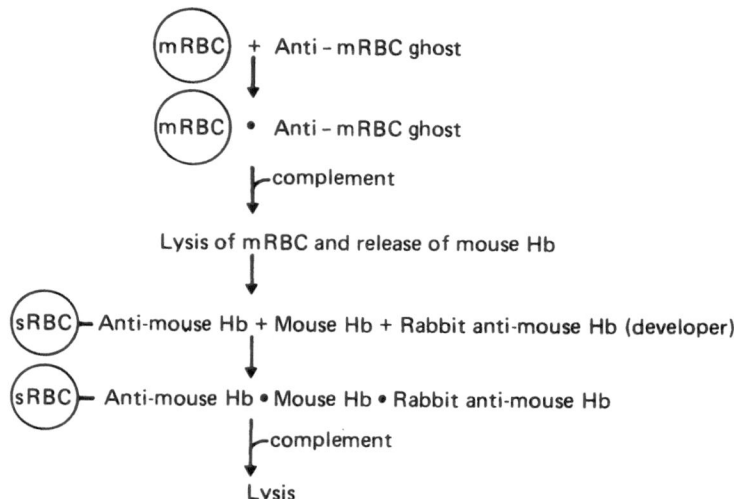

Figure 1. Schematic representation of the possible steps involved in the RBC–antibody plaque assay.

RBC carrying normal H2Hb + sRBC - Anti-H1Hb + Sheep Anti-mRBC ghost + Rabbit Anti-H1Hb
+ complement → No lysis of indicator sRBC (No Plaque)

RBC carrying mutant H2Hb + sRBC - Anti-H1Hb + Sheep Anti-mRBC ghost + Rabbit Anti-Hb
+ complement → Lysis of indicator sRBC around the mutant RBC (Plaque)

Figure 2. Use of RBC plaque assay to detect mutation in Hb. All sRBC in the vicinity of each mRBC are lysed, resulting in the formation of a clear zone or plaque.

immunological differences, then it may be possible to obtain an antibody that reacts only with the homologous antigen (say H1) and not with the heterologous antigen (H2). This specific antibody could be used for the detection of H1-carrying RBC in a population of H2-carrying RBC by the RBC plaque assay. If specific anti-H1-coated sRBC are plated with H2-carrying RBC, anti-RBC ghost, complement, and an appropriate developer, then the normal (H2-carrying) RBC would not form plaques. However, if a mutation in H2 has taken place such that it has acquired amino acid(s) normally present in H1 at specific position(s), then the RBC containing this Hb will form a plaque (see Figure 2). One mutant cell will thus form one plaque.

Potential applicability of the RBC plaque assay in the detection of mutation in Hb is demonstrated by the ability of the assay to distinguish between RBC from two inbred strains of mice, namely DBA/2 and C57BL/6, which carry two different variants of Hb.

At this stage some knowledge of structural and immunological properties of mouse Hb is required. Mouse Hb is a tetrameric protein consisting of two kinds of polypeptide chains, namely α and β, controlled by the Hba locus [5] and the Hbb[6] locus, respectively. Variants at both of these loci have been identified.[7-10] Four kinds of α chains—1, 2, 3, and 4—and four kinds of β chains—s, d_{maj}, d_{min}, and p_{min}—have been recognized. The α chains differ from each other by one to three amino acid residues at positions 25, 62, and 68,[8] while β chains may differ from each other by as many as 13 amino acid residues (Table I).[3]

TABLE I
Amino Acid Differences among Various Mouse β Chains[a]

	Amino acids at different positions in the β chain													
β Chain	9	13	16	20	22	23	58	72	83	76	77	80	109	139
s	Ala	Gly	Gly	Ala	Glx	Val	Ala	Ser	Asp	Asn	His	Asn	Met	Ala
d_{maj}	—	Cys	—	Ser	—	—	—	Asn	—	—	—	Ser	—	Thr
d_{min}	Ser	Cys	Ala	Pro	Glu	—	Pro	Asn	Glu	Lys	Asn	—	Ala	Thr
p_{min}	Ser	Cys	Ala	Pro	Ala	Ile	Pro	Asn	Glu	Lys	Asn	—	Ala	Thr

[a]The amino acid sequence of the s chain is taken as reference; a dash indicates the same amino acid as in the s chain at the particular residue position. (Modified from Ref. 12.)

While DBA/2 mouse Hb has d_{maj} and p_{min} β chains, C57BL/6 mouse Hb has s-type β chains. Besides the amino acid sequence differences (see Table I), the two types of Hb have been shown to differ immunologically.[11]

3. REAGENTS

The following reagents are needed for an RBC antibody plaque assay by which d Hb-carrying mouse RBC (mRBC; from DBA/2 mouse) can be distinguished from s Hb-carrying mRBC (from C57BL/6 mouse): (1) antibody against mRBC ghost; (2) a specific anti-d Hb antibody to be coupled to sRBC to obtain indicator cells (this antibody should bind only the DBA/2 Hb and not C57BL/6 Hb); (3) a polyspecific anti-mouse Hb antibody to be used as developer; (4) indicator cells; and (5) complement. Preparation of each of these reagents is described in the following sections.

3.1. Anti-Mouse RBC Ghost Sera

Anti-mRBC ghost serum is needed to lyse the test RBC in the assay mixture. It is essential that this antiserum is capable of fixing the complement and its specificity should be such that it could bind only the mouse RBC and not the indicator sRBC. The best approach is to immunize sheep with mRBC ghosts, although rabbit antisera have also been found satisfactory. To prepare mRBC ghosts, blood is collected from the mouse in the presence of an anticoagulant (e.g., 3.2% sodium citrate). RBC are isolated and washed three times with 0.11 M sodium phosphate buffer, pH 7.4, by centrifugation at 800g for 5 min at 4°C. The cells are lysed by suspending in 15 volumes of hypotonic sodium phosphate buffer (7×10^{-3} M, pH 7.4) overnight and the RBC ghosts are sedimented by centrifugation at 20,000g for 20 min at 4°C.[13] The supernatant is discarded and the ghosts are washed three times with the hypotonic buffer to remove any residual Hb bound to the ghosts and finally with 0.15 M NaCl. The final pellet is suspended in equal volume of 0.15 M NaCl.

Anti-RBC ghost antibody is raised in sheep by injecting each sheep intravenously with 1 ml of the 50% RBC ghost suspension once every week for 4 weeks. One week after the last injection, the sheep is bled. If the titer is adequate, then every week the sheep is bled and then injected with the same dose of the antigen for 6 more weeks. Activity of the antibody is determined by incubating mRBC with several dilutions of the antibody in the presence of complement and checking for lysis of the mRBC. Before use in the plaque assay, the anti-RBC ghost antiserum is absorbed on washed sRBC in cold for 1 hr (1 ml packed sRBC/10 ml of the antiserum) to get rid of any antibody that could cross-react with sRBC. The volume of antibody to be used in the plaque assay is determined experimentally.

3.2. Anti-Mouse Hb Antibodies

Two anti-mouse Hb antibodies are required for the RBC antibody plaque assay. One is used to coat the sRBC to obtain indicator cells and the other is used as the developer. The same antibody could also be used for both purposes. The two antibodies should meet the following criteria:

1. Either of the two antibodies must be capable of fixing complement.
2. At least one of the two antibodies should be monospecific for a particular variant of mouse Hb (d Hb in the present case) to be able to detect mutation; the other antibody could be polyspecific.
3. The antibody that is coupled to the sRBC should not lose its antigen binding activity after coupling.

Different kinds of approaches to preparing specific antibodies have been described elsewhere.[1] The best approach appears to be to inject one variant of mouse Hb into a mouse carrying another Hb variant, such as immunizing a d Hb-carrying mouse with s Hb and vice versa (alloimmunization). Accordingly, immunization of LP mice (d Hb-carrying) with s Hb from C57BL/6 mice produces an antibody that reacts only with C57BL/6 RBC and not with DBA/2 RBC.[3] Unfortunately, when this antibody is coupled to sRBC using different coupling reagents (see Section 3.3 for methods) it loses its antigen binding activity. Similar loss of activity on coupling to sRBC was also observed with mouse anti-mouse immunoglobulin allotype antibodies.[14] Another limitation with mouse anti-mouse antibodies is that they have poor complement-fixing activity and therefore they cannot be used as developer if the antibody that is coupled to the sRBC is also not capable of fixing the complement.

It therefore becomes necessary to raise antibodies against mouse Hb variants, say d Hb, in other species, such as rabbits, horses, and goats. Such antibody would cross-react with d Hb as well as with other mouse Hb variants because of the presence of some common antigenic determinants. However, the antibodies raised against the common antigenic determinants can be absorbed out using appropriate immunoabsorbents of mouse Hb variant and then the specific antibody could be recovered. For example, Schreiber et al.[15] isolated anti-human HbS antibody from an antiserum reacting with both HbS and HbA by first precipitating the cross-reacting antibody with HbA followed by absorption on HbA bound to CM-cellulose. The resulting antiserum was absorbed on HbS bound to CM-cellulose from which the specific bound antibody–HbS complex was eluted, dissociated, and separated by Sephadex gel filtration.

Another promising approach is to make hybridomas that can synthesize monoclonal antibodies of defined specificity against a mouse Hb variant. The two approaches are considered below.

3.2.1. Raising the Anti-Mouse Hb Antibodies in Horses, Rabbits, and Goats

3.2.1a. Immunization. Blood from several mice of one strain is pooled in 3.2% sodium citrate. RBC are obtained by centrifugation at 800g for 5 min, washed, lysed by suspending in water and passing carbon monoxide, and the hemolysate is frozen at $-20°C$ overnight. The frozen hemolysate is thawed and centrifuged at 20,000g for 1 hr in cold to remove cell debris and unlysed cells. The supernatant may be used for immunization directly or the Hb can be fractionated by DEAE–Sephadex A-50 chromatography using a linear pH gradient from pH 8.2 to 7.2 of 0.05 M Tris–HCl buffer.[16] Concentration of Hb is determined spectrophotometrically using an extinction coefficient $E_{1cm}^{1\%}$ of 8.4 at 540 nm.[17]

Shetland ponies are immunized by injecting intramuscularly at multiple sites 20 mg of Hb emulsified with complete Freund's adjuvant. After 2 weeks, two more injections of the same dose of the antigen in incomplete Freund's adjuvant are given 15 days apart. One week later an injection of 15 mg antigen in incomplete Freund's adjuvant is given, followed by two injections of 20 mg antigen in incomplete Freund's adjuvant after 4 weeks each. The animals are bled 1 week later.

Rabbits are injected subcutaneously at multiple sites and in hind-foot pad with 0.2 ml emulsion of unfractionated Hb (2 mg) in complete Freund's adjuvant at weekly intervals. Weekly bleedings before the injections are started after the fourth week. This rabbit antiserum contains antibodies against mouse Hb as well as against mRBC ghost.

For immunization of goats, the animals were injected intramuscularly at multiple sites with 1 ml of Hb (4.5 mg) emulsified with complete Freund's adjuvant (1 : 1.2) 2 weeks apart. Weekly injections of the same dose of Hb in incomplete Freund's adjuvant are given following the second injection for 13 weeks. The goats are bled every week after the fifth injection.

Sera are separated and stored at $-70°C$ until use.

We have observed that anti-mouse Hb antibodies raised in rabbits and horses lose their Hb-binding activity after they are coupled to sRBC. Avrameas *et al.*[18] have also reported similar observations with various rabbit and horse antibodies. Therefore, these two antibodies cannot be used to obtain indicator sRBC for the RBC antibody plaque assay. However, since rabbit antibodies are excellent complement activators, they could be employed as developer in the assay.

The antibodies raised in goats retain the antigen-binding activity after they are coupled to sRBC. However, goat antibodies do not have sufficient complement-activating property. Therefore, for the RBC–antibody plaque assay, specific anti-Hb antibody purified from goat antiserum can be used to prepare indicator sRBC and rabbit anti-Hb antibody can be used as developer.

3.2.1b. Purification of Specific Goat Anti-d Hb Antibody from the Antiserum. As expected, the antibodies raised in goats against *d* Hb from DBA/2 mice and *s* Hb from C57BL/6 mice cross-reacted with homologous (immunizing) as well as heterologous antigens. Theoretically, one should be able to isolate specific antibody from the antiserum that could react only with the immunizing antigen and not with its other variant(s) by negative (removal of antibody population of unwanted specificities) and positive (recovery of specific antibody) absorptions on appropriate immunoabsorbents.

Different steps involved in the isolation of monospecific antibody from goat anti-*d* Hb that reacts only with DBA/2 Hb and not with C57BL/6 Hb are described below.

Preparation of Cross-Linked Immunoabsorbents. Immunoabsorbents (proteins bound to CNBr-activated Sepharose beads) are widely employed for purification of specific, active antibodies or antigens from complex samples. However, a serious problem with such immunoabsorbents is that the bound proteins "leakout" during the elution with acidic buffer of the specific antibody from the immunoabsorbent.[19-23] This makes it necessary to perform another chromatographic step (gel or ion exchange chromatography) to separate the antibody from antigen that "leaked out" during the elution,[3,24-28] resulting in a significant loss of precious purified material. For the purification of anti-*d* Hb antibody, the Hb–Sepharose immunoabsorbents were therefore cross-linked with glutaraldehyde before use in order to prevent any significant leakage of Hb during elution of the antibody.[29]

Glutaraldehyde cross-linked immunoabsorbents are prepared as follows. First, Hb solution is dialyzed extensively against the coupling buffer (0.1 M $NaHCO_3$ buffer, pH 8.3, containing 1 M NaCl). Required amount (1 g for 35 mg of protein) of freeze-dried CNBr-activated Sepharose 4B (Pharmacia Fine Chemicals, Piscataway, NJ) is swollen and washed with 1 mM HCl on a sintered glass funnel. The gel is then washed with a small volume of coupling buffer and transferred quickly to the Hb solution in a suitable container. The mixture is shaken end-over-end for 2 hr at room temperature (25°C), after which excess buffer is decanted and any remaining reactive groups on Sepharose are blocked by suspending the gel in 0.5 M Tris–HCl buffer, pH 8.0, for 2 hr. The gel is washed to remove any physically adsorbed protein with coupling buffer followed by water, coupling buffer again, and then with carbon dioxide-saturated water (pH 4.0). The whole washing cycle is repeated five times. The washed gel is suspended in three volumes of 0.25 M $NaHCO_3$ buffer, pH 8.8. Glutaraldehyde solution is gradually added to the gel slurry to a final concentration of 0.005 M and the mixture is shaken at room temperature. After 1 hr, the liquid is removed and an equal volume of 1 M ethanolamine solution, pH 8.0, is added to the gel. After shaking for 1 hr at room temperature, the gel is washed with four cycles of coupling buffer followed by 0.1 M acetate buffer, pH 3.6, containing 1 M NaCl. Finally, the immunoabsorbent is washed with

0.01 M phosphate-buffered saline, pH 7.2, containing 0.02% sodium azide and stored at 4°C. Before use, the immunoabsorbent is washed first with eluting agent and then equilibrated with binding buffer.

Adsorption of Goat Anti-d Hb Antiserum on C57BL/6 Hb Immunoabsorbent. The antiserum is clarified by centrifugation and is absorbed first on washed sRBC (⅒₀ the total volume of the antiserum) in cold for 1 hr. Cross-linked C57BL/6 Hb (heterologous antigen) immunoabsorbent is washed with 0.1 M acetic acid, equilibrated with phosphate-buffered saline, pH 7.2, and the liquid removed by suction to form a "cake." The sRBC adsorbed antiserum is mixed with the immunoabsorbent (one-fifth packed volume) and shaken using an end-over-end mixer at 4°C overnight. The antiserum is recovered by filtration on a sintered glass funnel under vacuum. In order to ensure the quantitative removal of antibody molecules cross-reacting with C57BL/6 Hb, the absorption on C57BL/6 Hb immunoabsorbent is usually repeated two more times using fresh immunoabsorbent. The absorption time is reduced to 7 hr each time.

Isolation of Specific Anti-d Hb Antibody. After absorption on C57BL/6 Hb immunoabsorbent, the antiserum is incubated with freshly washed cross-linked DBA/2 Hb (homologous antigen) immunoabsorbent (one-fifth the volume of the antiserum) with shaking at room temperature for 1 hr. The slurry is then poured in an appropriate size chromatographic column at 4°C. After the column is packed, the effluent antiserum is recycled through the column. The column is washed with phosphate-buffered saline, pH 7.2, until the absorbance of the effluent at 280 nm is equal to zero. The bound specific antibody is eluted with 0.1 M acetic acid. Fractions of 1 ml are collected in tubes containing 100 μl of saturated disodium hydrogen phosphate solution. The protein-containing fractions are pooled, dialyzed against phosphate-buffered saline, and stored in small aliquots at −70°C.

3.2.2. Anti-Mouse Hb Antibody Production by Hybridomas

3.2.2a. Introduction. Hybridomas, first developed by Köhler and Milstein,[30] are the hybrids between a myeloma cell line and spleen cells and secrete monoclonal antibodies of defined specificity. Hybridomas that synthesize anti-mouse Hb antibodies specific for a particular variant of Hb could be produced. Several review articles deal with the methodology of the production of hybridomas.[31,32] As mentioned in Section 3.2.1, LP mice immunized with *s* Hb from C57BL/6 mice produce an antiserum that reacts specifically with *s* Hb and not with *d* Hb. Therefore, spleen cells from LP mice immunized with *s* Hb are used to fuse with myeloma cells. For immunization of the mice, three intraperitoneal injections of 1 mg Hb emulsified with complete Freund's adjuvant are given on days 0, 7, and 14. The animals are boosted by an intravenous injection of Hb (0.1 mg) in saline after 4 weeks of the last injection. After 3–4 days of the booster injection, which is the best time for fusion,[33] the mouse is killed, and its spleen is removed aseptically and placed in Hank's balanced salt solution (Flow Laboratories, McLean, VA). After rinsing with the solution several times, the cells are squeezed out and dispersed by passage through a pasteur pipette. The cell suspension is then transferred to a 50-ml centrifuge tube and allowed to stand for 5 min to let big clumps settle. The uniform suspension from the top is transferred to another tube and centrifuged at $400g$ for 5 min. The pellet is tapped loose and suspended in 10 ml of RBC lysing buffer (0.17 M NH_4Cl containing 0.01 M $KHCO_3$ and 0.1 mM disodium ethylenediamine tetraacetic acid). After 5 min, the suspension is centrifuged at $300g$ for 5 min and the cells are washed twice with Dulbecco's modified Eagle's medium (DMEM; GIBCO, Grand Island, NY). Finally, the spleen cells are suspended in 5 m DMEM and their number and viability determined by counting in the presence of 0.4% trypan blue solution. About 150 × 10^6 viable cells are obtained from one spleen.

Two myeloma cell lines, namely Sp2/0e5-P33, developed by recloning Sp2/o-Ag-14[34] and X63-Ag-8.653[35] are generally used for fusion. These cell lines do not produce their own immunoglobulins and therefore are ideal for fusion purposes. The myeloma cells are grown in standard medium (DMEM supplemented with 10% fetal bovine serum, 2% glutamine, and 1% antibiotic) containing 1.6 × 10^{-4} M 8-azaguanine. Three days and then 1 day prior to fusion, the myeloma cells are transferred to the standard medium without 8-azaguanine because for fusion the myeloma cells must be in the exponential phase of growth. On the day of fusion, the myeloma cells are harvested, washed twice with DMEM, suspended in 3 m DMEM, and their viability assessed, which should be more than 95% for proper fusion.

Polyethylene glycol is used as the fusing agent. A weighed amount of polyethylene glycol 1500 is sterilized by autoclaving. It is allowed to cool to about 50°C and then an appropriate volume of DMEM (2 ml for each gram of polyethylene glycol) is added. The contents are mixed by vortexing and the solution is kept at 37°C in an incubator.

For fusion, spleen cells and myeloma cells are mixed at a ratio of 2:1 or 5:2 in a 50-m tube and centrifuged at $400g$ for 5 min. The supernatant is removed, pellet is loosened by tapping, and then 0.5 ml of warm (37°C) polyethylene glycol solution is added. The contents are mixed by swirling the tube and centrifuged at $300g$ for 6 min. After additional 2 min, 10 ml of DMEM is added gradually with gentle tapping to suspend the cells. The cells are harvested by centrifugation at $300g$ for 6 min, suspended in 10 ml of selective HAT (hypoxanthine, amethopterin, thymidine) medium. After overnight incubation in a 100-mm petri dish in 37°C incubator having 7% CO_2 in the atmosphere, the cells are harvested, suspended in fresh HAT medium, and plated in 96-well Linbro microculture plates (10^4–10^5 cells per well). Unfused myeloma and spleen cells die in the HAT medium and only the hybrids that have acquired the growth capability of myeloma cells and antibody-synthesizing activity of spleen cells are able to survive. After making sure that all the unfused cells are dead, HAT medium is withdrawn. First, amethopterin is removed by growing the cells in the hypoxanthine–thymidine medium for a few days before replacing it with the standard medium. For feeding the cells, about half of the medium in a well is removed using a Titertek multichannel pipette (Flow Laboratories, McLean, VA) and replaced with fresh medium. In about 2–3 weeks, colonies of hybrid cells are visible. At this stage, the supernatant medium is screened for the presence of antibody.

After identifying the positive wells, the cells are cloned. In order to increase the cloning efficiency, microtitration plates containing normal mouse peritoneal cells[36,37] are prepared 1 day prior to the cloning. Peritoneal cells are collected by washing out the peritoneal cavity of mouse with 0.34 M sucrose solution. The cells are washed with standard medium and 2×10^4 cells[38] per well are plated in 96-well culture plates.

Hybrid cells from positive wells are harvested, counted, and plated at 10, 2.5, and 0.5 cells per well of the culture plate having the "feeder" cells. After the hybridoma cells are cloned, they may be grown on mass scale in culture or may be transferred to peritoneal cavity of mice [(LP $\times$ BALB/c) F_1] hybrids.

3.2.2b. Screening of Anti-Mouse Hb-Producing Hybridoma Cells. Prerequisites for a screening procedure are that it should be sensitive and quick to perform so that large number of assays can be performed in relatively short time. Enzyme-linked immunoabsorbent (ELISA) assay[39,40] is such a procedure that can be used to detect monoclonal antibodies.[41] First, flat-bottom microculture plates are coated with mouse Hb. To each well of the plate is added 100 μl of 0.1 mg/ml solution of Hb in 20 mM carbonate–bicarbonate buffer, pH 9.6. After overnight incubation at 4°C, the supernatant is removed and the plate is washed five times with buffer A (50 mM phosphate-buffered saline, pH 7.2, containing 1.5 mM $MgCl_2$, 2 mM 2-mercaptoethanol, 0.05% Tween 20, and 0.05% sodium azide). Culture supernatants (50 μl) are transferred to the wells of the antigen-coated plate and incubated for 2 hr at room temperature with constant shaking. The plate is washed three times with buffer A and then 50 μl of 1:200 diluted (with 1% bovine serum albumin) hybridoma screening reagent–β-galactosidase conjugated F(ab)$'_2$ fragment of sheep anti-mouse immunoglobulin (Bethesda Research Lab, Gaithersburg, MD) is added. After 2 hr of incubation, the plate is washed with buffer A as before. Finally, 50 μl of 1 mg/ml solution of enzyme substrate, *p*-nitrophenyl-β-D-galactopyranoside, prepared in 50 mM phosphate buffer, pH 7.2, containing 1.5 mM $MgCl_2$ and 100 mM 2-mercaptoethanol, is added to the wells. After incubation with constant shaking for 1 hr, the reaction is stopped by the addition of 50 μl of 0.5 M sodium carbonate. Development of yellow color indicates the presence of antibody in the culture supernatant. As a positive control, LP anti-s Hb antiserum is used. Normal mouse serum serves as negative control.

3.2.3. Testing of Specificity of the Purified Antibodies

Monospecificity of the antibody purified from antiserum or produced by hybridomas can be tested using the following tests.

3.2.3a. Fluorescent Bead Test. In this test [42] antibody preparation is allowed to react with different variants of Hb conjugated to Sepharose 4B. After washing off the unreacted antibody from the Sepharose beads, a second antibody, goat anti-mouse γ-globulin conjugated with fluorescein isothiocyanate, is added. The beads are washed again and then observed under a fluorescence microscope. An antibody preparation specific for d Hb should give a strong fluorescence with d Hb immunoabsorbent and little or no fluorescence with s Hb immunoabsorbent.

3.2.3b. Fluorescent Staining of Fixed mRBC. This test is performed essentially as described elsewhere.[3] Specificity of purified goat anti-d Hb for d Hb carrying mRBC is checked as follows. Washed RBC from DBA/2 and C57BL/6 mice are mixed separately with one volume of fetal calf serum and four volumes of phosphate-buffered saline, pH 7.2. Smears are prepared on microscope slides from each mixture and air dried for 1 hr at room temperature. RBC are then fixed by immersing the slides in a mixture of acetone, ethanol, and methanol (50:45:5) for 1 hr at room temperature followed by washing with phosphate-buffered saline for 30 min and then with water for 1 min. After drying, the cells are labeled with fluorochrome-conjugated antibody. In the so-called "sandwich technique," 10 μl of the purified goat anti-d Hb antibody is applied on the fixed smear at a marked position. The slides are shaken in a humid chamber for 2 hr, after which they are washed with phosphate buffered saline for 30 min and then with water for 1 min. The slides are dried again and a second antibody, fluorescein-conjugated goat anti-mouse γ-globulin, is applied on the same area where the first antibody was applied. The slides are again shaken for 1 hr in dark, washed with phosphate-buffered saline and water as before, dried, and observed under a fluorescence microscope. If the goat anti-d Hb antibody is monospecific, smears prepared from DBA/2 RBC should be fluorescent, while C57BL/6 RBC should show no or very little fluorescence.

Alternatively, the test antibody itself is labeled with the fluorochrome and the RBC smears are stained directly by transferring appropriate volume of the antibody into a very thin chamber prepared by separating the slide and a coverslip by two layers of scotch tape (Scotch tape no. 810, 3M Co., St. Paul, MN). The slides are shaken in a humid chamber. After about 4 hr, the coverslip is removed and the slides are immersed immediately into phosphate-buffered saline for 30 min and then washed with water and dried. Results obtained

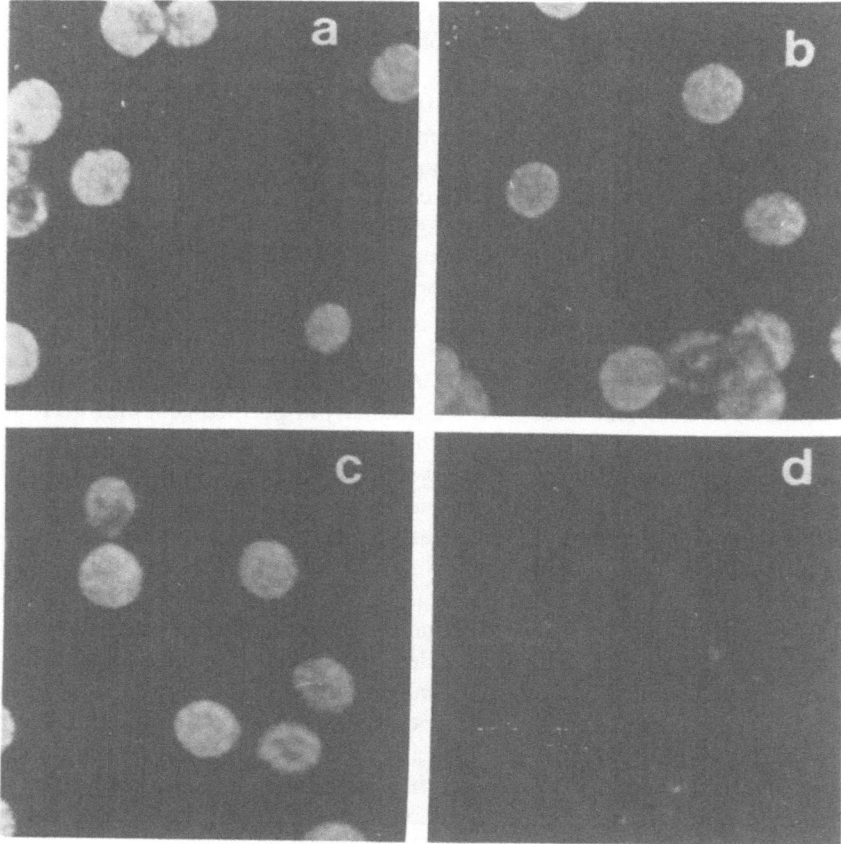

Figure 3. Direct immunofluorescent staining of mouse RBC with unpurified and affinity-purified goat anti-*d* Hb antibody conjugated with fluorescein isothiocyanate: (a) DBA/2 and (b) C57BL/6 cells stained with unpurified antibody; (c) DBA/2 and (d) C57BL/6 cells stained with the purified antibody.

with the fluorescein isothiocyanate-labeled unpurified and purified goat anti-d Hb antibody are shown in Figure 3. Both DBA/2 and C57BL/6 RBC are stained by the unpurified antibody (Figures 3a and b), while only the DBA/2 RBC are stained by the purified antibody (Figure 3c) and C57BL/6 RBC are not (Figure 3d).

3.3. Indicator Cells. Methods for Coupling Antibodies to Sheep RBC

Sheep RBC coated with appropriate antibody are used as indicator cells. Sheep blood is collected in Alsever's solution and is stored at 4°C for 1 week before use. For a set of experiments, blood from the same sheep should be used. Several sheep may have to be checked for best results. RBC are separated by centrifugation of the blood at 800g for 5 min and washed four times with 0.15 M NaCl. Instead of sRBC, goat RBC can also be used.

Several chemical reagents are used to coat sRBC with proteins. Commonly used methods are now described.

3.3.1. Chromium Chloride Method

Chromium chloride is the most widely used reagent to couple proteins to sRBC.[43–47] A stock 10 mg/ml solution of $CrCl_3 \cdot 6H_2O$ in 0.15 NaCl is prepared and stored at 4°C. Appropriate dilution of this stock solution is used in the coupling procedure. The procedure involves the mixing of one volume of packed sRBC with two volumes of protein solution (γ-globulin fraction of antiserum) in 0.15 NaCl and two volumes of appropriately diluted chromium chloride solution. After shaking at room temperature for 5–30 min, the cells are washed four times with Hank's balanced salt solution and suspended in five volumes of Hank's balanced salt solution containing 8% fetal calf serum. Optimal coupling of antibody to sRBC depends on (2) the concentration of antibody solution, (1) the concentration of chromium chloride solution, and (3) time of incubation. The optimal coupling conditions vary for different antibodies. Therefore, for determining optimal conditions of coating a particular antibody to sRBC, several combinations of antibody concentration (0.5–10 mg/ml), chromium chloride concentration (5- to 25-fold dilution of the stock solution), and incubation time should be investigated. Phosphate ions inhibit the coupling by chromium chloride and therefore should be kept from the reaction mixture. The coating of sRBC with antibody can be checked by performing the hemagglutination test. Best coupling of goat anti-d Hb to sRBC is obtained when 0.8 mg/ml solution of chromium chloride and 2 mg/ml solution of antibody are used and the mixture is incubated for 30 min.

3.3.2. ECDI Method

1-Ethyl-3-(3-dimethylaminopropyl) carbodiimide hydrochloride (ECDI) couples proteins covalently to sRBC. Sheep RBC are washed with phosphate-buffered saline, pH 7.2, and suspended to a 50% (v/v) suspension in the buffer. The γ-globulin fraction is isolated from the antiserum by 18% sodium sulfate precipitation, dialyzed against the buffer, and diluted to an appropriate protein concentration (10–20 mg/ml). Coupling is carried out[48–50] by mixing 0.1 ml of 50% sRBC suspension with 3 ml of the antibody solution and 0.5 m of 100 mg/ml ECDI solution in phosphate-buffered saline. The reaction mixture is incubated in cold for 1 hr with occasional shaking. The RBC are then centrifuged and washed three times with buffer containing 1% fetal calf serum. The ECDI method has drawbacks in that the reagent is comparatively expensive and requires large amounts of proteins, which limits its use with affinity-purified antibodies.

3.3.3. BDB Method

Bis-diazo-benzidine (BDB) has been successfully used for coating sRBC with proteins.[51–53] However, its use is limited due to the known carcinogenicity of benzidine. The method as used by Kapp and Ingraham[53] is described here. BDB is prepared by the method of Kabat and Mayer[54] and is stored in 1-ml aliquots in sealed glass tubes at −70°C. The coupling reaction is carried out at 0°C. Sheep RBC are washed with 0.005 M phosphate-buffered saline, pH 7.3, containing 0.5% dextrose and diluted to 50% suspension in the buffer. The desired amount of protein is dissolved in 18 ml of the buffer and mixed with 50% sRBC suspension in a 30-ml centrifuge tube. One aliquot of BDB is thawed in a cold bath and added to 2.8 ml of 0.1 M phosphate buffer, pH 7.4. Then 2.5 of this solution is added to the sRBC–protein mixture with shaking. The mixture is incubated for 30 min with occasional shaking. The cells are then washed with phosphate-buffered saline plus 0.5% dextrose.

Beside the methods described above, several other methods have been used, which employ tannic acid-treated sRBC,[52] p-benzoquinone,[55] glutaraldehyde,[18,56] and cyanuric chloride[18] for coupling proteins to sRBC.

3.4. Complement

The RBC plaque assay is very sensitive to the quality of complement. Guinea pig serum is generally used as the source of complement. Although fresh serum is considered better, lyophilized sera are also used with good results. However, sera from several commercial sources should be screened for their activity before selecting one. Lyophilized guinea pig complement from

Flow Laboratories, McLean, VA (Cat. No. 44-011-43), has worked best in our hands. Lyophilized complement is reconstituted with water and absorbed on washed sRBC (15:1) in cold for 1 hr and then small aliquots are frozen at -70°C. Before use, one aliquot is thawed and diluted as required. Optimal dilution of complement to be added to the assay mixture is determined experimentally.

4. EQUIPMENT

4.1. Plaque Chambers

Plaque chambers are prepared from glass microscope slides. Precleaned plain microscope slides (2.5 × 7.5 cm) are used. If ordinary slides are used instead of precleaned slides, they should be thoroughly cleaned to make them grease-free. This involves soaking the slides in chromic acid, and rinsing with tap water followed by distilled water and then with absolute ethanol. After the slides are dried, they are rubbed with a clean, lint-free cloth.

To make plaque chambers, the slides are laid adjacent to each other on a clean, flat surface (working bench) and are lined in a row vertical to the edge of the bench with the help of a ruler. Two-sided tape (¼-in. Scotch tape no. 410, 3M Co., St. Paul, MN) is then applied in three parallel strips—two along each of the ends of the slides and one along the middle. The slides are now fixed on the table and are cleaned by rubbing with a lint-free cloth wetted lightly with absolute ethanol. The backing of each strip of the two-sided tape is removed and a second row of slides, cleaned with an ethanol-wetted cloth, is placed over the first row, each slide going right over the bottom row slide. The top layer is pressed down firmly with the help of a plate sealing roller, the excess tape at the right end is cut, and the individual chambers are separated by bending them at the joint. The volume of a plaque chamber varies in the range 170–180 μl.

4.2. Additional Materials

Other materials needed for the RBC plaque assay are 96-well microculture plates, preferably with V-shaped wells, Pasteur pipettes, bulbs, 10-cm glass petri dish, candle wax, Vaseline petroleum jelly, hot plate, aluminum slide trays, and a small fluorescent lamp.

Hank's balanced salt solution (diluted from 10× solution obtained from GIBCO, Grand Island, NY) containing 8% fetal calf serum is used as the medium.

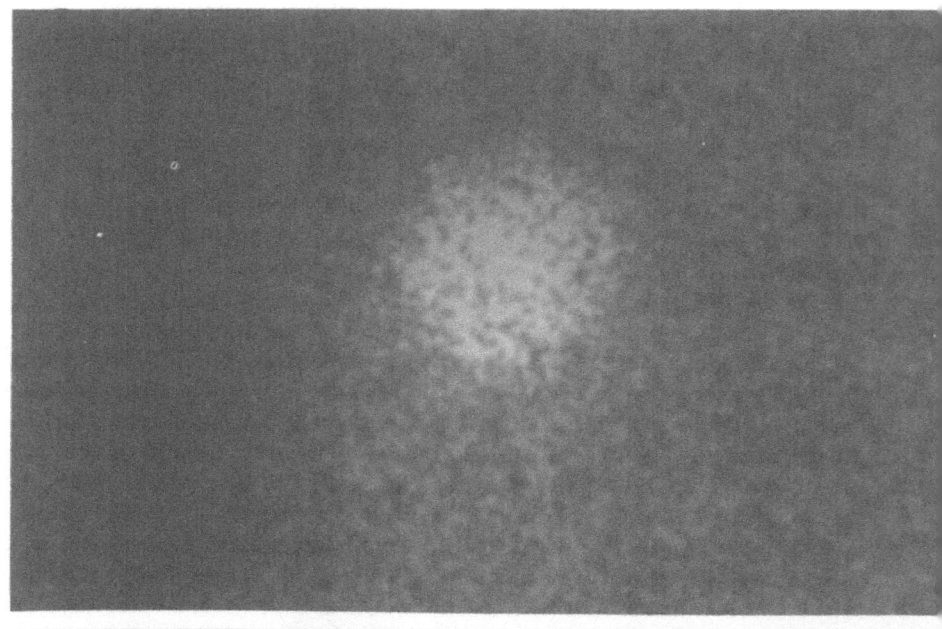

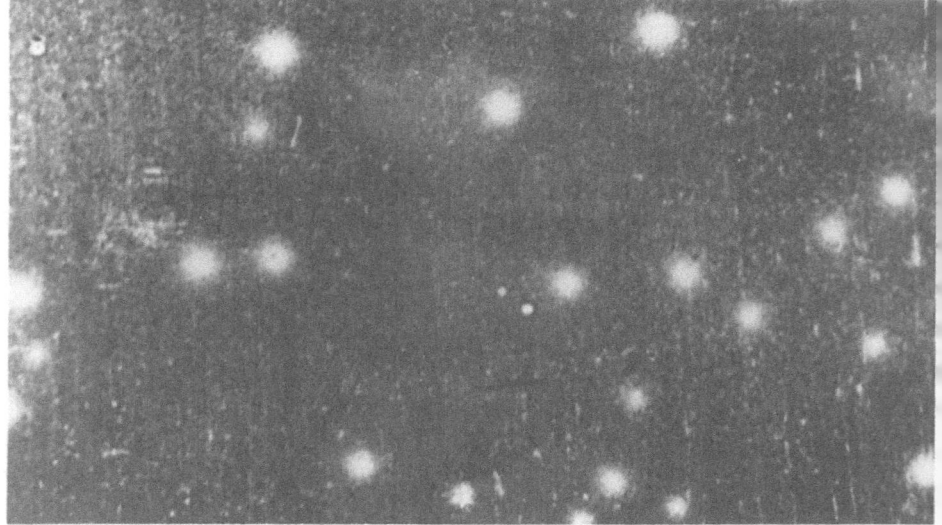

5. PROCEDURE FOR RBC-ANTIBODY PLAQUE ASSAY

A typical 170-μl plaque assay mixture is prepared by mixing the following reagents in the wells of a microculture plate: 85 μl of Hank's balanced salt solution containing 8% fetal calf serum, 25 μl of 16% suspension of indicator cells (sRBC coated with affinity-purified specific goat anti-d Hb) in the medium, known number of DBA/2 mouse RBC in 25 μl of the medium, 15 μl of a suitable dilution of developer (1.5 mg/ml solution of γ-globulins from a rabbit antiserum containing polyspecific antibodies against mouse Hb and mRBC ghost), and 20 μl of three times diluted guinea pig complement. The order in which the reagents are added is important to avoid lysis of mRBC before the assay mixture is poured into the plaque chambers. The components are mixed immediately by drawing and delivering through a Pasteur pipette and poured into a plaque chamber. The chamber is sealed by dipping its edges into a molten mixture of wax and petroleum jelly (1:1). The plaque chambers are then incubated at room temperature. After 3–4 hr, the plaques are fully developed. They can be identified and counted with the naked eye by holding the plaque chambers against a small fluorescent lamp. Photographs showing the RBC-antibody plaques are given in Figure 4.

5.1. Factors Affecting the RBC Plaque Formation

As has been mentioned earlier, plaque formation depends on the concentrations of anti-mRBC ghost antibody, developer (rabbit anti-mouse Hb), and complement. Therefore, optimal concentrations of these reagents should be determined experimentally by performing the assay at various concentrations of one while keeping the other variables constant in the assay mixture.

The number of indicator sRBC in the assay mixture also affects the development of RBC plaques. Most distinct plaques are obtained when about 100 million indicator sRBC are used in a total assay mixture of 170 μl. Increasing the number beyond 100 million results in a decrease of plaque size, while decreasing the number leads to the formation of poorly defined plaques that are not clearly visible and therefore make the scoring difficult.

5.2. Specificity of the RBC Plaque Assay

Table II shows the specificity of plaque formation by DBA/2 mouse RBC. The number of plaques increases with increase in the number of DBA/2 RBC in the assay mixture. Also, only inclusion of RBC from DBA/2 mouse in the assay mixture results in the formation of plaques, while RBC from C57BL/6 mouse does not form plaques. Plaques are not formed when the antibody-

Table II
Specificity of the RBC Plaque Formation

Description	Number of DBA/2 RBC added	Number of plaques formed
Standard assay mixture[a]	0	0
Standard assay mixture[a]	7	6
Standard assay mixture[a]	12	10
Standard assay mixture[a]	23	19
Standard assay mixture[a]	47	44
Antibody-coated sRBC replaced by uncoupled sRBC	132	0
No complement	132	0
No developer (rabbit anti-mouse Hb)	132	0
Standard assay mixture plus free DBA/2 Hb	235	0

[a]A total volume of 170 μl standard assay mixture consists of 85 μl of the medium (Hank's balanced salt solution containing 8% fetal calf serum), 25 μl of sRBC coupled with specific goat anti-d Hb, the desired number of test mRBC in 25 μl of the medium, 15 μl of 1.5 mg/ml solution of the γ-globulin fraction of rabbit antiserum containing antibodies against mRBC ghosts and mouse Hb, and 20 μl of three times diluted guinea pig complement.

coated sRBC are replaced by uncoated sRBC. Further, no plaque formation takes place when either the complement or developer is omitted from the assay mixture. Moreover, the plaque formation is inhibited when free DBA/2 Hb is included in the assay mixture.

The specificity and sensitivity of the plaque assay are further checked by performing the assay with a mixture of a known number of DBA/2 and C57BL/6 mRBC. The number of DBA/2 cells is kept constant while the number of C57BL/6 cells is increased. The number of plaques formed with the mixture is approximately the same as the number of plaques formed when the assay is done with the same number of DBA/2 cells alone. However, when the number of C57BL/6 cells is increased over 10^3, keeping the number of DBA/2 cells constant, plaques are not formed. A possible reason for this inhibition of plaque formation could be that the Hb released from the large number of C57BL/6 cells binds most of the developer, rabbit anti-mouse Hb, which is not monospecific, thus leaving little or no developer for Hb released from DBA/2 RBC. This binding is "nonproductive" because the C57BL/6 Hb–developer complex cannot bind to the indicator cells coated with an anti-Hb antibody, which is specific for DBA/2 Hb, and therefore plaques are not formed. This problem could be overcome probably by using a complement-fixing monoclonal antibody that is specific for DBA/2 Hb as developer.

6. RBC–PROTEIN A PLAQUE ASSAY

Staphylococcus aureus protein A is known to specifically bind the Fc region of most immunoglobulins.[57,58] This property of protein A has been exploited in lymphocyte plaque assay[59] by using protein A-coated sRBC as indicator cells. Such indicator cells can also be used for RBC plaque assay. However, an absolute requirement for the RBC–protein A plaque assay to be useful in mutation monitoring is that the developer, anti-mouse Hb antibody, should be specific for a particular variant of Hb and that it should be capable of fixing the complement. Protein A is coupled to sRBC using chromium chloride as coupling reagent.[59] Assay mixture for RBC–protein A plaque assay consists of 100×10^6 protein A-coated sRBC (25 μl), test mRBC (15 μl), appropriately diluted anti-mRBC ghost antibody (20 μl), specific antibody against mouse Hb (15 μl), and three times diluted guinea pig complement (20 μl). The volume is made up to 170 μl with the medium. The mixture is poured into plaque chambers and incubated at room temperature. After 3–4 hr, plaques similar to those shown in Figure 4 are developed.

What appears to happen is that the Hb from test RBC is released by the action of anti-RBC ghost antibody and complement. The released Hb binds to the anti-Hb antibody and the complex in turn binds to protein A present on the indicator sRBC. This complex activates the complement and results in the lysis of indicator sRBC to form a plaque.

7. CONCLUSIONS

The RBC plaque assay can be used to detect and quantitate cells carrying a particular variant of Hb, as demonstrated by its ability to distinguish between mRBC carrying *d* Hb and those carrying *s* Hb. In humans, RBC carrying sickle cell Hb can be detected by this method. Also, RBC carrying fetal Hb or HbC can be detected specifically, provided suitable monospecific antibodies against these hemoglobins are available.

REFERENCES

1. A. A. Ansari and H. V. Malling, in: *Chemical Mutagens: Principles and Methods for Their Detection* (A. Hollaender and F. J. deSerres, eds.), Vol. 7, pp. 37–93, Plenum Press, New York (1981).
2. A. A. Ansari, M. A. Baig, and H. V. Malling, *In vivo* germinal mutation detection with "monospecific" antibody against lactate dehydrogenase-X, *Proc. Natl. Acad. Sci. USA 77,* 7352–7356 (1980).

3. A. A. Ansari, M. A. Baig, and H. V. Malling, Development of *in vivo* somatic mutation system using antibody against hemoglobin, *Mutat. Res. 81*, 243–255 (1981).
4. N. K. Jerne and A. A. Nordin, Plaque formation in agar by single antibody-producing cells, *Science 140*, 405 (1963).
5. E. S. Russel, Announcement of linkage between *Hba* and *wa-2* (Chromosome 11, L. G. VII), *Mouse Newsl. 49*, 33 (1973).
6. R. A. Popp and W. St. Amand, Studies on the mouse hemoglobin locus, I. Identification of hemoglobin types and linkage of hemoglobin with albinism, *J. Hered. 51*, 141–144 (1960).
7. R. A. Popp, Hemoglobins of mice: Sequence and possible ambiguity at one position of the alpha-chain, *J. Mol. Biol. 27*, 9–16 (1967).
8. K. Hilse and R. A. Popp, Gene duplication as the basis for amino acid ambiguity in the alpha chain polypeptides of mouse hemoglobins, *Proc. Natl. Acad. Sci. USA 61*, 930–936 (1968).
9. R. A. Popp. Sequence of amino acids in the β-chain of single hemoglobins from C57BL, SWR and NB mice, *Biochim. Biophys. Acta 303*, 52–60 (1973).
10. R. A. Popp and E. G. Bailiff, Sequence of amino acids in the major and minor β-chains of the diffuse hemoglobin from Balb/c mice, *Biochim. Biophys. Acta 303*, 61–67 (1973).
11. A. A. Ansari, L. M. Bahuguna, M. Jenison, and H. V. Malling, Immunological comparison of mouse hemoglobins, *Immunochemistry 15*, 557–560 (1978).
12. J. G. Gilman, Hemoglobin beta chain structural variation in mice: Evolutionary and functional implications, *Science 178*, 873–874 (1972).
13. J. T. Dodge, C. Mitchell, and D. J. Hanahan, The preparation and chemical characteristics of hemoglobin-free ghosts of human erythrocytes, *Arch. Biochem. Biophys. 100*, 119–130 (1963).
14. M. A. Baig and A. A. Ansari, Studies of mouse immunoglobulin allotypes by reverse plaque assay: Detection of spleen cells secreting immunoglobulins with specific allotype in C57BL/6 mice, *Cell. Immunol. 66*, 164–170 (1982).
15. R. D. Schreiber, R. W. Noble, and M. Reichlin, Restriction of heterogeneity of goat antibodies specific for human hemoglobin S, *J. Immunol. 114*, 170–175 (1975).
16. A. M. Dozy, D. F. Kleihauer, and T. H. J. Huisman, Studies on the heterogeneity of hemoglobin, XIII. Chromatography of various human and animal hemoglobin types on DEAE–Sephadex, *J. Chromatogr. 32*, 723–727 (1968).
17. E. Antonini and M. Brunori, *Hemoglobin and Myoglobin in their Reactions with Ligands,* North-Holland, Amsterdam (1973).
18. S. Avrameas, B. Taudou, and S. Chuilon, Glutaraldehyde, cyanuric chloride and tetraazotized O-dianisidine as coupling reagents in the passive hemagglutination test, *Immunochemistry 6*, 67–76 (1969).
19. P. Cuatrecasas and C. B. Anfinsen, Affinity chromatography, *Annu. Rev. Biochem. 40*, 259–278 (1971).
20. J. H. Ludens, J. R. DeVries, and D. D. Fanestil, Criteria for affinity chromatography of steroid-binding macromolecules, *J. Biol. Chem. 247*, 7533–7538 (1972).
21. V. Sica, I. Parikh, E. Nola, G. A. Puca, and P. Cuatrecasas, Affinity chromatography and the purification of estrogen receptors, *J. Biol. Chem. 248*, 6543–6558 (1973).
22. I. Parikh, V. Sica, E. Nola, G. A. Puca, and P. Cuatrecasas, Estrogen receptors, *Methods Enzymol, 34*, 670–688 (1974).
23. I. Parikh and P. Cuatrecasas, in: *Immunochemistry of Proteins* (M. Z. Attasi, ed.), Vol. 2, pp. 1–44, Plenum Press, New York (1977).
24. G. Stamatoyannopoulos, W. G. Wood, Th. Papayannopoulou, and P. E. Nute, An analytical form of hereditary persistence of fetal hemoglobin in blacks and its association with sickle cell trait, *Blood 46*, 683–692 (1975).

25. W. G. Wood, G. Stamatoyannopoulos, G. Lim, and P. E. Nute, F-Cells in the adult: Normal values and levels in individuals with hereditary and acquired elevation of HbF, *Blood 46*, 671–682 (1975).

26. P. E. Nute, W. G. Wood, G. Stamatoyannopoulos, C. Olweny, and P. J. Failkow, The Kenya form of hereditary persistence of fetal hemoglobin: Structural studies and evidence for homogeneous distribution of hemoglobin F using fluorescent anti-hemoglobin F antibodies, *Br. J. Haematol. 32*, 55–63 (1976).

27. Th. Papayannopoulou, M. Brice, and G. Stamatoyannopoulos, Stimulation of fetal hemoglobin synthesis in bone marrow cultures from adult individuals, *Proc. Natl. Acad. Sci. USA 73*, 2033–2037 (1976).

28. Th. Papayannopoulou, G. Lim., T. C. MacGuire, V. Ahern, P. E. Nute, and G. Stamatoyannopoulos, Use of specific fluorescent antibodies for the identification of hemoglobin C in erythrocytes, *Am. J. Hematol. 2*, 105–112 (1977).

29. A. A. Ansari, M. A. Baig, and H. V. Malling, Purification of fluorescein-labeled specific anti-hemoglobin antibody using cross-linked immunoabsorbent, *J. Immunol. Methods 42*, 45–51 (1981).

30. G. Köhler and C. Milstein, Continuous cultures of fused cells secreting antibody of predefined specificity, *Nature 256*, 495–497 (1975).

31. J. W. Goding, Antibody production by hybridomas, *J. Immunol. Methods 39* 285–308 (1980).

32. S. F. St. Groth and D. Scheidegger, Production of monoclonal antibodies: Strategy and tactics, *J. Immunol. Methods 35*, 1–21 (1980).

33. V. T. Oi, P. P. Jones, J. W. Goding, L. A. Herzenberg, and L. A. Herzenberg, Properties of monoclonal antibodies to mouse Ig allotypes, H-2 and Ia antigen, *Curr. Top. Microbiol. Immunol. 81*, 115–129 (1978).

34. M. Shulman, C. D. Wilde, and G. Köhler, A better cell line for making hybridomas secreting specific antibodies, *Nature 276*, 269–270 (1978).

35. J. F. Kearney, A. Radbruch, B. Liesegang, and K. Rajewsky, A new mouse myeloma cell line that has lost immunoglobulin expression but permits the construction of antibody-secreting hybrid cell lines, *J. Immunol. 123*, 1548–1550 (1979).

36. P. Coffino, R. Baumal, R. Laskov, and M. D. Scharf, Cloning of mouse myeloma cells and detection of rare variants, *J. Cell. Physiol. 79*, 429–440 (1972).

37. W. Lernhardt, J. Andersson, A. Coutinho, and F. Melchers, Cloning of murine transformed cell lines in suspension culture with efficiencies near 100%, *Exp. Cell Res. 111*, 309–316 (1978).

38. H. Hengartner, A. L. Luzzati, and M. Schreier, Fusion of *in vitro* immunized lymphoid cells with X63Ag8, *Curr. Top. Microbiol. Immunol. 81*, 92–99 (1978).

39. B. K. Van Weemen and A. H. W. M. Schuurs, Immunoassay using antigen–enzyme conjugates, *FEBS Lett. 15*, 232–236 (1971).

40. E. Engvall and P. Perlamnn, Enzyme-linked immunoabsorbent assay (ELISA). Quantitative assay of immunoglobulin G, *Immunochemistry 8*, 871–874 (1971).

41. Y. Naot and J. S. Remington, Use of enzyme-linked immunoabsorbent assays (ELISA) for detection of monoclonal antibodies: Experience with antigens of *Toxoplasma gondii, J. Immunol. Methods 43*, 333–341 (1981).

42. A. A. Ansari and H. V. Malling, A rapid screening method for the detection of monospecific antibodies, *J. Immunol. Methods 24*, 383–387 (1978).

43. E. R. Gold and H. H. Fundenberg, Chromic chloride: A coupling reagent for passive hemagglutination reactions, *J. Immunol. 99*, 859–866 (1967).

44. G. N. Vyas, H. H. Fundenberg, H. M. Pretty, and E. R. Gold, A new rapid method for genetic typing of human immunoglobulins, *J. Immunol. 100*, 274–279 (1968).

45. G. H. Sweet and F. L. Welborn, Use of chromium chloride as the coupling reagent in modified plaque assay, *J. Immunol. 106*, 1407–1410 (1971).
46. J. W. Goding, The chromic chloride method of coupling antigens to erythrocytes: Definition of some important parameters, *J. Immunol. Methods 10*, 61–66 (1976).
47. G. J. V. Nossal, A. E. Bussard, H. Lewis, and J. C. Maize, *In vitro* stimulation of antibody formation by peritoneal cells, *J. Exp. Med. 131*, 894–935 (1970).
48. H. M. Johnson, K. Brenner, and H. E. Hall, Use of water-soluble carbodiimide as a coupling reagent in the passive hemagglutination test, *J. Immunol. 97*, 791–796 (1966).
49. A. M. Kaplan and M. J. Freeman, Enumeration of cells synthesizing antiprotein antibodies by a modified hemolytic plaque assay, *Proc. Soc. Exp. Biol. Med. 127*, 574–576 (1968).
50. E. S. Golub, R. I. Mishell, W. O. Weigle, and R. W. Dutton, A modification of the hemolytic plaque assay for the use with protein antigens, *J. Immunol. 100*, 133–137 (1968).
51. D. Pressman, D. H. Campbell, and L. Pauling, The agglutination of intact azoerythrocytes by antisera homologous to the attached groups, *J. Immunol. 44*, 101–105 (1942).
52. D. W. Dresser and H. H. Wortis, in: *Handbook of Experimental Immunology* (D. M. Weir, ed.), 1st ed., p. 1054, Blackwell Scientific Publications, Oxford (1967).
53. J. A. Kapp and I. S. Ingraham, Anti-protein plaque-forming cells detected with high efficiency by the use of red cells coupled to bovine serum glubulin through bis-diazo-benzidine, *J. Immunol. 104*, 1039–1042 (1970).
54. E. A. Kabat and M. M. Mayer, *Experimental Immunochemistry*, Charles C. Thomas, Springfield (1961).
55. T. Ternynck and S. Avrameas, A new method using *p*-benzoquinone for coupling antigens and antibodies to marker substances, *Annu. Immunol. (Inst. Pasteur) 127C*, 197–208 (1976).
56. S. Lemieux, S. Avrameas, and A. E. Bussard, Local hemolysis plaque assay using a new method of coupling antigens on sheep erythrocytes by glutaraldehyde, *Immunochemistry 11*, 261–269 (1974).
57. G. Kronvall, H. M. Grey, and R. C. Williams, Jr., Protein A reacting with mouse immunoglobulins, *J. Immunol. 105*, 1116–1123.
58. H. M. Grey, J. W. Hirst, and M. Cohn, A new mouse immunoglobulin: IgG3, *J. Exp. Med. 133*, 289–304 (1971).
59. E. Gronowicz, A. Coutinho, and F. Melchers, A plaque assay for all cells secreting Ig of a given type or class, *Eur. J. Immunol. 6*, 588–590 (1976).

4

Direct Assay by Autoradiography for 6-Thioguanine-Resistant Lymphocytes in Human Peripheral Blood

RICHARD J. ALBERTINI, PHILIP C. KELLEHER, AND DAVID SYLWESTER

1. INTRODUCTION

1.1. Human Mutagenicity Monitoring

There is great current interest in tests that may be useful for human mutagenicity monitoring. Mutagenicity monitoring, as contrasted with mutagenicity screening, is based on methods that detect evidence of genetic damage—whether germinal or somatic—that occurs *in vivo*. Most current short-term mutagenicity tests, however, have been developed for screening, i.e., for *in vitro* mutagenicity testing of chemicals or other agents with mutagenic potential.

Epidemiology provides the traditional methodology for human mutagenicity monitoring. For public health purposes, the enumeration of "affected" individuals for epidemiologic studies provides the most realistic indicator of human health hazards. However, the goal of human mutagenicity monitoring must be to find other, realistic measures of genetic damage occurring *in vivo* in humans. Direct mutagenicity tests that can quantify such damage occurring in somatic or germinal cells obtained directly from the body can provide these measures.

RICHARD J. ALBERTINI AND PHILIP C. KELLEHER • Department of Medicine, University of Vermont College of Medicine, Burlington, Vermont 05405.   DAVID L. SYLWESTER • Biometry Facility, University of Vermont College of Medicine, Burlington, Vermont 05405.

Several direct mutagenicity tests are available or under development. Standard cytogenetic tests,[1,2] tests of sister chromatid exchange,[3-6] measures of DNA damage or repair,[7] and the detection of double Y bodies[8] or morphological abnormalities in sperm,[9] may all be capable of measuring different aspects of genetic damage occurring *in vivo* in humans. To be included in this list are tests that detect specific-locus somatic-cell mutants arising *in vivo*. Two such test systems have been, or are being, developed. One is the mutant hemoglobin test.[10-12] The other, to be described in detail here, is the detection of mutant T-lymphocytes that arise *in vivo*. These cells are present in human peripheral blood.

1.2. 6-Thioguanine-Resistant (TG^r) Human Peripheral Blood T Lymphocytes (T-PBLs)

Normal, non-mutagen-exposed adults have in their peripheral blood-variant T lymphocytes that are resistant to TG at concentrations that kill normal T cells. The variant cells, as detected autoradiographically, are present at frequencies of $(1-10) \times 10^{-6}$. All lymphocytes from males with the Lesch–Nyhan (LN) syndrome are similar to these rare cells of normal individuals with respect to their TG resistance. The LN syndrome results from a naturally occurring mutation of the X-chromosomal gene for the enzyme hypoxanthine-guanine phosphoribosyltransferase (HPRT).[13-15] The TG resistance of LN cells is explained by the resultant deficiency of HPRT activity. HPRT is required to phosphorylate TG, causing it to become cytotoxic.[16,17] It is therefore assumed that the TG^r T-lymphocytes of normal, non-LN individuals arise from *in vivo* somatic cell mutation of this X-chromosomal gene.

Consistent with the mutational origin of TG^r T-PBLs in normal individuals is the observation that the frequency of these variant cells is elevated over controls in individuals knowingly exposed to mutagens, e.g., patients with cancer who are receiving chemotherapy.[18-20] Frequency elevations in such patients may be severalfold over controls—up to $(50-60) \times 10^{-6}$.[21] Also, we have recently been able to clone directly *in vitro* the TG^r T-PBLs of human blood under conditions where TG resistance must have arisen *in vivo*.[22] Characterization of the variant cells has shown that the resistant phenotype is maintained during long term *in vitro* culture, and that the TG^r cells are deficient in HPRT activity as expected.

1.3. Direct Enumeration of TG^r T-PBLs by Autoradiography

The TG^r T-PBLs may be detected by their ability to incorporate tritiated thymidine ([^{3}H]-dThd) following phytohemagglutinin (PHA) stimulation *in vitro* in the presence of cytotoxic concentrations of TG. The culture interval *in vitro* is sufficiently short so that cell division does not occur.[18] Thus, the TG-sensitive normal cells are inhibited by TG from incorporating [^{3}H]-dThd during their first DNA synthesis period (S period) *in vitro*, while the TG^r cells are resistant to the inhibition. Autoradiography allows the enumeration of the rare variant cells.[18]

Under basal conditions, the majority of lymphocytes in the peripheral blood are in an arrested G_0 stage of the cell cycle, and enter into cycle only following a stimulus. Then, when put into culture, the G_0 T-PBLs are induced by PHA to undergo a G_0 to G_1 transformation, with the acquisition of T-cell growth-factor receptors[23] on the transformed cells. After this, T-cell growth factors, elaborated by other cells in PHA-stimulated cultures, cause the transformed T cells to progress through G_1, to synthesize DNA, and to proliferate. The transformation itself is associated with profound metabolic shifts.[24,25] We believe that it is this transformation step, from G_0 to G_1, that is inhibited in normal resting T-PBLs in the short-term PHA cultures used in the autoradiographic assay, where TG-sensitive cells fail to incorporate [^{3}H]-dThd during their first *in vitro* DNA synthesis period.[26]

1.4. Phenocopies

In contrast to our more recent studies, the initial determinations of TG^r T-PBL variant frequencies V_f in normal, nonmutagen-exposed adults found these to be in excess of 10^{-4}.[18] However, a series of subsequent investigations demonstrated that these early values were grossly inflated by the scoring of "phenocopies," i.e., nonmutant cells that mimicked, under the conditions of assay that we were using, the "LN-like" TG^r mutant T-PBLs.[26]

Although, as stated, most T-PBLs *in vivo* are in G_0, a minority population is in cell cycle. The T-PBLs that are already in cycle *in vivo* have no need to undergo the G_0 to G_1 transformation *in vitro* as described. Then TG operates on different cell functions in this minority population of cycling cells than in the majority population of cells, which require transformation to G_1 *in vitro* prior to DNA synthesis. Spontaneously cycling cells are eventually inhibited by TG *in vitro*, but, because they do not require the profound metabolic alteration prior to DNA synthesis, they may accomplish this synthesis and even undergo cell division prior to arrest. We postulate that a fraction of these cells, although not mutants, become labeled (phenocopies) in the short-term cultures used for the autoradiographic assay for TG^r T-PBLs.

Elsewhere, we show that liquid nitrogen cryopreservation of T-PBLs in dimethylsulfoxide (DMSO) prior to testing in the autoradiographic assay appears to eliminate this "phenocopy effect."[26] Such treatment appears to move the spontaneously cycling T-PBLs that are capable of labeling in TG *in vitro* through the S phase (DNA synthesis) earlier in culture than is the case with fresh T-PBLs.[26,27] These cells then are not labeled when the usual assay procedure described below is followed. Thus, the cycling cells are not eliminated but simply are not scored as mutant cells. We feel that the TG^r T-PBL V_f determinations made with cryopreserved cells detect primarily the cells that are resistant to TG inhibition of in vitro PHA-induced G_0 to G_1 transformation, i.e., the "LN-like" mutant T-PBLs. Cryopreservation is now part of our standard autoradiographic assay.

2. AUTORADIOGRAPHIC TG^r T-PBL ASSAY METHOD

2.1. Cell Preparation

Blood is obtained by venipuncture using syringes coated with 0.1 ml heparin (beef lung, 1000 units/ml, benzyl alcohol preservative; Upjohn) per 10 ml blood. Syringes are rotated to mix the contents and may remain up to 18 hr at room temperature before separating mononuclear cells (MNC).

The MNCs are separated from whole blood by the Ficoll–Hypaque method,[28] using 50-ml, sterile glass, round-bottom centrifuge tubes. To each tube is added approximately 20 ml of sterile Ficoll–Hypaque (specific gravity 1.077) and an equal amount of heparinized blood. Blood is layered over the Ficoll–Hypaque and centrifuged at ambient temperature at $420g$ for 30 min. After centrifugation, the upper layer in the tubes is plasma, the MNC-containing layer is at the plasma/Ficoll–Hypaque interface, and the other components of the blood are at the bottom. The MNC layer is gently aspirated using a plugged pipette and transferred to conical centrifuge tubes, which are then filled with sterile phosphate-buffered saline (PBS). The plasma is removed with a plugged pipette and may be centrifuged at $1000g$ for 10 min and used immediately as a medium supplement, or frozen for future use. Tubes are centrifuged at ambient temperature at $210g$ for 10 min, the supernatant removed, and the PBS wash repeated. Following another centrifugation, the supernatant is removed, leaving the MNC pellet. Cells are then frozen. On average, each milliliter of blood drawn from an adult yields $(1-2) \times 10^6$ MNCs.

2.2. Cryopreservation

For freezing, the MNC pellet is suspended in RPMI 1640 medium containing 25 mM HEPES, 2 mM glutamine, 100 units/ml penicillin, 100 μg/ml streptomycin, and either 10% human AB serum or autologous plasma. Dimethylsulfoxide (DMSO) is added to a final concentration of 7.5%. The cell density is 10^7/ml. The procedure is done rapidly, as DMSO is toxic to cells at room temperature. One-milliliter aliquots of the MNC suspension are transferred into 1-ml Nunc ampules. The samples are then frozen in a Union Carbide biological freezer for controlled cooling according to manufacturer's instructions. Frozen cells are stored in the vapor phase over liquid nitrogen. Cells remain viable for many months.

2.3. Cell Culture

The frozen cells are rapidly thawed in 37°C water bath, added drop by drop to prewarmed (37°C) medium RPMI 1640 to a final dilution of at least 1:10, centrifuged at ambient temperature at 420g for 10 min, and the resultant pellet is resuspended in 10 ml of medium RPMI 1640. This washing step is repeated and the twice-washed cells are suspended in a small volume of RMPI 1640. An aliquot is removed, resuspended in PBS–0.04% trypan blue solution, and viability counts as determined by dye exclusion are made. Cells are added to complete medium (CM), which consists of medium RPMI 1640, supplemented with 25 mM HEPES, 2 mM glutamine, penicillin/streptomycin (100 units/ml and 100 μg/ml respectively; GIBCO), and 30% autologous plasma or 10–20% AB human serum (Biobee), counted and diluted in CM to 1.4 × 10^6 cells/ml. Cryopreserved cell recovery varies from 30 to 100%. Viability should be in excess of 90%.

Culture flasks (T25) are prepared to receive control (without TG) or test (with TG) cultures. Phytohemagglutinin (PHA-P, 4 μg in 0.2 ml per ml final culture volume; Burroughs Wellcome) is added to all culture flasks. For each person tested, one flask is prepared to receive the control culture and several flasks are prepared to receive test cultures. For control cultures, flasks receive, in addition to the PHA-P, medium RPMI 1640 that has been adjusted to the pH of the stock TG solution. For TG cultures, flasks receive, in addition to the PHA-P, stock 2 × 10^{-3} M TG solution. For both, additions are in 0.1-ml volumes per ml final culture. Finally, the MNC suspension as described (i.e., 1.4 × 10^6 cells/ml) is added to all flasks at 0.7 ml per ml final culture volume. Thus, all cultures are made to contain 5 × 10^6 or 10 × 10^6 MNCs in 5- or 10-ml final culture volumes, respectively.

Inoculated culture flasks with loosely applied screw tops are incubated in a humidified 5% CO_2 atmosphere at 37°C for 30 hr. At 30 hr, 5 μCi [^{3}H]thymidine (New England Nuclear, S.A. 6.7 Ci/mM) is added per ml culture. Cultures are incubated for an additional 12 hr and terminated.

2.4. Termination, Coverslip Preparation, and Autoradiography

2.4.1. Termination

Cultures are terminated by adding 4 ml of 0.1 M citric acid per ml of culture fluid to each flask. The cell suspensions are then transferred from flasks to conical glass centrifuge tubes. After mixing, the tubes are centrifuged at ambient temperature at 420g for 15 min. The supernatants are aspirated and put into radioactive waste. The pellets contain free nuclei and cytoplasmic fragments. Four milliliters of freshly made fixative containing seven parts methanol to 1.5 parts glacial acetic acid are added to each tube and the nuclei resuspended. Tubes again are centrifuged at ambient temperature at 420g for 15 min, supernatants are aspirated and put into radioactive waste, and the pelleted nuclei are resuspended in 0.2 ml of fixative. Tightly capped tubes are refrigerated at 4°C for at least 1 hr for fixation. Samples may be kept for several days at this stage.

2.4.2. Coverslip Preparation

Nuclei in fixative suspension are counted with a Coulter counter (ZBI model). We count the nuclei in 20 μl of the suspension and add the remainder, in carefully measured volumes, to 18 × 18 mm glass coverslips previously fixed with Permount to glass slides. The nuclei are drawn into a 1-ml tuberculin syringe fixed with a 25-gauge, 10-cm needle. Nuclei are resuspended between each addition by trituration. Coverslips are air-dried between additions of the suspension. Nuclei from the control culture are spread on two coverslips. Nuclei derived from each test-culture flask are spread on one coverslip. The suspension is allowed to spread evenly and care is taken that the sample does not run over the coverslip edge. The total number of nuclei added to a coverslip is calculated from the density of nuclei per microliter (Coulter count) times the number of microliters added to the coverslip. Coverslips so prepared are air-dried, immersed in filtered 1% aceto-orcein stain for 1 min, dipped in distilled water, rinsed in cold running tap water, and then air-dried.

2.4.3. Autoradiography

In complete darkness, dried, stained slides in holders are immersed for 10–15 sec in prewarmed (48°C, 4 hr) autoradiographic emulsion (NTB2; Kodak). Excess emulsion is drained off and the slideholders are stored in an opaque box during exposure. The box is wrapped in black plastic bags and sealed with tape and placed in a refrigerator (4°C) or freezer (−20°C) for a minimum of 24 hr (but may be kept in the freezer for several weeks before developing).

After exposure, slides in holders are removed from the holding box, again in total darkness, and immersed for 4 min in developer D-19 (Kodak), drained, placed in a stop bath for 10–30 sec, removed, again drained, and placed in fixer (Kodak) for 5 min. Finally, slides (no longer light-sensitive) are washed briefly in cold water and allowed to dry.

2.5. Enumeration of TG^r T-PBLs and Calculation of TG^r T-PBL Variant Frequency (V_f)

Coverslips with nuclei from cultures containing PHA-P and pH-adjusted RPMI 1640 medium without TG (controls) are viewed with a high-power microscope (970×). Twenty-five hundred nuclei chosen at random are counted on each of two coverslips (5000 nuclei counted) and the incidence of autoradiographically labeled (positive) cells determined. (All nuclei containing silver granules above background levels are considered positive.) The labeling index of control cultures LI$_{(c)}$ is determined:

$$LI_{(c)} = \frac{\text{Number of labeled nuclei in 5000 nuclei}}{5000}$$

Coverslips prepared from test cultures containing PHA-P and TG are scanned at low power (160×) so that all labeled nuclei on each coverslip are viewed. Labeled nuclei detected at low power are confirmed at high power (970×). The LI of test cultures LI$_{(t)}$ is calculated by dividing the number of all labeled nuclei on all test coverslips by the total number of nuclei on the coverslips, which is obtained from Coulter counts as indicated above. Thus

$$LI_{(t)} = \frac{\text{Labeled nuclei from all test cultures}}{\text{Total nuclei recovered from test cultures}}$$

The TG^r T-PBL V_f is calculated as the ratio of the test and control LI's:

$$V_f = \frac{LI_{(t)}}{LI_{(c)}}$$

3. SAMPLE RESULTS

3.1. TG^r T-PBL V_f Assay: Appearance of Slides

A microscopic field from a coverslip containing nuclei from a control culture (without TG) is shown in photomicrographs made at 160× (Figure 1A) and high-power oil immersion microscopy (970×; Figure 1B). When 5000 nuclei from the control culture were examined (see Section 2.5), the LI was determined to be 0.36. Labeled nuclei on slides made from test cultures have the same appearance (Figure 2).

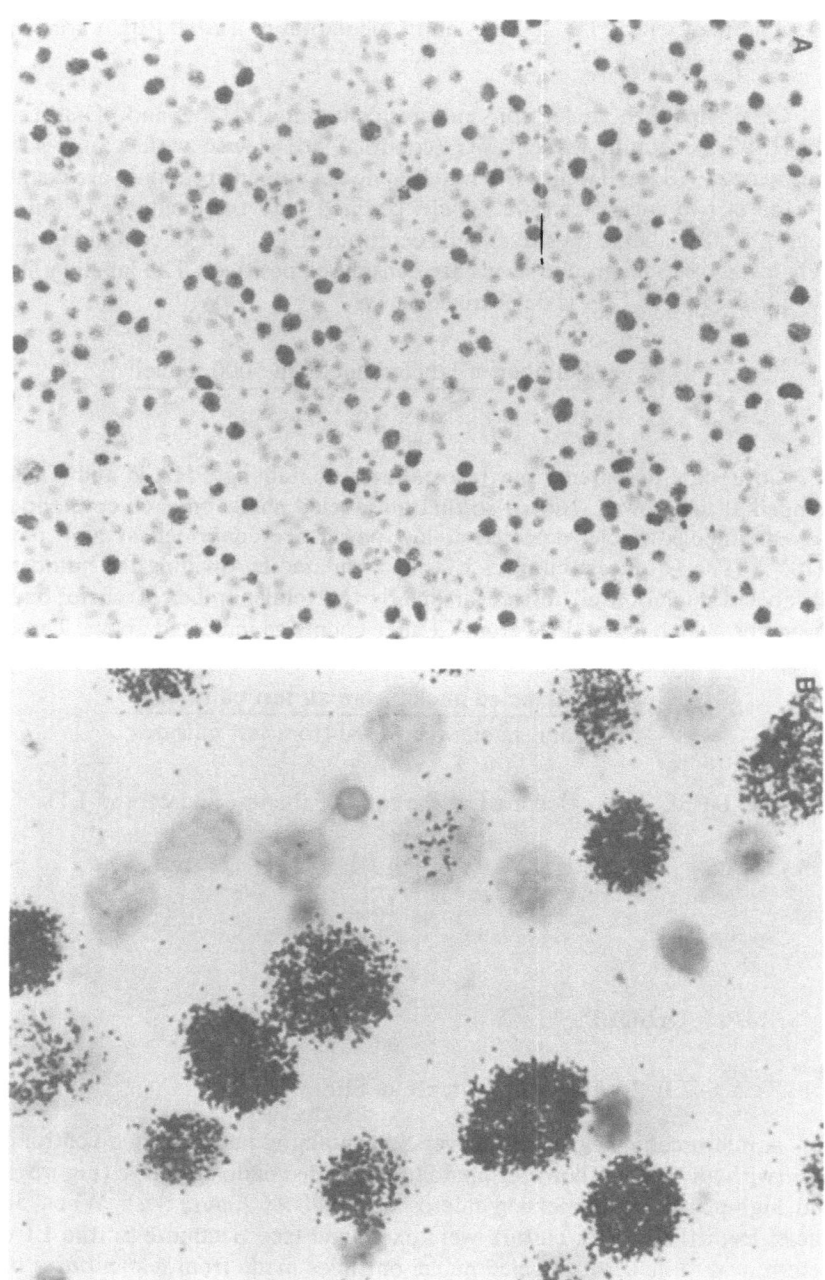

Figure 1. Appearance of nuclei from a control culture (top, ×72; bottom, ×440).

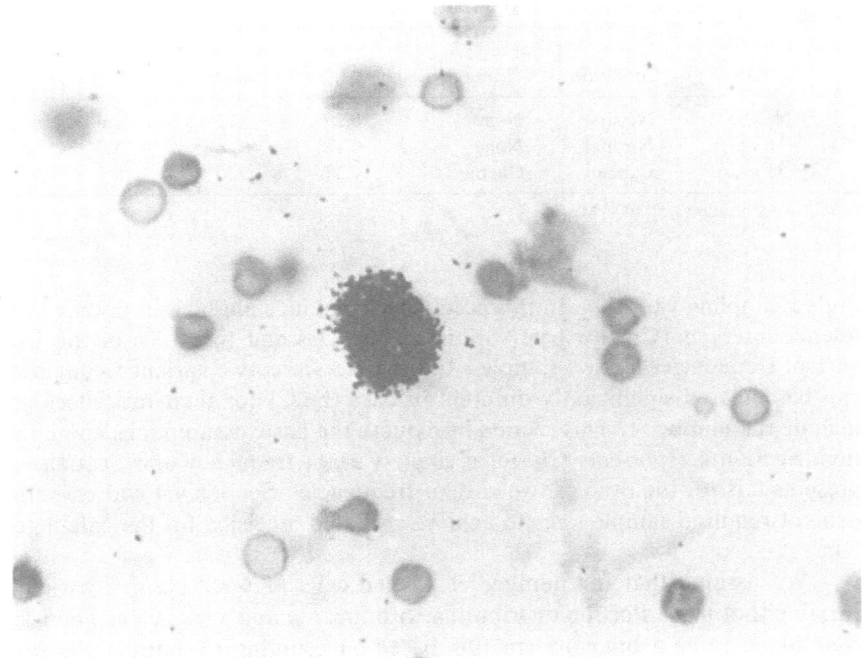

Figure 2. Appearance of a labeled nucleus in a test culture (×460).

3.2. TG^r T-PBL V_f Assay: Sample Data

Table I lists typical results obtained using cryopreserved cells. In general the V_f values of cord blood T-PBL are lower than in normal adults; however, occasional specimens have high V_f values. The high TG^r T-PBL V_f of subject 3 is encountered in approximately 40% of patients who have received chemotherapy for cancer.

4. STATISTICAL ANALYSIS METHODS

4.1. Notation and Basic Assumptions

Since the number of labeled cells scored in an autoradiographic assay is typically small, one must expect a relatively large amount of variation in results

Table I
6-Thioguanine-Resistant[a] Peripheral Blood Lymphocyte Variant Frequencies

Subject	Age	Condition	Mutagen	$LI_{(c)}$	Labeled nuclei	$V_f \times 10^{-6}$	95% CI $\times 10^{-6}$
1	Newborn	Normal	None	0.25	12	2.6	1.5, 4.6
2	21 years	Normal	None	0.18	8	3.7	1.8, 7.4
3	56 years	Cancer	ChemoRx	0.31	20	18.1	11.7, 28.1

[a]Thioguanine concentration 2×10^{-4} M.

due to sampling variation. In this section we introduce methods of finding confidence intervals (CI) for true variant frequencies and for ratios of the true variant frequencies for two samples. In the latter case, two variant frequencies can be declared significantly different in case the CI for their ratio does not include the number 1. This section introduces the basic assumptions and notation. Section 4.2 presents CIs for a single variant frequency and Section 4.3 presents CIs for the ratio of two variant frequencies. Section 4.4 addresses the issue of required sample sizes to achieve specified precision for the calculated CIs.

We assume that the number of labeled cells M is an observation on a variable that has a Poisson distribution with mean μ and variance ν. The $LI_{(c)}$ is assumed to be a binomial fraction based on counting C control cells with each cell having probability p of being scored positively. Thus $LI_{(c)}$ has a mean of p and a variance of $p(1 - p)/C$. The number N of evaluatable cells from the T cells in one set of test cultures is estimated by $N = T \times LI_{(c)}$. The number N is only approximately binomially distributed, since the fraction $LI_{(c)}$ is based on a different sample (the control sample). The mean and variance of N are calculated by using conditional means and variances.[29] The result is

$$E(N) = Tp \tag{1}$$

$$\text{Var}(N) = \frac{T^2 p(1 - p)}{C}\left(1 + \frac{C - 1}{T}\right) \tag{2}$$

$$\doteq \frac{T^2 p(1 - p)}{C}, \qquad \text{since } \frac{C - 1}{T} < 0.01 \tag{3}$$

(The symbol $\doteq$ denotes approximate equality.)

The estimated variant frequency V_f is simply $V_f = M/N$. Although both M and N are subject to random variation, we will treat N as a known constant since its coefficient of variation (CV) is much smaller than the CV for M, as the following estimates show:

$$CV(M) = \frac{[Var(M)]^{1/2}}{E(M)} \times 100 \doteq \frac{\sqrt{M}}{M} \times 100 = \frac{1}{\sqrt{M}} \times 100 \quad (4)$$

$$CV(N) \doteq \frac{[T^2 p(1-p)/C]^{1/2}}{Tp} \times 100 = \left(\frac{1-p}{Cp}\right)^{1/2} \times 100 \quad (5)$$

For values of M from 1 to 64, $C = 5000$, and $p \doteq LI_{(c)}$ with values from 0.10 to 0.50, we find that the $CV(M)$ ranges from 12% to 100%, while the $CV(N)$ ranges from only 1.5% to 4%.

4.2. Confidence Intervals for a Single Variant Frequency

Treating N as a known constant, we estimate the true variant frequency $\nu = \mu/N$ by $V_f = M/N$. Exact tables of CIs for the parameter μ of a Poisson variable are widely available for values of M from 0 to 100.[30] For example, if the observed $M = 11$, the 95% CI for μ is $(\mu_L, \mu_U) = (5.49, 19.68)$. For $N = 9.49 \times 10^6$, say, dividing the end points of the CI for μ by N gives the 95% CI for the variant frequency:

$$(\nu_L, \nu_U) = (0.579/10^6, 2.074/10^6 \text{ cells})$$

A convenient approximation for the CI for μ is available by taking advantage of the fact that the natural logarithm $Y = \ln(M)$ of a Poisson variable is approximately normally distributed with mean $\ln(\mu)$ and variance $1/\mu$. Thus an approximate 95% CI for $\ln(\mu)$ is the interval $[\ln(M) - 1.96/\sqrt{M}, \ln(M) + 1.96/\sqrt{M}]$. Taking antilogs gives a CI for μ; dividing the end points of the interval by N yields a CI for the variant frequency ν. The final result is

$$(\nu_L, \nu_U) = (V_f/\exp(1.96 M^{-1/2}), V_f \exp(1.96 M^{-1/2})) \quad (6)$$

For example, if $M = 11$ and $N = 9.49 \times 10^6$, then $V_f = 1.16/10^6$ cells and the 95% CI is $(\nu_L, \nu_U) = (0.642/10^6 \text{ cells}, 2.093/10^6 \text{ cells})$. Note that this approximate CI is quite close to the CI $(0.579/10^6 \text{ cells}, 2.074/10^6 \text{ cells})$ obtained using the exact CI tables for a Poisson variable.

If M is small, the approximate CI can be very different from the exact CI and moreover will be very wide, as the following example illustrates. Let $M = 3$ and $N = 945,100$. Then the estimated $V_f = 3.17/10^6$ cells and the approximate 95% CI is $(1.023/10^6 \text{ cells}, 9.844/10^6 \text{ cells})$, while the exact CI is $(0.655/10^6 \text{ cells}, 9.277/10^6 \text{ cells})$.

The approximate CIs have an upper bound that is within 5% of the exact upper bound in the case $M \geq 4$. For accuracy within 5% of the lower bound, one requires $M \geqq 20$. The value 1.96 in Equation (6) is the appropriate value from a normal table for a 95% CI. Other values may be used to obtain 99%, 90% or other levels of confidence, if desired.

4.3. Confidence Intervals for Ratios of Variant Frequencies

The comparison of two variant frequencies is most conveniently done as a ratio. The true ratio v_2/v_1 is estimated by the sample ratio V_{f2}/V_{f1}. If the sample ratio is close to 1.0, one cannot reject the possibility that the true variant frequencies are equal.

An approximate CI for the ratio is an easy extension of the approximate CI for v using the logarithm transformation. For two independent samples $\ln(M_2/M_1) = \ln(M_1) - \ln(M_1)$ is approximately normal with mean $\ln(\mu_2/\mu_1)$ and estimated standard deviation $s = (1/M_2 + 1/M_1)^{1/2}$. Taking antilogs yields a 95% CI for μ_2/μ_1:

$$[(M_2/M_1)/e^{1.96s}, (M_2/M_1)e^{1.96s}] \tag{7}$$

Dividing the interval end points by N_2/N_1 yields the approximate 95% CI for v_2/v_1:

$$[(V_{f2}/V_{f1})/e^{1.96s}, (V_{f2}/V_{f1})e^{1.96s}] \tag{8}$$

For example, if $M_1 = 15$, $N_1 = 5.123 \times 10^6$, $M_2 = 11$, and $N_2 = 9.490 \times 10^6$, then $V_{f2}/V_{f1} = 0.396$. The estimated standard deviation is

$$s = (1/11 + 1/15)^{1/2} = 0.3969$$

so that $e^{1.96s} = 2.177$. Then the approximate 95% CI for v_2/v_1 is (0.164, 0.922). Replacing 1.96 with other normal table values gives CIs with other levels of confidence.

An exact CI for v_2/v_1, which is especially appropriate for small values of M, is based on the fact that the conditional distribution of M_2 given the sum $T = M_1 + M_2$ is binomial with parameters T and

$$p = \mu_2/(\mu_1 + \mu_2) = v_2 N_2/(v_1 N_1 + v_2 N_2) \tag{9}$$

The parameter p is estimated by $M_2/(M_1 + M_2)$. One then uses CI tables for the binomial to obtain an exact CI for p from which an exact CI for v_2/v_1 can be obtained (by algebra), since Equation (9) is equivalent to

$$v_2/v_1 = N_1/[N_2(1/p - 1)] \tag{10}$$

For example, for the data given above $T = 11 + 15 = 26$ and p is estimated by $11/26 = 0.423$. From binomial CI tables the exact CI for p is (0.234, 0.631). Using these two interval end points in Equation (10) yields the exact 95% CI for ν_2/ν_1: (0.182, 0.862). The approximate CI found earlier has end points within 10% of the values for the exact CI. Neither the exact nor the approximate CI includes the value 1.0, so that in both cases we conclude that $\nu_2 \neq \nu_1$ with 95% confidence.

For small values of M the approximate CI can be very different from the exact CI and moreover will be very wide, as the following example illustrates. Let $M_1 = 4$, $N_1 = 840,000$, $M_2 = 3$, and $N_2 = 945,100$. Then the estimated ratio of the variant frequencies is $V_{f2}/V_{f1} = 0.667$. The approximate 95% CI is (0.149, 2.978), while the exact CI is (0.098, 3.942). Thus we cannot declare the true variant frequencies unequal based on either the exact or approximate CI calculations.

4.4. Sample Size Determinations

The percentage error of the CI relative to the mean can be defined as $100(\nu_U - \nu)/\nu$ for the upper limit and $100(\nu - \nu_L)/\nu$ for the lower limit. These errors can be approximated by replacing the ν's by the appropriate sample estimates: V_f for ν and $V_f \exp(\pm 1.96 M^{-1/2})$ for ν_U and ν_L respectively. The estimated percentage error is then $100[\exp(1.96 M^{-1/2}) - 1]$ for the upper limit and $100[1 - \exp(-1.96 M^{-1/2})]$ for the lower limit. For $M = 15$ the estimated upper percentage error is 66% and the estimated lower percentage error is 40%.

Usually, one first specifies the desired percentage error. One then needs to score sufficient cells to obtain (approximately) the required M. For example, if the upper limit percentage error is to be 40%, the solution to $40 = 100[\exp(1.96 M^{-1/2}) - 1]$ is $M = 34$. If the investigator has available estimates of LI and ν, then it is straightforward to calculate T, the approximate number of cells needed to yield a sufficiently large value of M, since $M \doteq \nu T \times LI$.

If information is not available for making an estimate of T, then one may use inverse sampling, in which an increasing number of cells are accrued until M positive cells have been scored. In that case M is a constant and T is a variable. The CI for ν under inverse sampling is based on the χ^2 distribution. Numerically, the CI obtained is very close to that obtained in Section 4.2 where T was fixed and M was the variable.[31]

Sample sizes required to confirm that two variant frequencies are unequal may be estimated by using Equation (8). For example, suppose it is desired to score sufficient cells so that if $\nu_2 = 2\nu_1$ the lower confidence bound will be larger than 1.0 (so that one declares $\nu_2 \neq \nu_1$). If we set $N_2 = N_1$, then from Equation (8) we obtain

$$1 < 2/e^{1.96s} \tag{11}$$

where $s = (1/M_2 + 1/M_1)^{1/2}$. If $v_2 = 2v_1$, then we will have $M_2 \doteq 2M_1$ and (11) may be solved for the unknown M_1. The solution is $M_1 \doteq 12$ and we may expect that $M_1 \doteq 24$. A more exact approach using Equation (10) leads to the solutions $M_1 \doteq 14$ and $M_2 \doteq 28$.[31]

As for the one sample case discussed first, one may use prior knowledge to estimate the number of cells that need to be tested to yield sufficiently large values for M_1 and M_2. Alternatively, one may carry out inverse sampling in which M_1 and M_2 are fixed and prespecified while T_1 and T_2 are increased until M_1 and M_2 positive cells are scored. The CI for v_2/v_1 is based on the F-statistic. Numerical values obtained under inverse sampling are very close to those obtained when the T's were fixed and the M's were variable.[31]

5. DISCUSSION

This chapter presents in detail our method for the autoradiographic detection of TG^r T-PBLs that arise *in vivo* in human peripheral blood. We believe that the majority of these cells arise *in vivo* by a process of somatic-cell mutation. Our recently achieved ability to clone TG^r T-PBLs under conditions where the resistance had to have developed *in vivo*, to propagate these clones *in vitro*, and to characterize the cells in terms of phenotypic stability and their HPRT activity allows us to conclude, based on standard criteria, that the variant cells recovered by cloning are mutant somatic cells.[22] Preliminary mutant frequencies (M_f) determined by cloning are in the range of V_f values determined autoradiographically, although parallel determinations in the same individuals have not yet been made.[22,27] Such parallel studies are being undertaken.

Whether the direct autoradiographic assay as presented here or the cloning assay described elsewhere[22] will ultimately be the one used for human direct mutagenicity testing remains to be determined. Cloning allows mutants to be recovered and characterized, will allow the use of markers other than TG resistance for specific-locus mutagenicity testing, and will allow the construction of *in vivo–in vitro* mutagenicity test systems. Alternatively, the direct autoradiographic method is more highly developed at present, and may be more easily automated. It does not require experience in long-term cell culture or the use of T-cell growth factors.

It must be remembered that determinations of TG^r T-PBL frequencies are probably determinations of mutant frequencies—not of mutation frequencies or rates. This, of course, is true for any direct mutagenicity test, but it does require consideration when interpreting results. Mutation is the event of interest in mutagenicity monitoring. While it is true that an increase in mutant frequency may be the result of an increase in mutation, changes in factors other than mutation may result in changes in mutant frequencies. Some of the factors may be the cell population affected by mutation (e.g., stem versus mature), *in vivo* selection for or against mutants, changes in cell pool distributions *in vivo* (e.g., sensitive versus resistant), etc. The methods developed for deriving mutation frequencies or rates from mutant frequencies *in vitro* are not strictly applicable to *in vivo* studies. Further work is clearly needed in this regard.

Despite this limitation, direct mutagenicity tests provide information for human mutagenicity monitoring that is not available from other sorts of mutagenicity tests. It may be possible empirically to correlate individual test results with health outcomes of the individuals tested—i.e., to link a laboratory test result with a health risk prediction. If so, then a laboratory test could be substituted for an "affected individual" as an indicator of the health hazard associated with a particular environment. As stated, this is the goal of human mutagenicity monitoring. The autoradiographic assay for TG^r T-PBLs of human blood is presented as a potential measure to achieve that goal.

REFERENCES

1. H. J. Evans and M. L. O'Riordan, Human peripheral blood lymphocytes for the analysis of chromosome observations in mutagen tests, in: *Handbook of Mutagenicity Test Procedures* (B. J. Kilbey, M. Legator, W. Nichols, and C. Ramel, eds.), pp. 261–274, Elsevier/North-Holland, Amsterdam and New York (1977).
2. A. Brogger, Chromosome damage in human mitotic cells after *in vivo* and *in vitro* exposure to mutagens, in: *Genetic Damage in Man Caused by Environmental Agents* (K. Berg, ed.), pp. 87–99, Academic Press, New York (1979).
3. P. Perry and H. J. Evans, Cytological detection of mutagen–carcinogen exposure by sister chromatid exchange, *Nature 258*, 121–125 (1975).
4. D. G. Stetka and S. Wolff, Sister chromatid exchange as an assay for genetic damage induced by mutagen–carcinogens. I. *In vivo* test for compounds requiring metabolic activation, *Mutat. Res. 41*, 333–342 (1976).
5. S. Latt, J. W. Allen, W. E. Rogers, and L. A. Juerglus, *In vitro* and *in vivo* analysis of sister chromatid exchange formation, in: *Handbook of Mutagenicity Test Procedures* (B. J. Kilbey, M. Legator, W. Nichols, and C. Ramel, eds.), pp. 275–291, Elsevier/North-Holland, Amsterdam and New York (1977).
6. S. Wolff, Sister chromatid exchanges, *Annu. Rev. Genet. 11*, 183–210 (1977).
7. R. W. Pero and F. Mitelman, Another approach to *in vivo* estimation of genetic damage in humans, *Proc. Natl. Acad. Sci. USA 76*, 462–463 (1979).
8. A. W. Kapp, Jr., D. J. Picciano, and C. B. Jacobson, Y-Chromosomal nondisjunction in dibromochloropropane exposed workmen, *Mutat. Res. 64*, 47–51 (1979).
9. A. J. Wyrobek and W. R. Bruce, The induction of sperm shape abnormalities in mice and humans, in: *Chemical Mutagens* (A. Hollaender and F. J. deSerres, eds.), Vol. 5, pp. 257–285, Plenum Press, New York (1978).
10. Th. Papayannopoulou, T. C. McGuire, G. Lim, E. Garzel, P. E. Nute, and G. Stamatoyannopoulos, Identification of hemoglobin S in red cells and normoblasts using fluorescent anti-Hb antibodies, *Br. J. Haematol. 34*, 25–31 (1976).

11. Th. Papayannopoulou, G. Lim, T. C. McGuire, V. Ahern, P. E. Nute, and G. Stamatoyan-nopoulos, Use of specific fluorescent antibody for the identification of a hemoglobin C in erythrocytes, *Am. J. Hematol. 2*, 105–112 (1977).

12. G. Stamatoyannopoulos, P. E. Nute, Th. Papayannopoulou, T. McGuire, G. Lim, H. F. Bunn, and D. Racknagel, Development of a somatic mutation screening system using Hb mutants. IV. Successful detection of red cells containing the human frameshift mutants Hb Wayne and Hb Cranston using monospecific fluorescent antibodies, *Am. J. Hum. Genet. 32*, 484–496 (1980).

13. M. Lesch and W. L. Nyhan, A familial disorder of uric acid metabolism and central nervous system function, *Am. J. Med. 36*, 561–570 (1964).

14. J. E. Seegmiller, F. M. Rosenbloom, and W. N. Kelley, Enzyme defect associated with a sex linked human neurological disorder and excessive purine synthesis, *Science 155*, 1682–1684 (1967).

15. M. Strauss, L. Lubbe, and E. Geissler, HG-PRT structural gene mutation in the Lesch–Nyhan syndrome as indicated by antigenic activity and reversion of the enzyme deficiency, *Hum. Genet. 57*, 185–188 (1981).

16. G. B. Elion and G. H. Hitchings, Metabolic basis for the actions of analogs of purine and pyrimidines, in: *Advances in Chemotherapy* (A. Goldin, F. Hawkins, and R. J. Schnitzer, eds.), Vol. 2, pp. 91–177, Academic Press, New York (1965).

17. G. B. Elion, Biochemistry and pharmacology of purine analogs, *Fed. Proc. 26*, 898–904 (1967).

18. G. H. Strauss and R. J. Albertini, Enumeration of 6-thioguanine resistant peripheral blood lymphocytes in man as a potential test for somatic cell mutation arising *in vivo*, *Mutat. Res. 61*, 353–379 (1979).

19. G. H. Strauss, R. J. Albertini, P. Krusinski, and R. D. Baughman, 6-Thioguanine resistant peripheral blood lymphocytes in humans following psoralen long-wave light therapy, *J. Invest. Dermatol. 73*, 211–216 (1979).

20. R. J. Albertini, Drug resistant lymphocytes in man as indicators of somatic cell mutation, *Teratog. Carcinog. Mutagen. 1*, 25–48 (1980).

21. R. J. Albertini, D. L. Sylwester, B. D. Dannenberg, and E. F. Allen, Mutation *in vivo* in human somatic cells: Studies using peripheral blood mononuclear cells, in: *Genetic Toxicology: An Agricultural Perspective*, (R. A. Fleck, ed.), pp. 403–424, Plenum Press, New York (1982).

22. R. J. Albertini, K. L. Castle, and W. R. Borcherding, T-Cell cloning to detect the mutant 6-thioguanine-resistant lymphocytes present in human peripheral blood, *Proc. Natl. Acad. Sci. USA 79:* 6617–6621 (1982).

23. A. L. Maizel, S. R. Mehta, S. Hauft, D. Franzini, L. B. Lachman, and R. J. Ford, Human T-lymphocyte/monocyte interaction in response to lectin: Kinetics of entry into S-phase, *J. Immunol. 127*, 1058–1064 (1981).

24. A. C. Allison, T. Hovi, W. E. Watts, and A. B. D. Webster, The role of *de novo* purine synthesis in lymphocyte transformation, in: *Purine and Pyrimidine Metabolism* (K. Elliot and E. W. Fitzsimmons, eds.), pp. 207–224, Elsevier/North-Holland/Excerpta Medica, Amsterdam (1977).

25. T. Hovi, A. C. Allison, K. O. Raivio, and A. Vaheri, Purine metabolism and control of cell proliferation, in: *Purine and Pyrimidine Metabolism* (K. Elliot and D. W. Fitzsimmons, eds.), pp. 225–248, Elsevier/North-Holland/Exerpta Medica, Amsterdam (1977).

26. R. J. Albertini, E. F. Allen, A. S. Quinn, and M. R. Albertini, Human somatic cell mutation: *In vivo* variant lymphocyte frequencies as determined by 6-thioguanine resistance, in: *Population and Biological Aspects of Human Mutation: Birth Defects Institute Symposium XI* (E. B. Hook and I. H. Porter, eds.), pp. 235–263, Academic Press, New York (1981).

27. R. J. Albertini, Studies with T-lymphocytes: An approach to human mutagenicity monitoring, in: *Banbury Conference Report 13, Indications of Genotoxic Exposure in Man and Animals* (B. A. Bridges, I. B. Weinstein, and V. K. McElheny, eds.) pp. 393–412, Cold Spring Harbor Laboratory, Cold Spring Harbor (1982).

28. A. Boyum, Separation of leukocytes from blood and bone marrow, *Scand. J. Clin. Lab. Invest. (Suppl. 97)* **21,** 51–76 (1968).

29. E. Parzen, *Modern Probability Theory and Its Applications,* Wiley, New York (1960).

30. K. Diem, *Documenta Geigy: Mathematical Tables,* Geigy Pharmaceuticals, Ardsley, New York (1962).

31. R. J. Albertini, D. L. Sylwester, and E. F. Allen, The 6-thioguanine resistant peripheral blood lymphocyte assay for direct mutagenicity testing in man, in: *Mutagenicity: From Bacteria to Man* (J. A. Heddle, ed.), pp. 130–145, Academic Press, New York (1981).

5

Application of Antibodies to 5-Bromodeoxyuridine for the Detection of Cells of Rare Genotype

HOWARD G. GRATZNER

1. INTRODUCTION

A current objective of research in the area of environmental mutagenesis is the development of automated methods of assessing *in vivo* and *in vitro* genetic damage.[1,2] The primary purpose of automating mutagen detection is to increase the speed and statistical reliability that is afforded by the instrumentation being recruited to this task, flow or image cytometry. In addition, this approach would eliminate the human bias and error characteristic of manual methods. In the case of *in vivo* assessment of mutagenesis, a method would be available to measure genetic variation in cells that either do not clone or clone at extremely low efficiencies.

The rationale for expanding effort toward the identification of individuals at genetic risk or for exploring new techniques for testing possible genotoxic substances has been discussed.[3-5]

Current techniques for the detection of mutation in mammalian systems that should be adaptable to automation fall into two categories: clonal selection, i.e., growth in culture to detect, for example, drug-resistant variants,[6] and cytochemical or immunocytochemical staining, to detect antigenically or enzymatically altered variants.[7,8] In this report, research has centered upon the former, that is, development of a method to enumerate drug-resistant variants on the basis of their growth in selective medium.

HOWARD G. GRATZNER • Institute for Cell Analysis and Department of Medicine, University of Miami School of Medicine, Miami, Florida 33124.

One promising assay for human *in vivo* mutagenesis utilizes peripheral lymphocytes and detects forward mutation for 6-thioguanine resistance (TG^r), presumably mutations at the HGPRT (hypoxanthine-guanine phosphoribosyltransferase) locus on the X chromosome (see Ref. 9 and this volume, Chapter 4).

The procedure we are developing, an extension of Albertini's method, consists in growing cells, PHA-stimulated peripheral blood lymphocytes in the case of *in vivo* mutagenesis, and human lymphoblast cell lines for *in vitro* studies, in short-term culture in the presence of a selective drug such as 6-thioguanine (TG) for the selection of HGPRT mutants, and then pulsing the cells with bromodeoxyuridine (BrdUrd)-containing medium before termination of the culture. The cells are then fixed and stained by fluorescent antibody techniques. The antibody utilized is highly specific for 5-bromodeoxyuridine. Cells that fluoresce will be distinguished and enumerated by flow cytometry (FCM). Those cells of the population are variants, that is, presumptive HGPRT mutants, that are capable of growing and replicating their DNA in the presence of thioguanine. Bromodeoxyuridine is an analog of thymidine, the normal precursor for DNA replication, and is incorporated into DNA in place of thymidine. Cellular fluorescence signifies DNA synthesis. Since the analysis is performed with individual cells, the fraction of those cells that are TG-resistant can be directly enumerated, eliminating the requirement of growing clones from individual cells, a procedure not feasible for the testing of peripheral lymphocytes for detection of *in vivo* mutations.

The chief emphasis of our current studies is to improve the signal-to-noise ratio between BrdUrd-labeled and non-BrdUrd-labeled cells. This is the prime importance, since one in 10^6 cells must be detectable for statistical significance in mutagenesis experiments. We hope to accomplish this objective through the production of monoclonal antibodies that are highly specific for BrdUrd.

1.1. Flow Cytometry

The technique of flow cytometry (FCM) permits the analysis and separation of cells in suspension. Cells flowing single file past a laser light source at rates approaching 300,000 cells/min can be analyzed for fluorescence and size by narrow-angle light scatter or electronic-cell volume.[10] One of the key features of this instrumentation is its multiparameter aspect. Several measurements, e.g., narrow-angle light scatter, which correlates with cell size, and several different fluorescence emission wavelengths can be measured concurrently and correlated for a single cell. Multiple-parameter analysis, together with a high flow rate, permits the discernment of subpopulations of cells not apparent by other methods, such as fluorescence microscopy. Another feature of flow cytometry that contributes to its versatility is the ability to distinguish subpopulations by parameter gating,[10] i.e., the ability to electronically subdivide a population of cells on the basis of size (light scatter) and then to analyze and sort the specific size range for a second parameter, such as a membrane antigen, by immunofluorescence.

1.2. The Use of 5-Bromodeoxyuridine for the Detection of Cell Proliferation

Several methods have been presented for detecting cycling cells in the various kinetic parameters by FCM. These methods involve the use of the base analog 5-bromodeoxyuridine, which is incorporated into DNA in place of thymidine to distinguish newly synthesized DNA. The incorporation of an appreciable amount of BrdUrd into DNA causes either a quenching or enhancement of fluorescence when specific dyes are bound to DNA. Quenching of fluorescence is exhibited by the dye 33258 Hoechst,[11] and enhancement of fluorescence by mithramycin.[12] Incorporation of BrdUrd into DNA in cells causes approximately a 25% increase in mithramycin fluorescence intensity after 48 hr growth in 30 μg BrdUrd /ml (CHO or tumor cells) and correspondingly less fluorescence enhancement with shorter pulses.

It is doubtful whether the dye-binding techniques can be employed for the detection of rare fluorescent cells, because of the small increase of fluorescence obtained; only 5% or greater of the total cell population could be detected, since there will be a large background of fluorescent, nonlabeled cells visible by FCM.

This chapter is a progress report of our efforts to detect a very small number of replicating (fluorescent) cells against a background of nonreplicating (nonspecifically fluorescent) cells.

A basic goal of these studies is to increase the signal–noise between the specifically fluorescent and nonspecifically fluorescent cells. This can be accomplished in several ways. One method is by the use of monoclonal antibodies[14] for BrdUrd, and we have found that little nonspecific staining occurs when monoclonal antibodies to BrdUrd when they are applied to immunofluorescent staining.[15] Cross-reactivity with thymidine has been eliminated.

The monoclonal antibodies also provide a defined reagent that will be available to any laboratory for many applications in which it is necessary to detect replicating cells.

2. MATERIALS AND METHODS

2.1. Cell Culture

The Chinese hamster cell line CHO was obtained from Los Alamos Scientific Laboratories and was maintained in Ham's F10 medium (GIBCO) buffered with HEPES buffer and supplemented with 10% fetal calf serum. The incorporation studies with BrdUrd were performed with minimal essential medium or F10 medium prepared without thymidine.

Cell synchrony and pulse labeling of the synchronous cultures have been described.[16] The human near-diploid cell line WiL2[13] was obtained from Dr. William Thilly, Massachusetts Institute of Technology. The cells were maintained in RPMI 1640 medium (GIBCO) with 10% newborn calf serum plus 25 mM HEPES (Sigma Chem. Co.), either in spinner flasks or in still culture in 100-ml serum bottles. Thioguanine-resistant cells were selected by cloning in RPMI 1640 plus 5 μg 6-thioguanine/ml.

2.2. Labeling with BrdUrd

The base analogue was added to medium to a final concentration of 10 μM. In addition, 1 μM fluorodeoxyuridine was also added in order to inhibit endogenous thymidylate synthesis. For radioactive labeling with [³H]-BrdUrd (New England Nuclear Corp.) 1 μCi/ml (27 mCi/mM) of the isotope was added to the nonradioactive BrdUrd.

2.3. Immunological Methods

2.3.1. Preparation of Conjugates

The antigen used to induce the formation of anti-BrdUrd antiserum consists of the hapten bromouridine coupled to bovine serum albumin (BSA).[17] Bromouridine is required instead of bromodeoxyuridine, since the coupling to BSA is by the 2′ and 3′ -OH groups of the ribose of bromouridine.

2.3.2. Immunization

The immunization of New Zealand rabbits was accomplished by the injection subcutaneously of an emulsion of 4 mg/ml in saline of bromouridine–BSA in an equal volume of complete Freund's adjuvant. Two milligrams per rabbit of this emulsion was injected every other week for 8 weeks. The first immunization was intraperitoneally, while subsequent injections, in incomplete adjuvant, were intramuscularly into the flank. The animals were bled after the second, third, and fourth injections. The serum from each bleeding was tested for antibody activity by immunodiffusion in agar,[18] or by immunofluorescent staining on slides, or by radioimmunoassay as described below.

2.3.3. Radioimmunoassay

The radioimmunoassay (RIA) was designed for measurement of the binding of anti-BrdUrd antibodies to either [³H]-BrdUrd or [¹²⁵I]-IdUrd, particularly for the determination of the degree of specificity of the antibody and cross-reactivity to other nucleosides such as thymidine and cytidine.[23] An assay mixture contained 100 μl of the diluted serum to be tested, 50 μl radioactive nucleosides ([^{3}H]-BrdUrd, 21.3 Ci/mM, or [^{125}I]-IdUrd, 2000 Ci/mM) obtained from New England Nuclear Corp.) and 800 μl borate buffer. The borate buffer consisted of 8.3 g boric acid, 37 mg EDTA, 0.8 g NaOH, 1% human serum albumin, pH 7.3, per liter. For hapten-inhibition studies the nonradioactive nucleosides to be tested were dissolved in the borate buffer (0.8 ml, so that the final volume of the incubation mix was 0.850 ml). Incubation of the mixtures was for 6–24 hr, at which time 0.5 ml of a mixture of charcoal and dextran was added. The charcoal–dextran mixture consisted of 2.5% charcoal and 0.25% dextran-70T (Pharmacia) in phosphate-buffered saline (PBS). The mixture was incubated for 5 min in an ice bath and centrifuged to remove the charcoal–dextran. The supernatant was removed and placed into scintillation vials with scintillation fluid (Riafluor or Aquafluor, New England Nuclear Corp.) and counted in a scintillation counter (or gamma counter in the case of [^{125}I]-IdUrd).

2.3.4. Immunological Staining on Slides

Cells to be stained with antibody were fixed in methanol–acetic acid (3 : 1) and then spread on clean microscope slides and air-dried. The chromatin was then denatured so that single-stranded regions of DNA were availabe for antibody binding. This was accomplished by heating slides in a formamide–saline-citrate (95% formamide, 0.15 M citric acid, and 0.15 M sodium chloride) solution for 1 hr at 65°C. Another method of denaturation, which yields somewhat more distortion but is more rapid, is to dip the slides into 0.07 M NaOH for 2 min, wash them twice in 70% ethanol, then once in 95% ethanol, and air dry.

Subsequent to the denaturation step, the slides were overlayered with goat serum for 5 min prior to incubation with a film of antiserum that had been serially diluted with a 1:5 mixture of PBS and goat serum. The incubation with anti-BrdUrd antiserum was for 1 hr in a humidified atmosphere (such as afforded by a Tupperware box). The slides were then washed on a platform-rocker in PBS three times for 1 min and stained with fluorescein-labeled secondary antibody or protein A. This second reagent was either goat anti-rabbit IgG coupled to fluorescein (Cappel Laboratories) diluted in PBS with 20% goat serum, or protein A coupled to fluorescein (Pharmacia), diluted in PBS with 3–4 mg BSA/ml. The incubation time with the goat antibody was 1 hr; incubation with protein A was for 30 min, due to the higher affinity of the protein A for IgG. Optimum concentrations of these immunological reagents is obviously dependent on the particular lot of antiserum or protein A employed and thus would require titration.

2.3.5. Immunoperoxidase Staining

Observation of BrdUrd incorporation with a conventional light microscope can be accomplished by secondary staining with goat antibody coupled to peroxidase and subsequent incubation of the slides with a substrate such as 3',3''-diaminobenzidine, which produces an insoluble product. For the conventional immunoperoxidase technique, the slides were incubated in goat anti-rabbit IgG coupled to horseradish peroxidase (Miles-Yeda) diluted approximately 1:250 to 1:500 in PBS, washed as described above, and then incubated in 0.003% H_2O_2 and 50 mg 3',3''-diaminobenzidine in 100 ml PBS. The slides were incubated in this solution for 5 min, or until satisfactory staining was observed by microscopic inspection.

In our experience, sufficient contrast in the BrdUrd-labeled nuclei and the background could be obtained with the immunoperoxidase method described; however, the unlabeled antibody techniques that employ the three-layer peroxidase–antiperoxidase technique of Sternberger[19] should increase the sensitivity of the system considerably.

2.3.6. Suspension Staining for Flow Cytometry

Cells are fixed subsequent to BrdUrd incorporation by slowly adding 100% ethanol with vortexing to the cells suspended in PBS to a final concentration of 70% ethanol. The cells were hydrolyzed for antibody binding by depurination with acid. We have found that depurination occurs at 1 N HCl and 0.2% dansyl hydrazine. Incubation in this solution causes the removal of adenines and enables the antibody to bind to the exposed bromouracil. The original purpose in using the dansyl hydrazine was to cause simultaneous staining of DNA to yield a feulgen-like quantitative DNA histogram for cell kinetic purposes, which should ultimately permit the coincident monitoring of both DNA replication and DNA content in the same cells by multiparameter analysis.

The cells were treated for all steps in 1.5-ml polypropylene centrifuge tubes designed for the Beckman microfuge. Use of this centrifuge facilitates the procedure, since centrifugation can be done in 5 sec at top speed, or about 12,000 rpm.

After 30 min incubation of the cells in the dansyl hydrazine–HCl, the medium was neutralized by the addition of a five-fold volume of PBS containing 0.05% Nonidet P40 (PBS/NP40), with an additional wash of 1 ml of PBS/NP40 before staining with the anti-BrdUrd antiserum. The antiserum was diluted 400-fold in PBS/NP40 3 mg/ml BSA, and cells stained for 1 hr, then washed in NP40/PBS twice with agitation for 5 min each wash. The secondary staining was the fluoresceinated protein A (1:200) for 30 min. After a second series of washes with PBS/NP40, the cells were resuspended in PBS/NP40 for flow analysis, since the NP40 was also found to maintain the single-cell dispersion necessary for accurate flow cytometric analysis.

2.4. Flow Cytometry

Measurements and sorting of the immunologically stained cells were performed with the EPICS IV cell sorter (Coulter Electronics), located at the Institute for Cell Analysis at the University of Miami School of Medicine. Fluorescein fluorescence was induced by excitation with the 488-nm line of a Lexel argon ion laser operating at an output of 200 mW to 1 W, dependent on the particular experiment. Data were transferred for analysis to a PDP 11/34 computer via serial line. In addition, some of the histograms were generated with a FACS III flow cytometer.

2.5. Hybridoma Production

Immunization of mice and cell fusion were performed as follows. Monoclonal antibodies against bromodeoxyuridine or iododeoxyuridine were produced by the fusion of spleen cells from BALB/c mice that had been immunized with approximately 200 μg/antigen mouse. The mice were injected intraperitoneally for 1 month with the antigen 5-iodouridine–ovalbumin, the conjugate synthesized by the procedure of Erlanger and Beiser.[17] Two hundred micrograms of the conjugate was injected in an emulsion with equal volume of complete Freund's adjuvant. Subsequent injections were made in incomplete adjuvant every 2 weeks, the final injection of IUrd–ovalbumin being made in saline, into the tail vein, three days prior to the fusion of spleen cells. Fusion of spleen cells from the immunized mice and the plasmacytoma line SP2/0 Ag 14[20] was performed by the method described by Gefter et al.[21]

The cells from the fusion were plated in four 96-well microculture plates (COSTAR) in Dulbecco's minimal essential medium (GIBCO) containing 15% fetal bovine serum. Twenty-four hours subsequent to the fusion and plating, medium containing hypoxanthine, thymidine, and methotrexate was added to each well, and the incubation continued for about 10 days. Colonies were first visible after 5 or 6 days. Cells from wells containing colonies were passed into 24-well microculture plates, and the media from these and the 96-well plates were assayed by an enzyme-linked immunosorbent assay (ELISA). The ELISA test was essentially the one presented by BRL Corporation in their newsletter.[22] Polyvinyl plates were coated with the hapten plus carrier (iodouridine–BSA) at a concentration of 500 ng/well, together with 10 μl/well of 1 mg/ml carbodiimide (EDAX, Biorad) in 0.1 M sodium carbonate, pH

9.6. The plates were incubated overnight and then washed with PBS four times and treated with 0.1 M NH$_4$Cl for 30 min in order to bind nonreactive groups. The wells of the microtiter plates were then washed with PBS and stored in PBS containing 0.05% sodium azide in the cold.

The supernatants from the wells of the hybridoma fusion plates were added to the wells of the microtiter plates containing the IUrd–BSA (at a volume of 100 μl/well) and incubated in the cold for 1 hr. After washing the wells free of the supernatants from hybridoma fusion, sheep F(ab)$_2$ anti-mouse Ig coupled to β-galactosidase was added (BRL) and the plates were then incubated for 2 hr at room temperature. The plates were then washed again with the solution PBS containing 0.05% Tween 20, 1.5 mM MgCl$_2$, and 2 mM mercaptoethanol; and the β-galactosidase substrate (p-nitrophenylgalactopyranoside diluted in 50 mM phosphate buffer, pH 7.2, plus 1.5 mM MgCl$_2$ was added and the plates incubated for an additional hour. After the addition of 0.5 M K$_2$CO$_3$, the plates were observed for the yellow color indicative of a positive reaction signifying the presence of anti-IUrd antibody. Quantitation was accomplished by means of a ELISA plate reader (Dynatech) at 415 nm. Positive cells from wells were recloned by limiting dilution and then recloned by plating single cells in agarose.

ELISA assay was also performed on 96-well microculture plates on which were grown monolayers of a cloned prostatic carcinoma cell line (UMS 1541 Q, obtained from Dr. David Reese, Department of Urology, University of Miami). The cells were grown in CMRL-1415 medium with or without 10 μM BrdUrd.

3. RESULTS

3.1. Determination of Antibody Specificity

Antiserum was raised against BrdUrd in rabbits and characterized by double diffusion in agar, as described previously.[18] Time course of the appearance of activity as determined by radioimmunoassay[22] is shown in Figure 1. Out of 10 animals immunized, three produced antibody specific for the BrdUrd. Our biggest problem was to make an antibody that did not cross-react with thymidine, which obviously would be the overwhelmingly predominant interfering molecule in DNA. Hapten-inhibition studies showed that antibody could be produced that cross-reacted less than 0.001% with thymidine.[23]

Attempts were made to produce antibodies that were more specific for BrdUrd. The most successful method was to employ affinity chromatography with bromouridine coupled to Sepharose 4B.[18] The immunoglobulin fraction of the serum, prepared by precipitation with 40% (NH$_2$)SO$_4$, was passed through the BrdUrd column, washed, and eluted with 0.1 M acetic acid–0.15

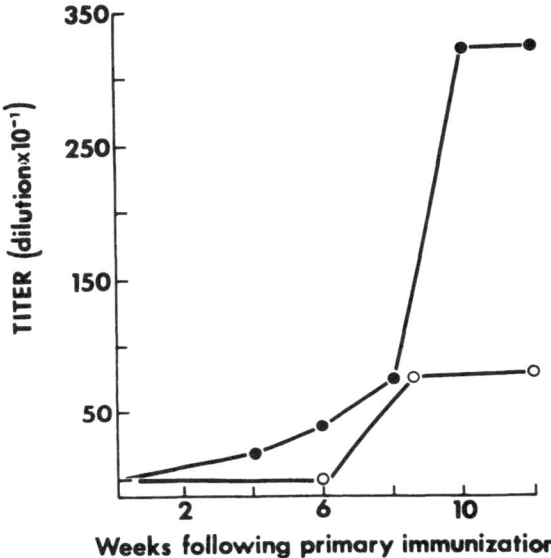

Figure 1. Time course of the appearance of antibody titer following immunization with the conjugate BrdUrd–bovine serum albumin. The anti-BrUrd activity of two animals was assayed by RIA, as described in Section 2.3.3. (From Gratzner et al.[23] with permission, PJD publications, Ltd.)

M NaCl solution. The antibody eluted from the column reacted specifically with only BrdUrd in Ouchterlony plates, and any precipitation band that formed with the unfractionated serum prior to chromatography was eliminated.

The more definitive test of specificity for BrdUrd was to stain cells that were grown in BrdUrd with antibody and compare the staining achieved with the labeled cells with those cells grown in medium without BrdUrd.

The nuclei of cells grown in the presence of BrdUrd stain specifically, whereas control cells grown in the absence of BrdUrd do not stain at the proper dilution of antiserum. However, at higher concentrations of antiserum, nonlabeled cells also stain, so titrations were performed to optimize the dilution of serum utilized for immunological staining.

In another test of specificity of anti-BrdUrd, we demonstrated that sister chromatids of chromosomes from cells grown in BrdUrd under the proper conditions could be differentially stained. For this experiment, CHO cells were grown for two generations (about 30 hr) in BrdUrd-containing medium and an additional generation in thymidine-containing medium. Subsequent to treatment of the cultures with colcemid, the cells were fixed, denatured, and stained

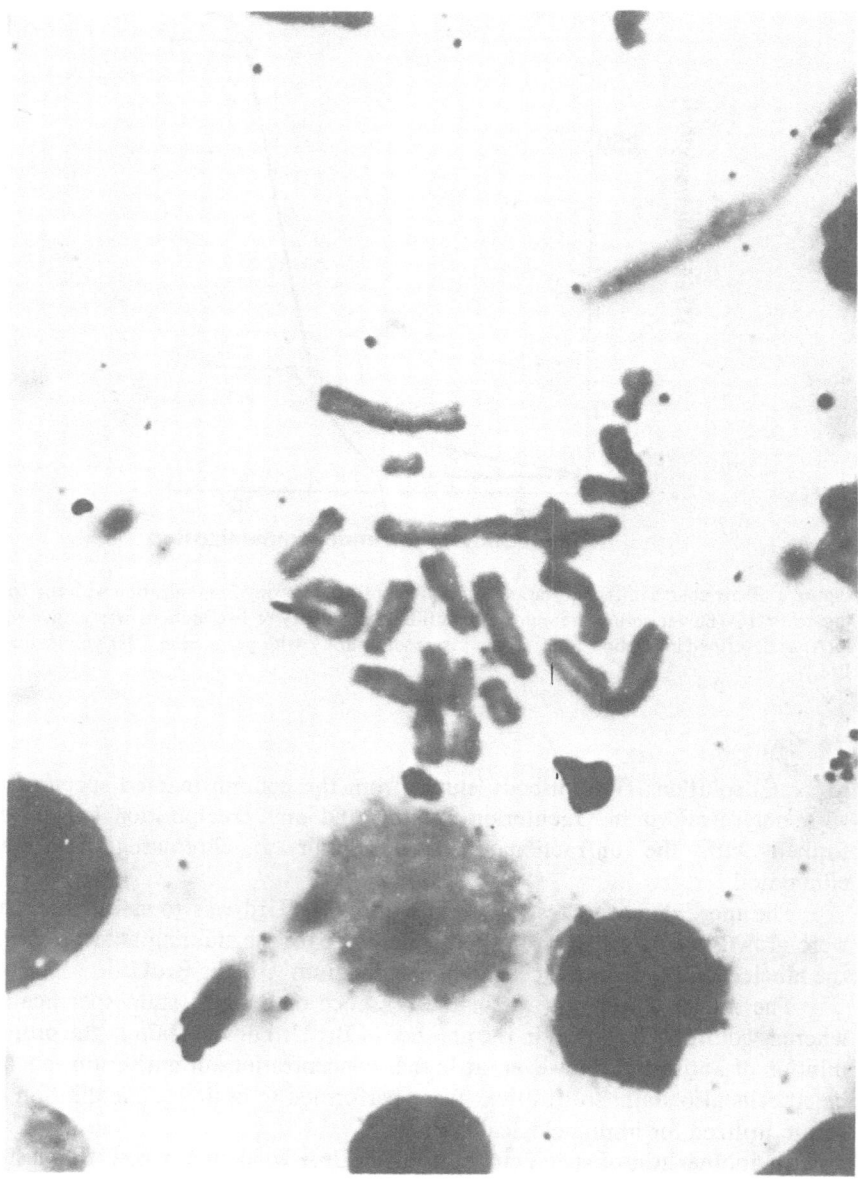

Figure 2. Specific sister chromatid labeling of chromosomes as detected by immunoperoxidase staining. CHO cells were incubated for two generations with BrdUrd and FdUrd, and an additional generation in thymidine-containing medium. The chromosomes were fixed and stained by the immunoperoxidase technique as described in Section 2.3.5. (From Gratzner et al.[18] with permission, Academic Press.)

by the indirect immunoperoxidase technique described in Section 2.3.5. As can be observed in Figure 2, the sister chromatids are differentially stained, as would be expected if one sister chromatid contained BrdUrd in one strand of the double helix. In addition, several sister chromatid exchanges are evident.

The anti-BrdUrd–immunoperoxidase technique can substitute for autoradiography as a way of measuring the percentage of cells undergoing DNA replication. It was shown that there was direct correlation between the percentage of cells that were labeled with [^{3}H]-BrdUrd after release of G_1 block either with autoradiography or the indirect immunoperoxidase technique for dectection of the incorporation of BrdUrd into DNA (Figure 3).

3.2. Flow Cytometric Method for Immunofluorescent Detection of DNA Replication

The original objective of these studies was to develop a method by which replicating cells could be distinguished by flow cytometry. Staining of the nuclei of single cells in suspension by immunological techniques was not as

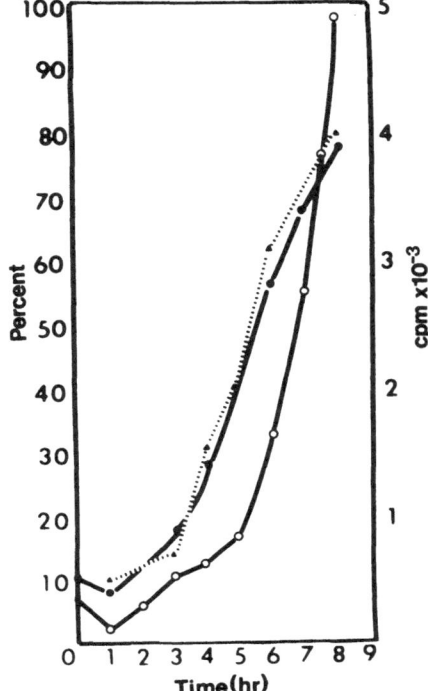

Figure 3. A comparison of the labeling index determined by immunoperoxidase–anti-BrdUrd (|▲|) and autoradiographic (-●-) techniques. At least 500 nuclei were counted for each time point. The cells were synchronized by the isoleucine deprivation method. (From Gratzner et al.[16] copyright by Elsevier North-Holland, Inc.) Open circle represents [^{3}H]-BrdUrd incorporation as measured by scintillation counting.

simple as performing DNA staining with a dye in order to generate the conventional DNA histogram, a task that can be performed in less than 15 min. For immunofluorescent staining of BrdUrd-labeled DNA, antibodies must penetrate into the nucleus and bind to single-stranded DNA. Thus, a convenient method must be available that denatures the DNA, but does not destroy the cells. We also decided to utilize whole cells instead of isolated nuclei for the suspension staining, in order that we could ultimately exploit other parameters of the cell, such as surface antigens and cell size (by immunofluorescence and light scatter, respectively). Another more pragmatic reason for using whole cells was that nuclei are difficult to work with—they clump during antibody staining—and a large percentage of the nuclei are lost during the repeated centrifugations necessary for the washing steps between the various antibody treatments. For staining whole cells, the best fixation proved to be 70% ethanol, as described in Section 2.3.4.

In order to expose the BrdUrd-containing DNA to the antibody, depurination was accomplished by hydrolysis with 1 N HCl. The cells can be dually stained for both DNA *replication* and DNA *content,* by staining with propidium iodide.[23a] The purpose of the dual staining is to apply the anti-BrdUrd technique to cell kinetic analysis: we can follow cohorts of cells through the cell cycle by multiparameter techniques. The dual stain enables labeled cells to be identified during their traverse through S phase. The dual staining might also be useful for mutagenesis analysis, as a means of "gating" specific variant cells in several dimensions together with cell size.

The hydrolytic technique proved to be successful for specifically staining the BrdUrd-labeled cells, and the secondary staining for DNA content has been successfully accomplished.

A problem that had to be overcome was nonspecific cytoplasmic staining: since conventional flow cytometric analysis is a "zero resolution" technique, no discrimination can be made between nuclear and cytoplasmic fluorescence. Thus it was required that some means be found to reduce any cytoplasmic fluoresence. This was accomplished by pretreating the cell suspension with solutions containing the nonionic detergent NP40 and a high concentration of some protein such as BSA or goat serum. The detergent also served to permit penetration of antibodies into the nucleus.[24]

While it would have been more convenient to employ a direct staining method in which the fluorescein was attached directly to the anti-BrdUrd antibodies, indirect techniques of immunostaining substantially amplify the fluorescence signal. For this reason a secondary fluorescent tag, protein A coupled to fluorescein, was employed. The protein A was chosen because of its high affinity for IgG and its relatively low molecular weight, which presumably should facilitate its transport into the cell.

Using the protocol described in Section 2.3.4 and outlined in Figure 4, it was found that detection of cells pulsed with BrdUrd for relatively short periods of time was possible. With antibodies produced in rabbits, titers of 1:500 could produce substantial fluorescence discrimination between labeled and unlabeled cells, as shown in Figure 5. While a certain degree of nonspecific fluorescence was observed, separation could be achieved between the non-BrdUrd-labeled and BrdUrd-labeled cells by multiparameter flow cytometry. Figure 6 shows a scatter plot of fluorescence versus light scatter of cells pulsed for 1 hr in BrdUrd. A "cloud" of labeled cells is well separated from the unlabeled cells.

An important consideration in these studies is whether one can determine, at the single-cell level, the rate of DNA replication. This appears to be the case, inasmuch as the amount of BrdUrd incorporated into the cells is a function of the time of incubation in BrdUrd-containing medium. When [^{3}H]-BrdUrd was used to label the cells, there was a linear relationship between the amount of acid-soluble counts incorporated and the fluorescence intensity. By electronic sorting of cells according to increasing fluorescence intensity into scintillation vials[25] it was found that there was a direct relationship between the fluorescence intensity of individual cells and BrdUrd incorporation (Figure 7). The

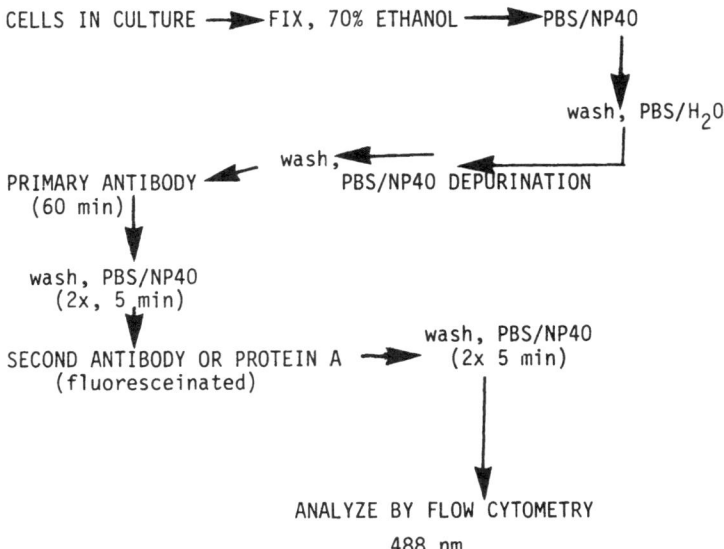

Figure 4. Flow diagram of protocol for immunofluorescent anti-BrdUrd staining of cells in suspension for flow cytometry. "Secondary antibody" is fluoresceinated goat anti-mouse Ig when staining with monoclonal anti–BrdUrd antibody.

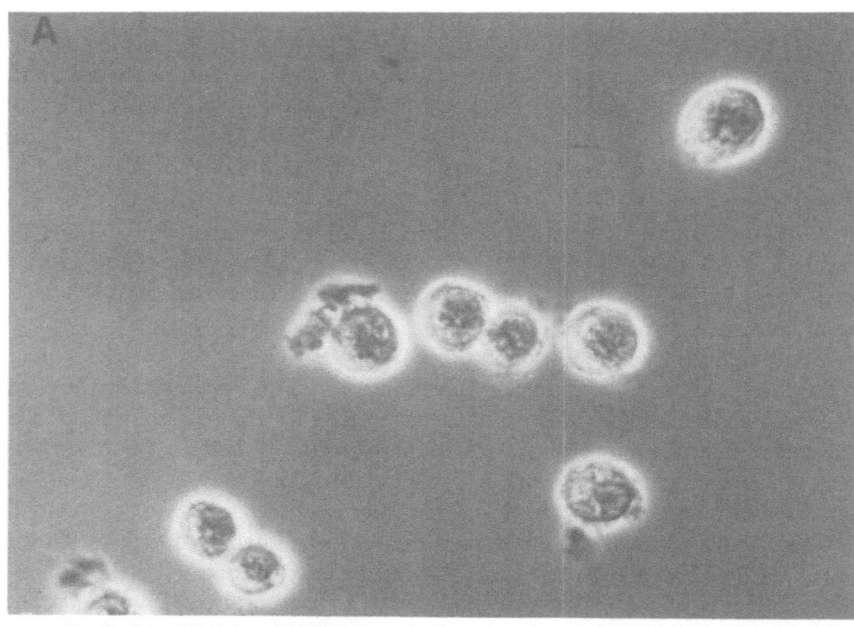

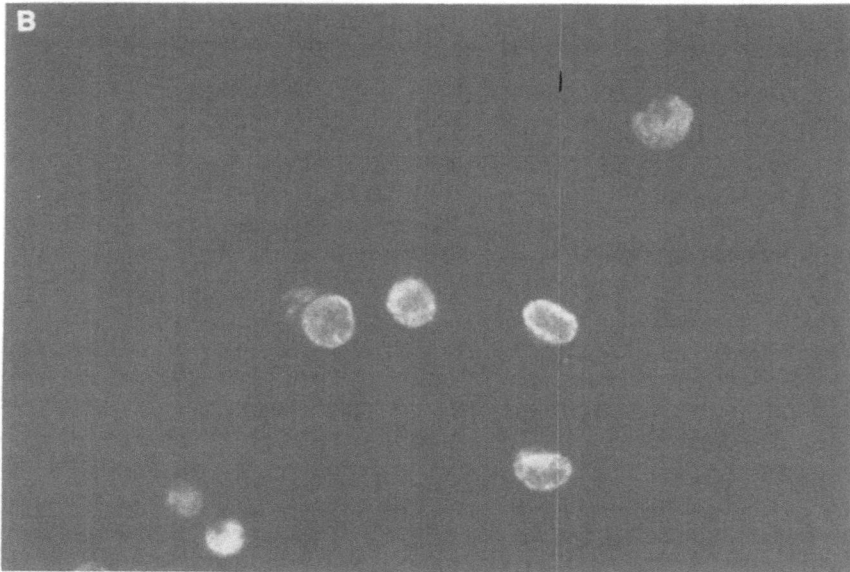

Figure 5. Suspension staining of human lymphoblast cells with anti-BrUrd antibody. WiL2 cells were grown for 3 hr in BrdUrd-containing medium and fixed and stained with anti-BrUrd antiserum and fluoresceinated protein A as described in Section 2. Photomicrography was with high-speed Ektachrome 400 film. (A) Phase contrast; (B) fluorescence micrograph of same field.

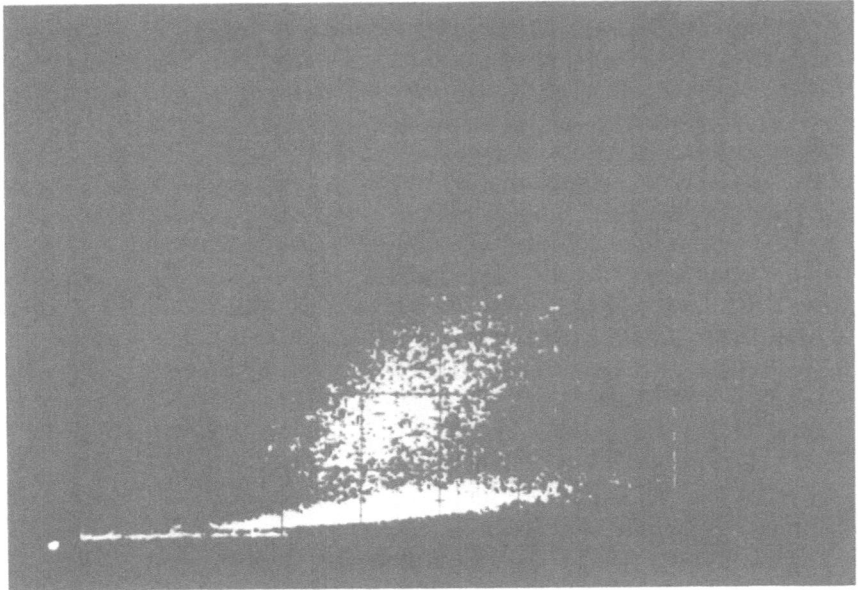

Figure 6. Immunofluorescence determination of BrdUrd incorporation in cultured lymphoid cells. Two-parameter dot plot: fluorescence (vertical) versus light scatter (horizontal). WiL2 cells were pulsed for 1 hr in spinner culture with 10 μM BrdUrd and 1 μM FdUrd. The cells were stained with 1:800 dilution of anti-BrdUrd antiserum, then 1:80 dilution of goat anti-rabbit IgG biotin conjugate, and then with fluoresceinated avidin D. The lower, elongated cluster represents non-BrdUrd-labeled cells, the upper cluster, BrdUrd-labeled cells. (From Gratzner and Leif[25] with permission, Society for Analytical Cytology.)

linear relationship is more dramatically demonstrated in Figure 10, as discussed in Section 3.3.

3.3. Application of the Flow Immunofluorometric Anti-BrdUrd Technique to the Assessment of DNA Damage

We are exploiting this technique of measuring DNA synthesis by flow immunofluorescence to assess damage to the DNA synthetic apparatus. The method is analogous to that developed by Painter.[26] However, whereas Painter's technique employs radioisotopic analysis of DNA synthesis, the anti-BrdUrd immunofluorescence method can analyze the effects of agents on DNA replication at the single-cell level.

It was anticipated that a method that analyzed DNA replication in unbro-

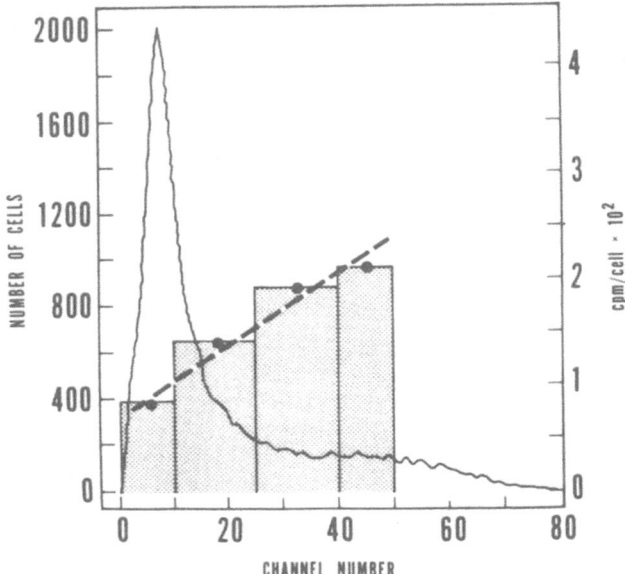

Figure 7. The relationship of [³H]-BrdUrd incorporation to fluorescence intensity, as demonstrated by cell sorting. WiL2 cells were incubated in culture medium containing [³H]-BrdUrd (1 mCi/ml, 10 mM) for 24 hr, after which time they were fixed in 70% ethanol, stained by the anti-BrdUrd fluorescein procedure. The cells were then sorted into scintillation vials with the EPICS IV cell sorter, according to the sort windows indicated by the vertical lines. (From Gratzner and Leif[25] with permission, Society for Analytical Cytology.)

ken cells on a cell-by-cell basis would be superior to the methods currently employed, i.e., autoradiography is tedious and has low statistical reliability, while scintillation counting will only measure gross synthesis in whole population of cells, but not discriminate the amount synthesized per cell (both methods also obviously suffer from introducing an environmental hazard themselves).

The flow immunofluorometric method using anti-BrdUrd antibodies has definite advantages over the aforementioned techniques: (1) Hundreds of thousands of cells can be measured in several minutes, providing great statistical reliability, and (2) computer interpretation of results, particularly when coupled with *multiparameter* analysis, might define subpopulations by combining the immunofluorescent replication data with a cell marker such as an antigen or indicator of cell cycle stage (DNA content). The latter would enable one to follow the *cohorts* of the cells through the cell cycle.

The method was applied to a study of the effects of the fungicide captan

(Figure 8) since there is evidence that it is mutagenic.[27] Cells were treated with various concentrations of captan and subjected to the immunofluorescence methodology to produce the dose curve shown in Figure 8.

When the cells were monitored for viability, it was found that the higher concentrations of captan were too cytotoxic; the succeeding experiments were thus conducted at 0.1 μM captan. For these studies, the cells were treated for 3 hr in captan, washed, and cultured in BrdUrd-containing medium. Aliquots of the cultures were removed at 1, 2, and 3 hr, fixed, stained with anti-BrdUrd

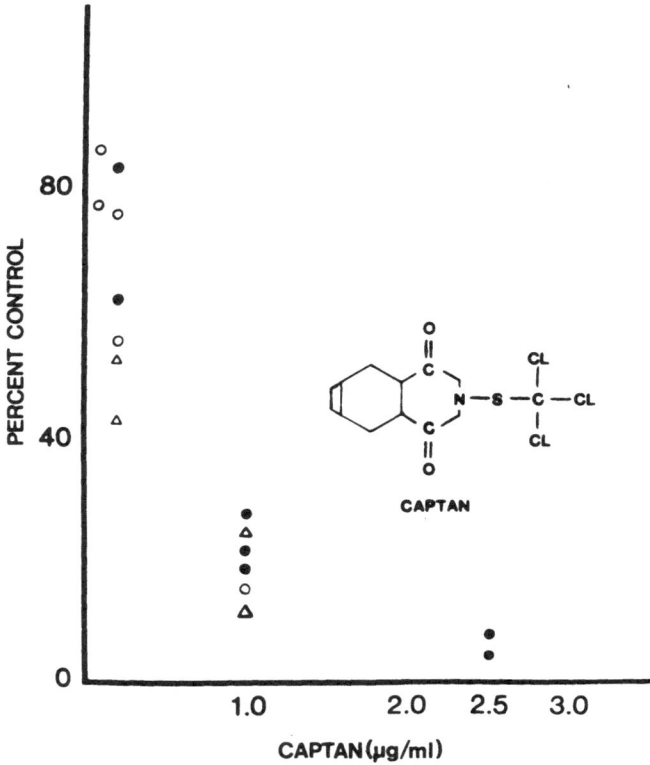

Figure 8. The effect of captan on BrdUrd incorporation in WiL2 human lymphoblast cells. In the experiments indicated, cells were incubated for 14 hr in captan and then in 10 μM BrdUrd for an additional 8 hr. The ordinate refers to the inhibition (percentage of fluorescent cells) caused by the captan. The percent fluorescent cells in the controls (without captan but with BrdUrd) was 40% and 52%. A total of 100,000 cells were counted for each concentration 0.05, 0.1, and 2.5 μg/ml of captan.

antibody, and analyzed by flow cytometry. Figure 9 shows the results of this experiment, which demonstrates the traverse of the replicating cells through S phase. The *treated* cells incorporate BrdUrd into DNA, but appear to be retarded in their traverse. Examination of the histograms leads to the speculation that possibly the treated cells have *initiated* replication, but *elongation* is inhibited. Such conclusions obviously await further studies with drugs that inhibit elongation and a molecular technique to confirm the present observations.

A more quantitative representation of the histograms of Figure 9 is shown in Figure 10. These data were produced by use of a computer program that subtracted the histogram generated by analyzing non-BrdUrd-labeled cells from the labeled cells at each time point on a channel-by-channel basis and multiplying the difference by its specific channel number. Note that the curves produced by this procedure are linear for the untreated cells and extrapolate near the origin. Thus, weighted values can be assigned to a fluorescence histogram that appears to accurately represent the behavior of the population.

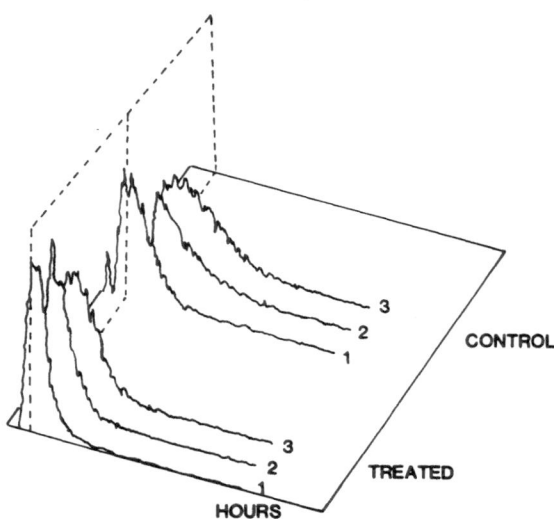

Figure 9. Time course traverse of S-phase cells traced with captan, 0.1 μM. Cells were treated for 3 hr with captan, washed, resuspended in medium with 10 μM BrdUrd + 1 μM FdUrd. Aliquots were removed from treated and control cultures at hourly intervals, fixed, and stained. The peaks represent the differences between BrdUrd-labeled and nonlabeled control cell histograms, subtracted channel-by-channel. The plane passes through the peak of the 1-hr-treated cells in order to depict the displacement of the other peaks. Y axis: number of fluorescent cells; X axis: fluorescent channel number.

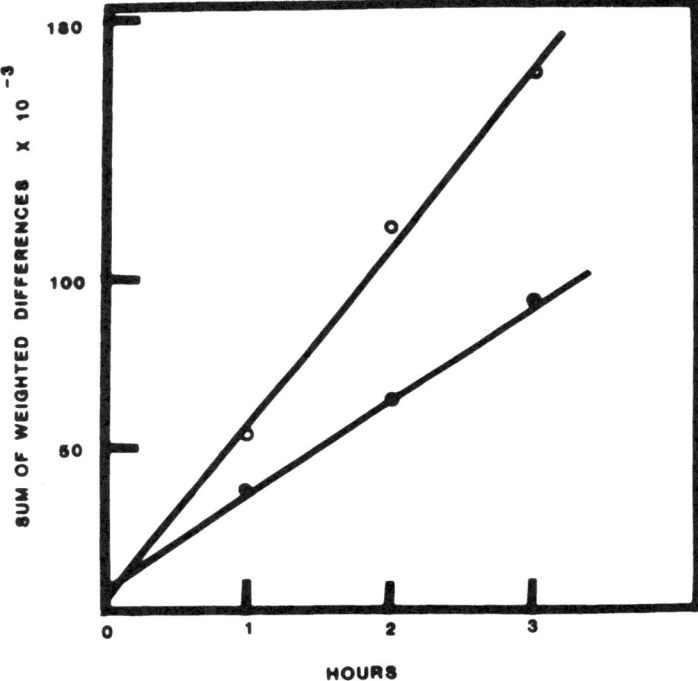

Figure 10. Effect of captan on S-phase traverse, as determined by computer analysis of Fig. 8 by the "sum of weighted differences" program. Open circles: control cells; closed circles, captan-treated cells. Conditions are described in Figure 8.

3.4. Reconstruction Experiments for the Detection of Thioguanine-Resistant Variants by the Immunofluorescent Anti-BrdUrd Method

In order to ultimately apply the flow immunofluorescent technique to the detection of rare variant cells, it is necessary to conduct reconstruction studies in which a minute number of known thioguanine-resistant cells (TG^r) are added to a large background of sensitive (TG^s) cells. Resistant variants of WiL2 cells were selected by growth on 5 μg/ml thioguanine. Table I shows the results of incubating both resistant and sensitive strains with and without 6-TG. Conditions must be found where the thioguanine-sensitive cells in a muta-genesis experiment incorporate no BrdUrd and the very small population of resistant cells do incorporate the analog. In practice, it appears that the wild-type (TG^s) cells will also incorporate some BrdUrd unless conditions are chosen such that the cells are blocked in cycle by thioguanine prior to the addition of

Table I

The Inhibition of Thioguanine-Sensitive and -Resistant Variants of WiL2
Lymphoblast Cells, As Determined by Immunofluorescent Measurement
of BrdUrd Incorporation

	Percent fluorescent cells		
Variant strain	+TG, BrdUrd	−TG, +BrdUrd	−TG, BrdUrd
WiL2$^+$ (TG^s)	4.6	27.6	1
TGR-1 (TG^r)	29.6	38.4	—
TGR-4 (TG^r)	25.3	29.3	—

BrdUrd. If the two compounds are added simultaneously, BrdUrd is incorporated to some extent, since DNA synthesis has not been arrested.

In a series of experiments, wild-type (TG^s) cells were incubated (a) with both thioguanine and BrdUrd and (b) with thioguanine, and resuspended in medium containing only BrdUrd 12 hr later. When the cells are first incubated in thioguanine and then resuspended in BrdUrd, the cells presumably block in S and G$_2$M,[28] and very little BrdUrd is incorporated in comparison to the case where they are both added together. However, a far greater than acceptable amount of BrdUrd was incorporated in terms of percentage of cells if one were to apply the technique to the enumeration of resistant cells in a mutagenesis experiment. It may be that the cells that incorporate thioguanine are thioguanine-resistant cells in the population of sensitive cells, since the cells are not passed through HAT medium for several generations to eliminate thioguanine-resistant cells prior to these studies. We are continuing the experiments for varying times of incubation in order to attain the ideal conditions for resistant cell selection. An additional problem that arose is the fact that WiL2 cells are quite sensitive to the cytotoxic effect of thioguanine in the medium, as opposed to the observations of Strauss and Albertini.[9] The cells that are sensitive to growth inhibition by thioguanine degenerate, and may not be recognizable by FCM as "cells" subsequent to fixation in ethanol. This toxicity is obviously not a problem in the usual growth selection methods of mutation enumeration, since one only is interested in the thioguanine-resistant cells that clone in the selective medium and are then counted as colonies. In the procedure to be developed in this work, the sensitive cells must appear to the flow cytometer as a "cell" by its light scatter characteristics or electronic-cell volume. The cells are analyzed by setting a light scatter or volume gate and counting only those cells that fall within a specific window. Since narrow-angle light scatter is a function of the cell's diameter, if a "dead" cell appears and is below the scatter gate, it will appear as debris and will not be counted, and spurious data will result. In our preliminary experiments with these cells, either heat killing or azide poisoning affect the apparent cell size by 30–50% as determined by light scatter immediately after the treatment. Therefore, times of exposure of the cells to thioguanine, and also their residence in culture medium subsequent to thioguanine treatment, must be important considerations in the development of a mutagenic technique based on FCM.

Studies were performed to determine whether it was feasible to detect small numbers of fluorescent, BrdUrd-labeled cells by the methods discussed above. Cells were grown in BrdUrd and added to nonlabeled cells, and the cells were stained by the methods described in Section 2. About 13,000 BrdUrd-labeled cells were added to suspensions of 1.6×10^6 unlabeled cells; the cells were stained by the immunofluorescence method described, and subjected to flow analysis. Figure 11 shows the results of this kind of experiment. Practically all of the cells fall into the unlabeled peak, but it is possible to distinguish the labeled cells in the sample to which they were added, within the limits of sampling errors accompanying the addition of the small number of cells as well as only counting 100,000 cells by FCM. One problem encountered with these studies is the fact that it is impossible to discern a distinct cutoff between unlabeled and labeled cells; cells with a very low level of fluorescence contribute to

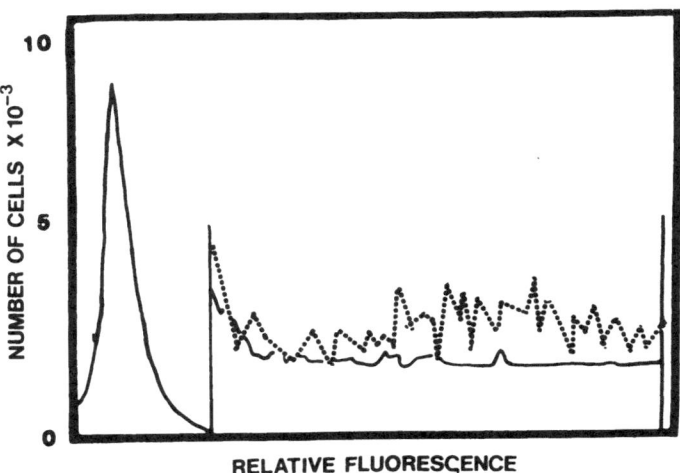

Figure 11. Discrimination of BrdUrd-labeled cells from nonlabeled cells by the flow immunofluorescence anti-BrdUrd method. In a reconstruction experiment, approximately 1350 and 13,500 BrdUrd-labeled WiL2 cells ($\pm 10\%$) were added to tubes that contained 1.6×10^6 nonlabeled cells; the cells were processed for immunofluorescence by means of anti-BrdUrd antibody technique and analyzed by flow cytometry. The left peak represents the unlabeled cells; the area between the vertical lines represents the labeled cells with the scale expanded $10\times$. Dashed line, 13,500-cell experiment (integrated $= 583/10^5$ cells, gated from channel 30).

the tail of the control curve. Another problem is the fact that the nonlabeled cells display a number of false positive cells. For these reasons we chose an arbitrary channel (channel 30 in Figure 11) and determined the number of cells from that channel to the last channel of the histogram (channel 127). It appears that it is possible to recover very small numbers of fluorescent cells from a large background of nonlabeled cells, subtracting the cells of a nonlabeled population. It is also obvious from these studies that an improved signal-to-noise ratio (fluorescence intensity of labeled cells) needs to be achieved in order to separate the nonlabeled from labeled cells.

3.5. Preparation of Monoclonal Antibodies against 5-Bromodeoxyuridine or 5-Iododeoxyuridine

Hybridomas were selected by growth in HAT subsequent to fusion of the spleen cells from mice that were immunized with the IUrd–ovalbumin. Wells with clones were screened for anti-IUrd activity by the ELISA technique. Since we had previously shown that IdUrd cross-reacts with BrdUrd by RIA,[23] the mice were immunized and clones screened with IUrd coupled to ovalbumin and bovine serum albumin, respectively.

The screening of supernatants was performed by replica plating the supernatants into 96-well microtiter plates coated with IUrd-BSA. Antibody activity was assayed by the ELISA technique described in Section 2.5. Twenty-four of 170 clones that were selected by their growth in HAT medium were positive for IUrd–BSA binding. The cells from positive wells were recultured in 24-well microculture plates and reassayed, and positive clones were then passed to tubes and recloned by limiting dilution. Positive cultures from the limiting dilution cloning were recloned by growth in soft agar, and subsequent expansion of the cultures for ascites production in BALB/c mice.

Initial characterization of clones was performed by hapten-inhibition, using the ELISA technique. Six of the clones were analyzed. Serial dilutions of the culture medium were added to microtiter wells together with 50 μg IdUrd/well. The results of one series of experiments is shown in Figure 12. It can be seen that the soluble nucleoside analogue competes with IUrd–BSA. On the other hand, *thymidine* does not compete for the *clone B44* antibody, which demonstrates the specificity for IdUrd. Three of the six clones tested in this manner gave a similar result. We have also tested the products of these clones against BrdUrd-substituted cell monolayers, by the ELISA method. The B44 clone reacts with BrdUrd-incorporated nuclei but not with control, non-substituted nuclei. We have determined that cells on slides and in suspension can be specifically stained with the monoclonal antibody, and the signal to noise ratio is greater than 12:1 when BrdUrd-labeled WiL2 cells are pulsed for 15 min in BrdUrd and stained by the usual method[15] (Figure 13).

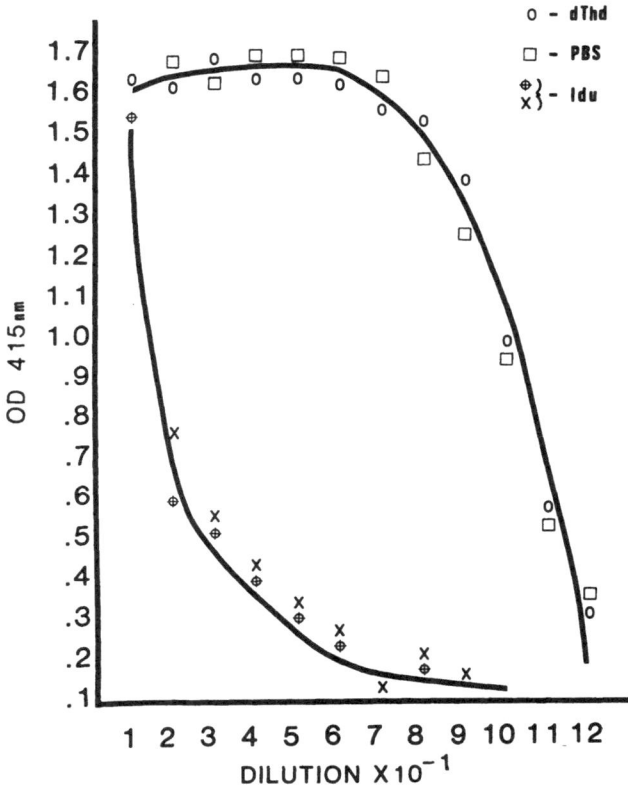

Figure 12. The specificity of anti-IdUrd antibody produced by mouse hybridoma clone B44. Supernatants from hybridoma cultures were assayed by the ELISA test described in Section 2.5. Iododeoxyuridine and thymidine were added at 50 μg/well of the microtiter plate.

The specificity of the monoclonal antibody for BrdUrd was dramatically demonstrated when we stained control, nonlabeled cells with undiluted, dialyzed 50% (NH₄)SO₄ precipitates of antibody-producing hybridoma cultures (20 mg/ml): virtually no fluorescence was visible by fluorescence microscopy.

4. DISCUSSION

This chapter is a report of work in progress toward the development of a method for the enumeration of variant cells. The method employs anti-BrdUrd antibodies and flow cytometry. More remains to be done in order to arrive at

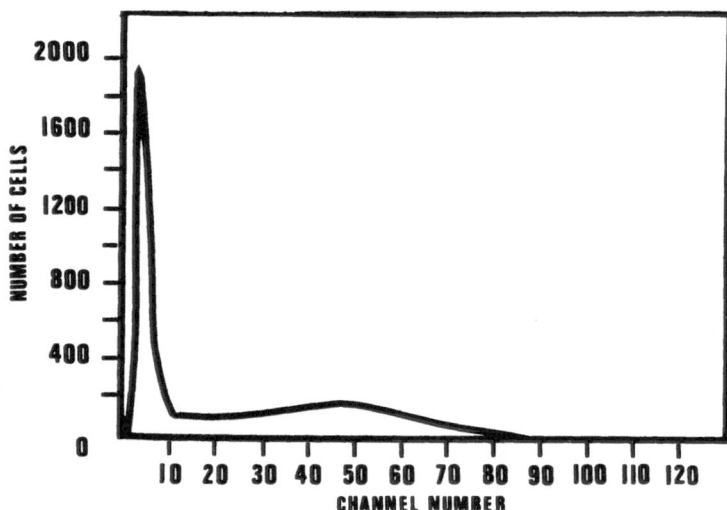

Figure 13. Flow histogram, staining of WiL2 cells with monoclonal antibody subsequent to 15-min BrdUrd pulse; 10 μM BrdUrd. Procedure for suspension staining was as diagramed in Figure 4. Peak at channel 4 represents control, unlabeled cells.

an assay that can be applied to the routine analysis of mutagenesis. We have, however, demonstrated that we can directly detect replicating cells by FCM and immunofluorescence techniques employing a highly specific monoclonal, anti-BrdUrd antibody. A spinoff of our studies has been the development of a technique for monitoring DNA damage, the efficacy of which has been demonstrated by its application to a study of the effects of the pesticide captan on DNA synthesis in human lymphoblast cells.

In order for this immunofluorometric method to function for the enumeration of rare fluorescent cells, we must accomplish at least two things: (1) we must increase the signal to noise ratio between BrdUrd-labeled and nonlabeled cells and (2) we must establish conditions in which only the thioguanine-resistant cells incorporate fluorescently detectable quantities of BrdUrd. Approaches to the former include the employment of indirect immunofluorescence techniques, such as the avidin–biotin method, which amplifies the fluorescence intensity.[25] The second approach is to produce monoclonal antibody that is highly specific for the single determinant, i.e., 5-bromouracil or iodouracil, and does not contain other components that would bind nonspecifically to either cytoplasmic or nuclear antigens. In addition, since there is no detectable competition found with thymidine, the nonspecific fluorescence with heteroclonal rabbit antibodies at lower titers is eliminated. It was an exciting result to exploit the hybridoma technology for the production of a consistent reagent[27] that can be applied to cytological detection of DNA replication.

The results were even better than anticipated, since the use of the monoclonal antibody resulted in virtual elimination of cytoplasmic and nonspecific nuclear fluorescence.

While the affinity-purified rabbit antibody[18] was effective for immunofluorescent staining, the recovery of high-affinity antibody from affinity columns resulted in low yields because of degradation, and would vary from rabbit to rabbit.

The hybridoma technique enables one to produce unlimited amounts of antibody by injecting the cells into mice to produce ascites tumors. In our hands, the titers of unfractionated ascites fluid (by ELISA) is 10^6-fold higher than unconcentrated medium from cell cultures.

The greatest impediment to the application of this immunofluorescent technique for enumeration of TG^r cells is the problem of phenocopies, that is, TG^s cells that incorporate BrdUrd and are thus fluorescent when stained with the anti-BrdUrd antibody. We are attempting to establish conditions whereby the cells are only exposed to BrdUrd subsequent to the point where TG^s cells are blocked in DNA replication by thioguanine. Perhaps the multiparameter aspect of flow cytometry can be exploited for this task. Since the fluorescence intensity is proportional to the amount of DNA replicated, it should be possible to gate only on cells that have traversed S phase a certain distance and thus have synthesized a specific quantity of DNA, which makes that cell eligible for counting. Another possibility is to simultaneously stain cells for *replication* and DNA *content* by staining with a DNA-specific dye and analyzing two colors in dual-parameter mode, as we have previously suggested for application of this immunofluorescence technique to cell kinetics.[25] Another consideration might be to *synchronize* the cells prior to pulsing with BrdUrd to ensure that all cells arrive at S phase simultaneously, and thus are subjected to the toxic effects of the thioguanine at the same point in time.

5. SUMMARY

This chapter is a review of the methodology that has been applied in our attempt to develop an automated system for detecting DNA damage and mutation in mammalian cells. The system is based upon the immunofluorescent detection of BrdUrd incorporation into DNA by means of specific antibodies. Cells that are resistant to a drug, e.g., 6-thioguanine, will replicate their DNA in the presence of the drug and thus will incorporate BrdUrd, which can then be detected by immunofluorescence and flow cytometry.

Monoclonal antibodies that can serve as consistent reagents can be produced and are applicable to the enumeration of replicating cells in many other areas of biology.

Conditions are being established whereby only variant cells will incorporate BrdUrd in the presence of the inhibiting drug.

REFERENCES

1. M. L. Mendelsohn, W. L. Bigbee, E. W. Branscomb, and G. Stamatoyannopaulos, The detection and sorting of rare sickle-hemoglobin containing cells in normal human blood, *Flow Cytom. IV*, 311–313 (1980).
2. B. Holtkamp, M. Cramer, H. Lemke, and K. Rajewsky, Isolation of a cloned cell line expressing variant H-2K$^+$ by fluorescence-activated cell sorting, *Nature 289*, 66–68 (1981). .
3. P. Howard-Flanders, Mutagenesis in mammalian cells, *Mutat. Res. 86*, 307–327 (1981).
4. Committee 17, Environmental mutagenic hazards, *Science 187*, 503–514 (1975).
5. B. N. Ames, Identifying environmental chemicals causing mutations and cancer, *Science 204*, 587–593 (1979).
6. A. Abbondandolo, Prospects for evaluating genetic damage in mammalian cell culture, *Mutat. Res. 42*, 279–298 (1977).
7. P. E. Nute, Th. Papayannopaulou, B. Tatsis, and G. Stamatoyannopoulos, Towards a system for detecting somatic-cell mutations. V. Preparation of fluorescent antibodies to hemoglobin Hasharon, A human a chain variant, *J. Immunol. Methods 42*, 5–44 (1981).
8. G. Stamatoyannopoulos, P. E. Nute, Th. Papayannopoulou, T. Mcguire, G. Lim, H. F. Bunn, and D. Ruchnagel, Development of a somatic mutation screening system using Hb mutants. IV. Successful detection of red cells containing the human frameshift mutants Hb Wayne and Hb Cranston using monospecific antibodies, *Am. J. Hum. Genet. 32*, 484–496 (1980).
9. G. Strauss and J. Albertini, Enumeration of 6-thioguanine-resistant peripheral blood lymphocytes in man as a potential test for somatic cell mutations arising *in vivo*, *Mutation 61*, 353–379 (1979).
10. W. Herzenberg and L. Herzenberg, Analysis and separation using the fluorescence activated cell sorter (FACS), in: *Handbook of Experimental Immunology* (D. M. Wier, ed.), Vol. 2, pp. 22.1–22.2, Blackwell, Oxford (1978).
11. S. A. Latt, Microfluorometric determination of deoxyribonucleic acid replication in human metaphase chromosomes, *Proc. Natl. Acad. Sci USA 70*, 3395–3398 (1973).
12. D. E. Swartzendruber, A bromodeoxyuridine (BrdUrd) mithramycin technique for detecting cycling and non-cycling cells by flow microfluorometry, *Exp. Cell Res. 109*, 439–443 (1977).
13. E. E. Furth, W. G. Thilly, B. W. Penman, H. L. Liber, and W. M. Rand, Quantitative assay for mutation in diploid human fibroblasts using microtiter plates, *Anal. Biochem. 110*, 1–8 (1981).
14. G. Kohler and C. Milstein, Continuous cultures of fused cells secreting antibody of predefined specificity, *Nature 256*, 495–497 (1975).
15. H. G. Gratzner, Monoclonal antibody to 5-Bromo and 5-Iododeoxyuridine: a new reagent for detection of DNA replication, *Science, 28*, 474–475 (1982).
16. H. G. Gratzner, A. Pollack, D. J. Ingram, and R. C. Leif, Deoxyribonucleic acid replication in single cells and chromosomes by immunologic techniques, *J. Histochem. Cytochem. 24*, 34–39 (1976).

17. B. F. Erlanger and S. M. Beiser, Antibodies specific for ribonucleosides and ribonucleotides and their reaction with DNA, *Proc. Natl. Acad. Sci USA 52*, 68–74 (1964).
18. H. G. Gratzner, R. C. Leif, D. J. Ingram, and A. Castro, The use of antibodies specific for bromodeoxyuridine for the immunofluorescent determination of DNA replication in cells and chromosomes, *Exp. Cell Res. 95*, 88–93 (1975).
19. O. A. Sternberger, *Immunocytochemistry*, Prentice-Hall, Englewood Cliffs, New Jersey (1974).
20. M. Shulman, C. D. Wilde, and G. Kohler, A better cell line for making hybridomas secreting specific antibodies, *Nature 276*, 269–270 (1978).
21. M. L. Gefter, D. L. Margulies, and M. Scharff, A simple method for the polyethylene glycol-promoted hybridization of mouse myeloma cells, *Somatic Cell Genet. 3*, 231–236 (1977).
22. Anon, Preparation of antigen coated plates for use in enzyme-linked immunoassays. *Hybrlines I*(5), 5 (1980).
23. H. G. Gratzner, N. Ettinger, and D. J. Ingram, Immunochemical studies of 5-bromodeoxyuridine, *Res. Commun. Chem. Pathol. Pharmacol. 20*, 539–598 (1978).
23a. F. Dolbeare, H. G. Gratzner, M. Pallavicini, and J. W. Gray, Flow cytometric measurement of total DM content and incorporated bromodeoxyuridine. *Proc. Nat. Acad. Sci USH* (1984), in press.
24. P. Laurila, I. Virtanen, J. Wartiovaara, and S. Stenman, Fluorescent antibodies and lectins stain intracellular structures in fixed cells treated with non-ionic detergent, *J. Histochem. Cytochem. 26*, 251–257 (1978).
25. H. G. Gratzner and R. C. Leif, An immunofluorescent method for monitoring DNA synthesis by flow cytometry. *Cytometry 1*, 385–389 (1981).
26. R. B. Painter, Rapid test to detect agents that damage DNA, *Nature 265*, 650–651 (1977).
27. C. Clark, The mutagenic specificities of pentachloronitrobenzene and captan, two environmental mutagens, *Mutat. Res. 11*, 247–248 (1971).
28. L. L. Wotring and J. L. Roti Roti, Thioguanine-induced S and G_2 blocks and their significance to the mechanism of toxicity, *Cancer Res. 40*, 1458–1562 (1980).
29. R. H. Kennett, T. J. Mckearn, and K. B. Bechtol, eds., *Monoclonal Antibodies. Hybridomas: A New Dimension in Biological Analyses*, Plenum Press, New York (1980).

6

Cytogenetic Abnormalities as an Indicator of Mutagenic Exposure

R. JULIAN PRESTON

1. INTRODUCTION

Chromosome aberrations can essentially be studied in any cycling cell population, or in any cell population that can be stimulated by a mitogenic agent to cycle. In animals there are several cell types that fit these criteria, but for humans there are to all intents and purposes only two types that are practically suitable. These are the bone marrow cells, which are a cycling population, and peripheral lymphocytes, which are normally noncycling, but can be stimulated to enter the cell cycle by *in vitro* culturing with a mitogen such as phytohemagglutinin. Because of ease of obtaining blood samples in contrast to taking bone marrow samples, the majority of studies on the induction of chromosome alterations in humans have been with the lymphocyte assay. This chapter will concentrate on this assay, with some additional comments on the bone marrow assay where appropriate.

In the 25 years since Moorhead *et al.*[1] demonstrated that normally noncycling peripheral lymphocytes could be stimulated to enter the cell cycle and subsequent mitotic cells analyzed, a vast array of experiments utilizing the lymphocyte assay have been reported.[2] Chromosome abnormalities in a wide variety of species have been studied following *in vivo* or *in vitro* exposure to many different chemical and physical agents. At the same time a considerable amount of basic information has also been obtained on the lymphocyte assay.

R. JULIAN PRESTON • Biology Division, Oak Ridge National Laboratory, Oak Ridge, Tennessee 37830.

It is not the intention of this chapter to review all the available data, but rather to choose specific information to address the questions of how useful is the lymphocyte assay for determining exposure to a clastogenic or mutagenic agent, and what limitations and pitfalls are associated with the assay.

A discussion of this type seems to be particularly appropriate at this time, because it has become a rather common practice to measure chromosome aberration frequencies in potentially exposed groups of people and either compare these frequencies to the frequencies in a control or unexposed group or use historical controls to decide whether or not the group was exposed to a clastogenic agent. Such an approach can be fraught with difficulties and the conclusions drawn should be considered with much greater caution than is often the case. The conclusions are, of course, of particular significance, and so no doubts should be raised by the experimental approach or the results themselves. This unfortunately is far from the case. The discussion here is not intended to provide a panacea, but rather an indication of the types of methodological approaches that will perhaps avoid a misinterpretation or overinterpretation of available data.

2. LYMPHOCYTE ASSAY METHODOLOGY

This section will be fairly brief because much of the information can readily be found elsewhere,[2-4] and many components of methods are optional and are dependent upon individual preference. Those that are more invariable will be stressed.

2.1. *In Vitro* Cultures

It appears to be somewhat advantageous to set up cultures from freshly drawn blood samples. However, this is not always possible, usually because samples are taken at some distance from the laboratory and have to be shipped, but it is still possible to achieve good growth from samples taken several days before culturing. It is also advantageous to maintain the samples at about 4°C during shipping or storage.

A large number of different tissue culture media have been successfully used, and the choice is a matter of personal preference. This is also true for the serum type used, with the added proviso that it should be virus-free. Several different mitogens are also suitable, but it is most common to use phytohemagglutinin.

An important additional consideration is the difference in mitogenic stimulation and subsequent cycle time of lymphocytes under different growth conditions. It appears that this can be quite variable, depending on the type of mitogen, culture medium, and serum used and, or course, culturing temperature (most often 37°C in a 5% CO_2/95% air environment). As will become apparent from later sections, it is most important to analyze cells at their first *in vitro* mitosis, and so each investigator should determine the optimum time for the specific growth conditions used when the great majority of analyzed cells are at the first metaphase in culture. This can be readily checked as described in Section 2.2.

It is possible to establish cultures from whole blood (approximately 0.5 ml) or buffy coats where either is suitable. If a large number of samples are to be handled at one time it is clearly advantageous to use whole blood. Also, for buffy coat cultures it is preferable to use the white cell layer from about 3 ml of centrifuged whole blood, and so larger total blood samples are needed in this case. One of the major advantages of buffy coat cultures is that the cell fixation procedure is not hampered by the large volume of red cells present in whole blood cultures, which are often rather difficult to disperse. A possible disadvantage of whole blood cultures is that small quantities of the agent whose effects are being studied, or another contaminating agent, could be carried over with the donor's serum. However, this would seem to provide a very small probability of influencing the results, and thus would certainly not negate the use of whole blood cultures.

It is also necessary to set up cultures in duplicate as a precautionary measure against culture failure or inadequacy of subsequent cell preparations.

2.2. Sampling Time

It is essential that the cells to be analyzed are at their first metaphase of *in vitro* culture, in order that a measure of induced aberration frequency is obtained. The reasons for this will be discussed later. The selection of a time at which the majority of the analyzable mitotic cell population is in its first division, with little contamination from second division cells, will vary from individual to individual and, as mentioned in Section 2.1, with culture conditions. In a population study where no previous information is available on the individuals being studied, it is not possible to select a fixation time that will guarantee a very high proportion of first-division cells. As a general rule most samples show greater than 80% of first divisions for fixation times of 42–48 hr. Before a laboratory decides upon a fixation time preliminary experiments should be performed.

The technique for differentially staining chromatids for sister chromatid exchange analysis[5-7] following the incorporation of bromodeoxyuridine (BrdUrd) into the DNA can be applied to cell-cycle analysis. The concentration of BrdUrd used varies from laboratory to laboratory, and in our case 25 μM is added to our regular culture medium. The chromosomes of cells that have progressed through one DNA replication in the presence of BrdUrd, and are in the metaphase of this first cycle, will not show differential staining of the chromatids when prepared by any one of the various staining techniques.[5-7] Chromosomes that have passed through two DNA replications in the presence of BrdUrd, and are in their second *in vitro* metaphase, will be differentially stained. Similarly cells in their third or subsequent metaphase can also be identified. Blood cultures from several different individuals should be set up using the particular laboratory's standard protocol and growth conditions, with BrdUrd added to the medium. Fixations should be performed over a range of about 42–54 hr and the proportions of first and second-division metaphases determined by differential staining. A fixation time that provides a high proportion of first division cells in all or the majority of samples should be selected.

It is also advantageous to include a culture containing BrdUrd in any study involving individuals for whom there has not been and cannot be any previous information. These samples should be fixed at the same time as the non-BrdUrd samples, and the proportions of first and second division cells determined. If there is a high proportion of second division cells (greater than, say, 20%) in any of these, then a decision has to be made on the appropriateness of analyzing this sample further for chromosome aberrations. It should also be appreciated that BrdUrd can increase the cell cycle time somewhat, and so the proportion of first-division cells in a BrdUrd-containing culture is likely to represent a slight overestimate of the proportion in a non-BrdUrd culture. The decision can be not to include such individuals, or to include them with the stipulation that the aberration frequency will be an underestimate of the induced value. A further possibility is to analyze the BrdUrd-containing sample, and analyze only those cells that are shown by the lack of differential staining to be in their first division. The argument has been made that the presence of BrdUrd could influence the aberration frequency either by itself or by interacting with DNA damage induced by a chemical agent. This is a valid argument for which no data are available to substantiate or refute the suggestion.

It is possible to analyze the frequency of aberrations in BrdUrd cultures without regard to whether the cells were in their first or second division, and compare this to the frequency in non-BrdUrd cultures. If these frequencies are not significantly different, then it would seem quite reasonable to take the aberration frequency in the first-division cells of the BrdUrd culture as a measure of the induced frequency.

The way that the decision on selecting or rejecting samples with high proportions of second divisions is handled is optional, but should at least be consistent. If resampling is possible, then this should be done, using an earlier fixation time than for the first sample.

There is also a slight possibility that at the selected fixation time there are insufficient analyzable mitotic cells as a result of an unusually long cell cycle, either inherent or induced. The only solution here is to resample and use a later fixation time.

2.3. Fixation and Slide Preparation

There are many different methods available for obtaining metaphase preparations, and essentially any one that produces well-spread, complete metaphases is acceptable. There is little likelihood of this step of the assay influencing the results.

2.4. Analysis of Cells

From a survey of the published literature it is apparent that there are many different schemes for classifying aberrations. While it is also clear that many of these are suitable, it is equally clear that many are not, either because they are ambiguous or in some cases inaccurate. Any classification scheme should include all possible aberration types, and these should be recorded separately. Examples of suitable schemes can be found in Refs. 8 and 9. In the context of population monitoring, it is particularly important to note that chromatid-type aberrations induced in lymphocyte precursor cells will appear as derived chromosome-type aberrations in peripheral lymphocytes as a consequence of cell division and the subsequent DNA replication.

The results for any sample should be presented as the aberration frequency per cell for each aberration type, or the frequency of aberrant cells for each aberration type. It is not appropriate to express them as total aberrant cells or total breaks per cell, as this method of presentation can hide important facets of the data. For the statistical analysis of data it is legitimate to combine aberration classes into the general categories of chromatid-type deletions, chromosome-type deletions, chromatid exchanges, and chromosome exchanges. Occasionally cells are seen with multiple aberrations, and an attempt should be made to analyze such cells completely, and not to record them simply as "multiple aberrations," since this latter classification will mean a loss of information. If it proves impossible to analyze the cells it should be recorded in a category of "too many aberrations to analyze" but not included in the total of cells scored.

The selection of cells to be analyzed is particularly important in order to prevent observer bias, which can result in either a higher or lower measure of the unbiased aberration frequency, depending on the nature of the selection.

The generally accepted method of cell selection is to scan slides at low magnification, and to analyze cells that appear to be suitable at higher magnification. Once a cell is observed at high magnification, there are only a small number of specific reasons why it can then be rejected: (1) if the cell cannot be analyzed because of the number or complexity of the aberrations when it should be appropriately recorded, but not included in total cells analyzed; (2) if the cell is not sufficiently well spread when seen at high magnification, and the overlap of chromosomes prohibits an accurate analysis; (3) if nonchromosomal material, such as dirt or stain crystals, not discernible at low magnification, prevents complete analysis; (4) if the cell contains fewer centromeres than the observer's acceptable cutoff point, which for some allows for analysis of cells with 46 ± 2 centromeres and for others only cells with 46 centromeres—either is acceptable provided that the criterion is consistent.

It is particularly important in population monitoring studies for the samples to be analyzed under code, such that the observer is unaware of the identity of the sample. There are also strong arguments in favor of at least two individuals in any one laboratory and two separate laboratories being responsible for the analysis, in order to remove possible individual or laboratory scoring bias that could influence the results. In order to provide further consistency it is advantageous for any cell classified as aberrant by one individual to be confirmed by a second, and also to keep a photographic record of all confirmed aberrant or otherwise suspect cells.

The number of cells to be analyzed from any sample cannot be fixed with any special justification, because it can be argued that this number can depend on the aberration frequency, and thus is retrospective. A general suggestion would be to analyze 200 cells from each sample.

Discussions of the pros and cons of analyzing banded preparations have been frequent, and do not warrant repetition here. The amount of time expended in the preparation and analysis of banded samples does not seem to be warranted by the increase in sensitivity of the analysis for those aberration types where detection would be improved by banding. Furthermore, in order to analyze banded preparations essentially all cells must be well banded, there should be little or no chromosome overlap, and in any cell all chromosomes have to be banded. These requirements introduce additional conditions for cell selection, and could provide an inaccurate measure of aberration frequency. However, the choice of scoring conventially stained or banded preparations should be at the discretion of each laboratory.

There are other features of the analysis and classification of chromosome abnormalities that are peculiar to each laboratory, but since they would not be likely to influence the aberration frequencies observed, it would seem to be unnecessary to discuss all of these.

3. CHROMOSOME ABERRATION ANALYSIS FOLLOWING RADIATION OR CHEMICAL EXPOSURE

3.1. The Sensitivity of the Lymphocyte Assay

In order to appreciate the limitations of the lymphocyte assay for detecting chromosome alterations in potentially exposed individuals or populations and the relevance of using these values to predict exposure, there are several aspects of the assay itself and the nature of aberration induction by different agents that have to be considered.

In terms of utilizing the lymphocyte assay for monitoring exposed or possibly exposed individuals or populations, by far the greatest amount of information has been obtained for situations where the exposure was to radiation. Initially this was because the clastogenic potential of chemical agents had not been considered. In retrospect this was a fortunate choice, because the mode of action of radiation in inducing chromosome aberrations is different from that of almost all chemical agents, and the frequency of observed aberrations is very directly related to radiation exposure. Subsequent studies on populations possibly exposed to chemical agents, either occupationally or environmentally, have confirmed that these differences in aberration induction characteristics for chemical and radiation impose problems in terms of the sensitivity and applicability of the lymphocyte assay for population monitoring in nonradiation exposure situations.

Although there is no complete understanding of the mechanism of induction of aberrations by radiation or chemicals, sufficient information is available to allow some discussion, particularly with relevance to the sensitivity of the lymphocyte assay following exposure to different types of agents.

Radiation and a small number of chemical agents (e.g., bleomycin, streptonigrin, cytosine arabinoside, and 8-methoxy caffeine) induce aberrations in all stages of the cell cycle—chromosome-type aberrations in G_1 and chromatid-type aberrations in S and G_2. The frequencies of aberrations vary in different parts of these cell cycle stages. In contrast, the majority of chemical agents induce aberrations only when the cell is in the S phase at the time of treatment, or when it passes through the S phase between treatment and observation at mitosis. The aberrations induced are of the chromatid type, and appear to be produced either at the time of DNA replication or as the result of a postreplication event. The frequencies of aberrations induced will vary as a function of the cell-cycle stage in which the cells reside at the time of treatment. The reasons for this will be apparent from later discussions.

These observations have led to the classification of radiation and the small number of truly radiomimetic chemicals as producing aberrations by an S-independent mechanism, and all other chemical agents as being S-dependent in action. Recent studies in this laboratory have indicated that this is not a valid classification, and that the spectrum of aberration types produced by different agents represents a difference in probability of inducing aberrations in the various cell-cycle stages as a consequence of the rate of repair of the DNA damage that can be converted into aberrations.[10,11]

These observations have an important bearing on the sensitivity of the lymphocyte assay for detecting chromosomes aberrations following radiation or chemical exposures. The peripheral lymphocyte remains in a noncycling G_1 stage of the cell cycle (normally referred to as G_0) until it is stimulated *in vitro* to reenter a cycling phase by a mitogenic agent such as phytohemagglutinin. If such cells are exposed to radiation, then chromosome-type aberrations will be induced directly in these G_0 cells. The frequency of aberrations observed at the first mitotic division in culture will thus be the induced frequency, and will be proportional to the exposure. For this reason it is possible to analyze aberrations, usually dicentrics, because of the reliability with which these can be scored, in the peripheral lymphocytes of individuals or populations who have been exposed to radiation, and determine the exposure with a reasonable degree of accuracy. This has been done in many cases, and in those where a physical estimate of exposure can be ascertained there is a good agreement between this measure and that obtained from a biological estimate.[12–14] It should be added that this can only be done reliably in cases where blood samples are taken fairly soon after exposure—within about 6 weeks.[13]

When samples have to be taken at much longer times after exposure, as was the case with the atomic bomb survivors in Hiroshima and Nagasaki, several factors have to be considered when attempting to determine the exposure. Similar considerations have to be taken into account when the effects of chronic radiation exposures are studied. When the time interval between exposure and sampling is long, the effects of turnover of the lymphocyte population become important. Aberrant and nonaberrant cells will be lost from the peripheral lymphocyte population, probably with equal probability, since no selective disadvantage has been ascribed to aberrant cells that are in G_0. This in itself would not alter the aberration frequency, but the repopulating cells will tend to be those that do not contain dicentrics or acentric fragments, and thus the aberration frequency will be reduced in samples taken some time after exposure. There will tend to be a continuous reduction in frequency with increasing sample time as more and more of the analyzed lymphocytes are those that are newly arisen rather than those that were present at the time of exposure. There will be a small proportion of lymphocytes remaining in the circulating population at 20 years or more after exposure,[15,16] as a proportion of lymphocytes are very long-lived.

The reason that the lymphocyte precursor cells that provide the repopulation of the peripheral blood are largely the nonaberrant ones involves the probability of transmission for different aberration types. The majority of observed chromosome-type aberrations (dicentrics, rings, and acentric fragments) are cell-lethal, either as the result of the loss of the acentric fragment at division or as a result of a mechanical interference with division. Lymphocyte precursor cells containing aberrations will not usually produce viable peripheral lymphocytes. Reciprocal translocations and inversions are generally nonlethal events, and so they can be transmitted with a high probability. Thus their frequency should show less decline with time after exposure, and it would seem sensible to analyze these types. Unfortunately, the frequency with which these can be detected is of the order of 50%, even when banded preparations are analyzed. It should also be remembered that the frequency of reciprocal translocations and inversions will show some decline with time after exposure if the exposure was rather high and the induced aberration yields high, since cells will have a finite probability of containing a cell-lethal aberration in the same cell as a translocation or inversion.

In the case of long-term chronic exposures, aberrations can be induced in G_0 lymphocytes and will accumulate in the long-lived lymphocyte population, and the frequency can be used to indicate an exposure.[17] However, there will be a continuous loss from and repopulation of the peripheral lymphocyte population, and the discussion above of the effect of this on aberration frequency will apply here also. The observed aberration frequency will be proportional to exposure, but not necessarily a direct measure of exposure as in the case of acute exposures with samples taken shortly after exposure.

The fact that aberrations are induced in G_0 lymphocytes by radiation, that is, at the same cell cycle stage as that which is exposed and where the DNA damage is induced, means that the lymphocyte assay can be a sensitive indicator of an exposure, and under the right set of circumstances a reliable indicator of the radiation dose.

The situation following chemical exposures is more complex, and the potential sensitivity of the lymphocyte assay for detecting exposure less well understood. As discussed above, the majority of chemical agents induce measurable frequencies of aberrations only when the cell passes through an S phase between treatment and observation. The peripheral lymphocyte is a G_0 cell, and so the first S phase it will pass through is that *in vitro* following mitogenic stimulation. There is considerable evidence showing a relationship between DNA repair, or perhaps more correctly "misrepair," and chromosome aberration induction.[10,11,18-20] Thus, it can be argued that the frequency of chromatid-type aberrations observed following exposure of G_0 will be related to the amount of the DNA damage, whose repair or replication results in aberration formation, that remains at the time of replication. This in turn will be influenced by several factors. It will, of course, be influenced by the amount of the specific DNA damage that results in aberrations, which will be dependent upon the agent and the exposure. It will be influenced by the amount of repair that can take place in G_0 and G_1 following stimulation with a mitogen. The amount of repair in G_0 will be dependent upon the rate of repair and the time between exposure and sampling—the longer the time, the more the repair. The amount of repair in G_1 will likewise be dependent upon the rate of repair and the length of G_1 *in vitro*.

The time between exposure and sampling is clearly even more important following exposure to chemical agents than following radiation exposure. This can be clearly demonstrated in situations where individuals receiving chemotherapeutic treatments have high aberration frequencies from samples taken during or shortly after the therapy, but essentially no induced aberrations in samples taken some 2 months after the cessation of therapy.[21]

Since the aberrations observed are not induced in the treated cell population at the time of treatment and several factors operate to reduce the aberration frequency by reducing the amount of DNA damage present at replication, the lymphocyte assay is far less sensitive for determining whether an individual or population has been exposed to a chemical agent than it is for radiation exposures. Furthermore, it is very unlikely that the observed aberration frequency will be directly related to exposure as it is for acute radiation exposures, although it might have a proportional relationship. It should also be added that an observed aberration frequency in a possibly radiation-exposed individual that is not significantly different from the background frequency can be used to rule out an exposure of some specific magnitude—the size of which, of course, can depend upon the number of cells analyzed. On the other hand, if the aberration frequency in an individual or population possibly exposed to a chemical agent is not significantly different from the background frequency, it is not possible to estimate a maximum possible exposure. It is in fact preferable not to draw any specific conclusions.

It can also be seen from the same arguments that the lymphocyte assay is not at all reliable for indicating chronic chemical exposures. The reason for this is that during the course of the chronic exposure repair can be taking place in the G_0 lymphocyte, resulting in less damage being present at the *in vitro* S phase, and also there will be a further reduction in aberration frequency as the result of lymphocyte turnover, as discussed above for acute exposure. The consequence is that the induced aberration frequency will be very low, and the likelihood is small of demonstrating a significant difference from the background frequency.

It should be stressed that all these factors should be taken into account before a decision is made to utilize the lymphocyte assay in situations where an occupational or environmental exposure is suspected. It is not sensible to rush into a population monitoring study thinking that a clear-cut answer will be obtained—the complexity of the assay necessitates caution.

3.2. Background Aberration Frequencies and "Matched" Control Groups

In order to determine whether or not chromosome aberrations have been induced by exposure of an individual or population to a chemical or physical agent, the frequency must be compared to that in an unexposed group. For suspected radiation exposures this is rather simple. The aberrations induced are of the chromosome type, and one of them, the dicentric, is usually used for estimating dose, because of the reliability with which it can be ascertained. The frequency of dicentrics in control populations is very low (about one per 1000 cells), and so the effect of even small radiation doses can be shown. Furthermore, most other environmental factors that could alter the background aberration frequency will be expected to induce chromatid-type aberrations, which would not be a factor when comparing control with radiation-exposed groups. There is also a large volume of data for chromosome-type aberrations in a variety of control groups (see review by Lloyd et al.[22]).

In contrast, the majority of chemicals induce chromatid-type aberrations, and so environmental factors that can influence their frequency in control or exposed groups will be of significance. First of all, there is very little data on the background frequency of chromatid-type aberrations. Second, it is not at all clear what factors can affect the background frequency.

In order to attempt to demonstrate an increase in aberration frequency in a possibly exposed group as a result of the specific exposure, it is usually recommended that the study group be compared to a "matched" control that is similar for age, sex, social background, occupation, geographical location, and often a variety of other miscellaneous factors. However, since it is not known what factors account for variations in background aberration frequency, it is currently very difficult if not impossible to provide a "matched" control. Pertinent data are very definitely a priority.

In cases where exposure is occupational, clearly the best controls are the individuals themselves, where blood samples are taken and chromosome analysis performed prior to the individuals' working in the potentially hazardous environment. To date, this type of control information is almost completely unavailable, because preoccupational analysis has not been performed.

There is also the possibility that specific individuals or population subgroups exist that are more sensitive to aberration induction than others. The upper extremes, such as individuals with xeroderma pigmentosum or ataxia telangiectasia, have been discussed in detail,[23,24] but these individuals are rare and clearly identified. It is possible that there are cases of less dramatic but still clearly increased sensitivity,[25] and these are of special concern. However, the information on the existence of such groups is sparse, largely because they have not really been looked for. This is an area of research that appears to have a priority.

There are many published reports of individuals or populations exposed environmentally or occupationally to radiation where the data are reliable, and the dose estimates derived from the aberration frequencies agree very closely with physical dose estimates, when these were available. In contrast, there is almost a complete lack of reliable studies for chemical exposures. This is due to the lack of appreciation of the sensitivity of the assay, the inadequacy or lack of appropriate control data, and the use of inappropriate sampling times or protocols. A very small number of reliable studies have been performed (e.g., Refs. 2, 26, and 27), and from these it can be seen that significant increases in aberration frequencies compared to controls can be observed, probably as a result of the exposure. The lymphocyte assay is applicable if the limitations and basic knowledge are taken into account.

4. THE ANALYSIS OF BONE MARROW SAMPLES

As mentioned in the introduction, it is also possible to analyze chromosome aberrations in bone marrow samples. However, the use of this assay can never be considered as routine, because of the problems associated with obtaining bone marrow samples, and also because of the difficulties in interpreting the results.

Bone marrow cells are a cycling population, in contrast to the peripheral lymphocyte population. Thus, at the time of an acute exposure, cells will be present in all stages of the cycle. For a radiation exposure this means that chromosome-type aberrations will be induced in G_1 cells and chromatid-type aberrations in S and G_2 cells, and these will be observed as such at the first mitosis after exposure, with the particular type being dependent upon the sampling time, and hence the exposed population being analyzed. However, if some time elapses between exposure and sampling (longer than about 24 hr), the analyzed population will be in its second or subsequent division after exposure, due to the fact that bone marrow cells are normally cycling. The aberration frequency measured will thus not represent the induced frequency but rather the transmitted frequency. It will be much less than the induced frequency, because of cell killing as the result of loss of acentric fragments at division or the mechanical inhibition of division by dicentrics. Also, chromatid-type aberrations will be converted into derived chromosome types as the result of division and subsequent replication. The only types likely to be transmitted with a high probability are reciprocal translocations, induced as the chromosome type, and inversions. The efficiency of analyzing these is not particularly high even with banded preparations. Thus the bone marrow assay is not recommended in radiation exposure situations unless very early samples are taken and specific information of effects in bone marrow cells is required. It can also be noted that it is inappropriate to use the bone marrow assay for chronic radiation exposures.

Following chemical exposures similar arguments will apply. Only chromatid-type aberrations would be expected to be induced, irrespective of treated cell cycle stage. Again, early samples analyzed at the first mitosis after exposure are necessary to measure the induced frequency. At later times derived chromosome-type aberrations would be produced from the induced chromatid aberrations, and cell killing would result from division of aberrant cells, resulting in a decreased aberration frequency. Also, the probability of transmission of an induced chromatid-type reciprocal translocation is lower than that for an induced chromosome-type reciprocal translocation.

However, if an early sample can be taken, the bone marrow assay is more sensitive for detecting a chemical exposure than is the lymphocyte assay. This is due to the fact that some proportion of the bone marrow cells will be in the S phase at the time of exposure, and aberrations can be produced in these cells, in contrast to the lymphocyte assay where the exposed peripheral lymphocytes are in G_0. Also, since the G_1 in bone marrow cells is much shorter than the first *in vitro* G_1 in lymphocytes, it is expected that nonrepaired DNA damage induced in these G_1 cells will still be present by the S phase, and aberrations could be formed. Thus a fairly high proportion of bone marrow cells have the potential to contribute to the aberrant cell population, whereas only a small proportion of lymphocyte cells have this same potential, as discussed previously. Studies on persons receiving chemotherapy tend to support this argument.[28,29] However, this should not be taken as a suggestion that routine bone marrow samples be taken. It should only be considered under particular circumstances, and preferably only when early postexposure samples can be taken. It will be apparent that it would be virtually impossible to draw conclusions from bone marrow assays in cases where the chemical exposure was chronic, because of the cycling of the cell population during the exposure.

5. THE PLAUSIBILITY OF ESTIMATING GENETIC OR CARCINOGENIC RISK FROM ABERRATION FREQUENCIES IN LYMPHOCYTES

On the assumption that an increase in aberrations is observed in the lymphocyte assay for an individual or a population, is it possible to interpret this observation in terms of future health effects?

In order for chromosome alterations to present a potential genetic hazard they have to be induced in germ cells and be transmissible. An increase in chromosome aberrations in lymphocytes can indicate that there is a possibility of their being induced in germ cells, on the assumption that the agent is able to reach the germ cells. The frequency of aberrations induced in germ cells compared to that in lymphocytes will, of course, be a function of the relative doses in the different cell types. For radiation exposures, where dosimetry is considerably more straightforward, the relationship has been established between the frequency of aberrations induced in lymphocytes and the frequencies of heritable aberrations, specifically translocations, recovered in the F_1 of the mouse, both for males and females. It is clear that only a small fraction of the induced translocations are recovered in the male following treatment of spermatogonial stem cells, and an even lower proportion for treated maturing or mature oocytes.[30-32] A small amount of data for humans relating aberration frequencies in lymphocytes to translocation frequencies in spermatocytes following exposure of spermatogonial stem cells indicate that similar relationships would occur in humans.[33] These studies were all for acute, relatively high-dose exposures. For low dose chronic exposures—the more likely human exposure—the relationship between aberration frequencies in lymphocytes and translocation recovery in the F_1 would be similar, but the induced aberration frequencies would be much lower.[34] This means that at low aberration frequencies in lymphocytes the probability of inducing a translocation that could be transmitted to the F_1 would be very low. Thus the presence of induced aberrations in the lymphocytes of an exposed individual does indicate the possibility of inducing heritable translocations, but the probability of recovery in the F_1 is likely to be very low.

Following chemical exposure the probability of transmission of translocations induced in spermatogonial stem cells is even lower. Without presenting the arguments, it can simply be stated that this is due to the fact that chromatid-type aberrations are induced, and to the fact that the aberrations tend to be formed during the S phase.[35] This latter point also is applicable to treated oocytes, since these will not pass through an S phase until after fertilization and the length of the time for DNA repair is thus generally rather long. If aberrations are observed in the lymphocytes of chemically exposed individuals or populations, then this can be considered as an indication of exposure, but it is not possible at this point to calculate the genetic risk with any degree of certainty. However, it is reasonable to say that the probability of a risk from low induced aberration frequencies is very low indeed.

There appear to be relationships between mutagenicity or clastogenicity and carcinogenicity. Also, there are some cases where a specific chromosomal change is associated with a specific tumor.[36] This does not in any way imply that chromosomal alterations are a cause of cancer. It is possible that they could be, but no direct evidence is available. Thus an increase in aberrations in lymphocytes following chemical exposure in an individual does not allow for a prediction that that individual has an increased risk of cancer. Such a prediction cannot even be made for radiation exposure. However, at the population level, an increased aberration frequency in lymphocytes might indicate the potential for an increased cancer risk in the population. However, again it will not predict this.

6. CONCLUDING REMARKS

This chapter does not attempt to cover a discussion or listing of all studies where the lymphocyte assay has been used to detect or estimate exposure to physical or chemical agents. It is rather an attempt to define the limitations and the advantages of the assay. It also serves to point out that the apparent ease with which possibly exposed individuals can be monitored makes such an assay open to abuse or misinterpretation. It would be intolerable to have situations where an inadequate assay was conducted, either because of the protocol or the control population, a slight increase in aberrations observed, and the conclusion drawn that the group assayed had an increased cancer risk. I hope that the increased interest in cytogenetic population monitoring will not lead to this.

ACKNOWLEDGMENT. Research sponsored by the Office of Health and Environmental Research, U.S. Department of Energy, under contract W-7405-eng-26 with the Union Carbide Corporation.

REFERENCES

1. P. S. Moorhead, P. C. Nowell, W. J. Mellman, D. M. Battips, and D. A. Hungerford, Chromosome preparations of leukocytes cultured from human peripheral blood, *Exp. Cell Res.* 20, 613–616 (1960).
2. R. J. Preston, W. Au, M. A. Bender, J. G. Brewen, A. V. Carrano, J. A. Heddle, A. F. McFee, S. Wolff, and J. S. Wassom, Mammalian *in vivo* and *in vitro* cytogenetic assays: A report of the U. S. EPA's Gene-Tox Program, *Mutat. Res. 87*, 143–188 (1981).
3. H. J. Evans and M. L. O'Riordan, Human peripheral blood lymphocytes for the analysis of chromosome aberrations in mutagen tests, *Mutat. Res. 31*, 135–148 (1975).
4. Report of Panel I, in: *Guidelines for Studies of Human Populations Exposed to Mutagenic and Reproductive Hazards* (A. D. Bloom, ed.), pp. 1–35, March of Dimes Birth Defects Foundation, New York (1981).
5. S. A. Latt, Microfluorometric detection of deoxyribonucleic acid replication in human metaphase chromosomes, *Proc. Natl. Acad. Sci. USA 70*, 3395–3399 (1973).
6. P. Perry and S. Wolff, Giemsa method for the differential staining of sister chromatids, *Nature 25*, 156–158 (1974).
7. K. Goto, T. Akematsu, H. Shimazu, and T. Sugiyama, Simple differential Giemsa staining of sister chromatids after treatment with photosensitive dyes and exposure to light and the mechanism of staining, *Chromosome 53*, 223–230 (1975).
8. H. J. Evans, Chromosome aberrations induced by ionizing radiations, *Int. Rev. Cytol. 13*, 221–321 (1962).
9. J. R. K. Savage, Classification and relationship of induced chromosomal structural changes, *J. Med. Genet. 12*, 103–122 (1975).
10. R. J. Preston, The effect of cytosine arabinoside on the frequency of X-ray-induced chromosome aberrations in normal human lymphocytes, *Mutat. Res. 69*, 71–79 (1980).

11. R. J. Preston and P. C. Gooch, The induction of chromosome-type aberrations in G_1 by methly methanesulfonate and 4-nitroquinoline-N-oxide and the non-requirement of an S-phase for their production, *Mutat. Res. 83*, 395–402 (1981).

12. M. A. Bender and P. C. Gooch, Somatic chromosome aberrations induced by human whole-body irradiation: The "Recuplex" criticality accident, *Radiat. Res. 29*, 568–582 (1966).

13. J. G. Brewen, R. J. Preston, and L. G. Littlefield, Radiation-induced human chromosome aberration yields following an accidental whole-body exposure to ^{60}Co γ-rays, *Radiat. Res. 49*, 647–656 (1972).

14. D. C. Lloyd, R. J. Purrott, J. S. Prosser, G. W. Dolphin, P. A. Tipper, E. J. Reeder, C. M. White, S. J. Cooper, and B. D. Stephenson, The study of chromosome aberration yield in human lymphocytes as an indicator of radiation dose, VI. A review of cases investigated, 1975, NRPB-R41, National Radiological Protection Board, Haswell (1976).

15. K. E. Buckton, G. E. Hamilton, L. Paton, and A. O. Langlands, Chromosome aberrations in ankylosing spondilitis patients, in: *Mutagen-Induced Chromosome Damage in Man* (H. J. Evans and D. C. Lloyd, eds.), pp. 142–150, Yale University Press, New Haven (1978).

16. A. A. Awa, T. Sofumi, T. Honda, M. Iton, S. Neriishi, and M. Otake, Relationship between the radiation dose and chromosome aberrations in atomic bomb survivors of Hiroshima and Nagasaki, *J. Radiat. Res. (Tokyo) 19*, 126–140 (1978).

17. H. J. Evans, K. E. Buckton, G. E. Hamilton, and A. Carothers, Radiation-induced chromosome aberrations in nuclear dockyard workers, *Nature 277*, 531–534 (1979).

18. H. J. Evans, Molecular mechanisms in the induction of chromosome aberrations, in: *Progress in Genetic Toxicology* (D. Scott, B. A. Bridges, and F. M. Sobels, eds.), pp. 57–74, Elsevier/North-Holland, Amsterdam (1977).

19. H. G. Griggs and M. A. Bender, Photoreactivation of ultraviolet-induced chromosomal aberrations, *Science 179*, 86–88 (1973).

20. R. J. Preston, DNA repair and chromosome aberrations: Interactive effects of radiation and chemicals, in: *Progress in Mutation Research*, Vol. 4 (A. T. Natarajan, G. Obe, and H. Altmann, eds.), pp. 25–35, Elsevier/North-Holland, Amsterdam (1982).

21. A. Schinzel and W. Schmid, Lymphocyte chromosome studies in humans exposed to chemical mutagens. Validity of the method in 67 patients under cytostatic therapy, *Mutat. Res. 40*, 139–166 (1976).

22. D. C. Lloyd, R. J. Purrott, and E. J. Reeder, The incidence of unstable chromosome aberrations in peripheral blood lymphocytes from unirradiated and occupationally exposed people, *Mutat. Res. 72*, 523–532 (1980).

23. R. H. C. San, W. Stich, and H. F. Stich, Differential sensitivity of xeroderma pigmentosum cells of different repair capacities towards the chromosome breaking action of carcinogens and mutagens, *Int. J. Cancer 20*, 181–187 (1977).

24. A. M. R. Taylor, J. A. Metcalfe, J. M. Oxford, and D. G. Harnden, Is chromatid-type damage in ataxia telangiectasia after irradiation at G_0 a consequence of defective repair?, *Nature 260*, 441–443 (1976).

25. M. C. Paterson, A. K. Anderson, B. P. Smith, and P. J. Smith, Enhanced radiosensitivity of cultured fibroblasts from ataxia telangiectasia heterozygotes manifested by colony forming ability and reduced DNA repair replication after hypoxic γ-irradiation, *Cancer Res, 39*, 3725–3734 (1979).

26. M. Kucerova, V. S. Zhurkov, Z. Polivkova, and J. E. Ivanova, Mutagenic effect of epichlorhydrin. II. Analysis of chromosomal aberrations in lymphocytes of persons occupationally exposed to epichlorhydrin, *Mutat. Res. 48*, 355–360 (1977).

27. I. F. H. Purchase, C. R. Richardson, D. Anderson, G. M. Paddle, and W. G. F. Adams, Chromosomal analyses in vinyl chloride-exposed workers, *Mutat. Res. 57*, 325–334 (1978).

28. P. Goetz, R. J. Sram, and J. Dohnalova, Relationship between experimental results in mammals and man. I. Cytogenetic analysis of bone marrow injury induced by a single dose of cyclophosphamide, *Mutat. Res. 31,* 247–254 (1975).

29. M. Krogh Jensen and A. Nyfors, Cytogenetic effect of methotrexate on human cells *in vivo.* Comparison between results obtained by chromosome studies on bone-marrow cells and blood lymphocytes and by the micronucleus test, *Mutat. Res. 64,* 339–343 (1979).

30. J. G. Brewen and R. J. Preston, The use of chromosome aberrations for predicting genetic hazards in man, in: *Radiation Research—Biomedical, Chemical and Physical Perspective* (O. F. Nygaard, H. I. Adler, and W. K. Sinclair, eds.), pp. 926–936, Academic Press, New York (1975).

31. J. G. Brewen, H. S. Payne, and R. J. Preston, X-ray-induced chromosome aberrations in mouse dictyate oocytes. I. Time and dose relationships, *Mutat. Res. 35,* 111–120 (1976).

32. A. G. Searle and C. V. Beechey, Cytogenetic effects of X-rays and fission neutrons in female mice, *Mutat. Res. 24,* 171–186 (1974).

33. J. G. Brewen, R. J. Preston, and N. Genzozian, Analysis of X-ray-induced chromosomal translocations in human and mormoset spermatogonial stem cells, *Nature 253,* 468–470 (1975).

34. J. G. Brewen, R. J. Preston, and H. E. Luippold, Radiation-induced translocations in spermatogonia. III. Effect of long-term chronic exposures to γ-rays, *Mutat. Res. 61,* 405–409 (1979).

35. J. G. Brewen and R. J. Preston, Chromosome aberrations as a measure of mutagenesis: Comparisons *in vitro* and *in vivo* and in somatic and germ cells, *Environ. Health Perspect. 6,* 157–166 (1963).

36. J. D. Rowley, Chromosome abnormalities in human leukemia, *Annu. Rev. Genet. 14,* 17–39 (1980).

7

Sister Chromatid Exchange Analysis in Lymphocytes

James W. Allen, Karen Brock, James Campbell, and Yousuf Sharief

1. INTRODUCTION

Sister chromatid exchanges (SCEs) are generally considered to arise from breakage and recombination of sister chromatid segments at homologous loci.[1] Although the fundamental nature of SCE is not well understood, interests in its frequency have been central both to historical and current studies. Early autoradiographic techniques used to detect this phenomenon were applied for a variety of investigations into its spontaneous and irradiation-related incidences in somatic and germ cells.[2,3] Nearly a decade ago technically simpler bromodeoxyuridine (BrdUrd)-differential staining methodology was developed in a cultured human lymphocyte system and shown to provide much superior resolving power.[4] Chemical mutagens were clearly demonstrated to induce SCEs at significantly lower doses than those required to cause chromosome aberrations.[5,6] This observation coincided with timely autoradiographic determinations of mutagen action in SCE formation[7,8] and set a new course of emphasis—SCE induction stemming from exposure to environmental agents. The BrdUrd methodology has since been extended to a wide variety of *in vitro* and *in vivo* cellular systems, and hundreds of SCE induction trials have implicated numerous chemical, physical (i.e., UV irradiation), and biological (i.e., virus) agents in the production of this effect.[9,10] A recent summary eval-

James W. Allen • Genetic Toxicology Division, Health Effects Research Laboratory, U.S. Environmental Protection Agency, Research Triangle Park, North Carolina 27711. Karen Brock, James Campbell, and Yousuf Sharief • Northrop Services, Inc., Research Triangle Park, North Carolina 27709.

uation of accumulated results has concluded that most chemical carcinogens induce SCEs, the test being particularly sensitive to agents that cause DNA adducts.[1]

The molecular mechanism of SCE formation is uncertain. Although SCEs bear some cytological likeness to meiotic crossover products and to certain forms of chromosome aberration and are biochemically close to various steps or consequences of DNA repair, there is no strong evidence in support of close, direct relationships to these processes.[9-12] On the contrary, SCE is generally viewed as a unique DNA event, which, when induced, arises from some small fraction of the actual number of lesions.[10,13] Its mechanics of formation apparently occur during DNA synthesis regardless of when the lesion was induced.[7] Evidence and theories favoring critical involvement of the replication fork are mounting. (For review, see Stetka [12]) Painter[14] has proposed an attractive model, which depicts SCEs as arising from unrepaired damage at junctions between replicon clusters. These sites are suggested to be especially susceptible to double-strand breakage, with subsequent recombination between parent and daughter strands leading to SCE. An alternative model,[15] with supporting evidence, depicts SCEs as arising from breakage following progression of the replication fork: Errors on the part of enzymes involved in replicated DNA unraveling processes then lead to sister chromatid recombinations.

The biological significance of SCE to the cell is also uncertain. SCEs are almost always detectable in control samples (although these may arise from the techniques used in the study), and increases in their frequency due to mutagen exposure are not known to directly affect cell viability or function. A linear relationship between induced SCEs and gene mutations (HPRT locus) in mammalian cells has been shown.[16-18] However, the relative efficiencies of these genetic end points (and of chromosome aberrations as well) are chemical-specific and may vary widely with different modes of chemical–DNA interaction.[16-19] Nevertheless, SCE remains an extraordinarily sensitive measure of DNA alteration by most mutagenic chemicals and is recognized as usually paralleling clastogenic and gene mutation events. Consequently, SCE both in its own right and in signalling the potential for more classical forms of genetic damage to which it is often a corollary, has become a major indicator of the genotoxic potential of chemicals.

Within experimental and human monitoring contexts, lymphocytes provide a convenient and relevant tissue for SCE analyses. They are easy to obtain and grow in culture, and in the laboratory have proven metabolically competent to activate certain mutagens to induce SCEs.[20,22] Expectations are high that SCE analyses of lymphocytes removed from individuals in various occupational settings may serve as monitors of preventable hazardous chemical exposures in much the same way that chromosome aberration analyses have been useful for determining irradiation exposures.[9,23-25] (SCE is only weakly responsive to ionizing radiations.[6] The enormous complexity of monitoring chemical exposures has not been underestimated: Problems such as diverse confounding exposures, chemical interactions, specific modes of action, and inherent weaknesses in lymphocyte cytogenetic tests (mentioned below) have been addressed. Nonetheless, SCE analyses, along with chromosome aberration tests, may well represent the most feasible and sensitive approaches to this end.

The basic differential staining procedure for assessing SCE in lymphocytes has changed little since its original development.[4] However, the scope of application has been broadened, and particular strengths and weaknesses are now more clearly appreciated. Details concerning the nature of SCE and the general utility of its analysis have been extensively reviewed elsewhere.[1,9,10] The intent of this chapter is to focus on methodological considerations that appear to be important to the general understanding and effective application of SCE studies, specifically in lymphocytes. A short discussion of some selected results is also provided.

2. METHODOLOGY

2.1. Background

2.1.1. Differential Staining for SCE Analysis

SCEs do not appear to involve inequalities in amounts of exchanged material, and there is no gross morphological evidence of their occurrence. Thus, some means of differentiating the sister chromatids is typically required for detecting these exchanges. Using [³H]thymidine as a DNA label, and following its semiconservative pattern of distribution through successive replication periods, Taylor et al.,[27] first delineated SCEs in second division metaphase cells. The exchanges appeared as sites of coincident alternation in grain patterns between the sister chromatids. Higher resolution differential staining methodology, which has now largely supplanted autoradiography for SCE analysis, relies upon the substitution of BrdUrd for thymidine in the DNA. Labeling over both, or alternatively only the first, of two consecutive DNA synthesis periods results in an equal distribution of BrdUrd to the sister chromatids of first subsequent metaphase stages and in an unequal distribution at second metaphase stages (Figure 1). This asymmetric presence of analogue in second metaphase sister chromatids causes their differential appearance when chromosomes are stained with a BrdUrd-sensitive dye. For example, BrdUrd quenches the fluorescence of 33258 Hoechst dye such that the more heavily substituted chromatid appears dull in contrast to the brighter chromatid with

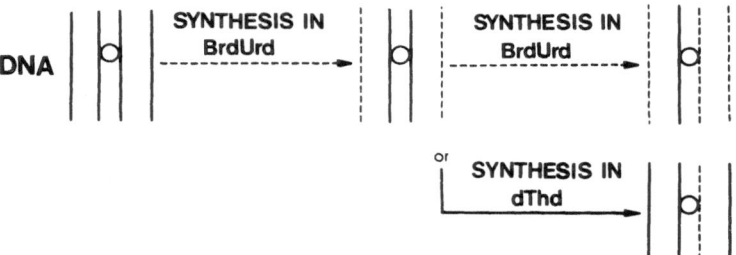

Figure 1. Diagrammatic representation of asymmetric BrdUrd substitution in sister chromatids as achieved by alternative labeling procedures over two consecutive DNA synthesis periods. BrdUrd incorporation (- - -) during the first replication period gives rise to first division chromosomes, which are unifilarly substituted in both chromatids. An additional replication with BrdUrd leads to unifilarly versus bifilarly substituted second division sister chromatids. In the absence of BrdUrd label during the latter replication, endogenous deoxythymidine is utilized (——),[1] and only one of the resulting sister chromatids will contain the analog (unifilarly substituted.)

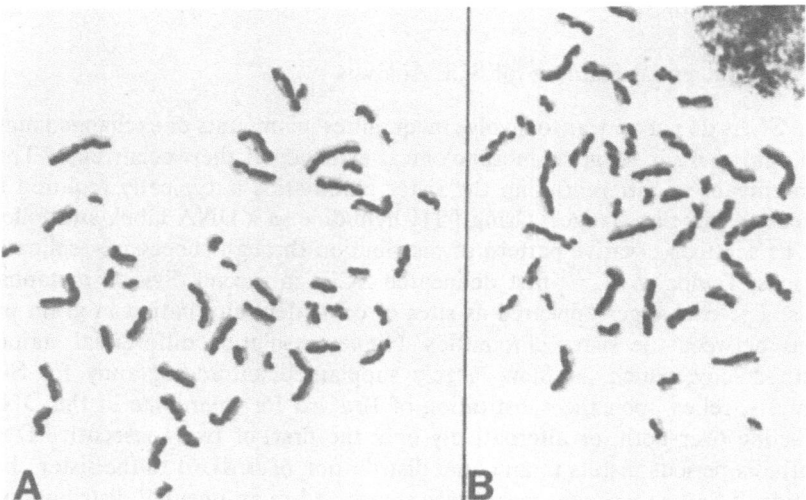

Figure 2. Human lymphocyte chromosomes substituted with BrdUrd and showing differential Giemsa staining. (A) Control example showing eight SCEs (evident as reciprocal discontinuities in staining). (B) A culture exposed to 0.1 mg/ml of vinyl carbamate; shows a moderate elevation in the incidence of SCE. Approximately 40 SCEs are evident.

relatively less analogue substitution.[4] SCEs are then clearly detectable as reciprocal staining discontinuities. However, since most fluorescence methods suffer from rapid fading, SCE analysis is more often performed on cells that are additionally processed through photolysis and Giemsa overlay steps[28,29] to become permanent differential staining preparations (Figure 2). Mean SCE frequencies for treatment groups of cells are statistically compared with those of control cell samples. Details concerning preparative and analytical methods for SCE analysis are comprehensively provided in a number of reviews,[1,9,10,23] and examples are given below. Although cell tolerance of BrdUrd uptake and escape from toxic effects may be somewhat variable among somatic, germ, and certain embryo tissues, this is not generally a problem in lymphocyte protocols. Rather, the basic concern in the latter tissue is simply the occurrence of sufficient cell division for the sequential steps of DNA labeling, cell cycling, and chromosome staining to be carried out.

2.1.2. Lymphocytes: *in Vivo* and *in Vitro*

Comprehensive reviews of lymphocytes and their activation characteristics are provided by Ling and Kay[30] and Greaves *et al.*[31] Aside from peripheral blood, lymphocytes are enmassed in a number of organs: spleen, thymus, bone marrow, lymph nodes, gastrointestinal tissue, tonsils, and appendix. In rodent experimental systems, several of these tissues have been analyzed for SCE[32]; the very high mitotic index of hematopoietic cell types in bone marrow has made it an especially routine tissue choice. The accessibility of peripheral blood primarily accounts for its selection as the usual source of lymphocytes for human cell experimentation and monitoring (and is similarly advantageous for experimental animal studies). In human blood, multigram quantities of lymphocytes are circulating throughout the body[30] and to various organs where specific genotoxic metabolites may be generated. These are, for the most part, marrow-derived, differentiated cell types in the nondividing G_0 cell-cycle stage except when involved in immune reactions. Their life span in blood is variable—up to many years. If plant lectins or other agglutinating mitogens of cultured lymphocytes are delivered *in vivo,* there is not a reliable increase in the yield of recoverable dividing cells. On the contrary, leukopenia may result from splenic corralling of the affected cells.[30]

SCE analyses in lymphocytes rely upon *in vitro* cell cycling and BrdUrd incorporation. Several such studies have utilized lymphoblastoid cells,[33–36] usually of permanent cell lines derived from patients with lymphoproliferative disorders. Systems employing exogenous metabolic activation have included the use of rat liver S-9 mix[35] and the implantation of diffusion chambers of lymphoblastoid cells into mice.[33] Lymphocytes from normal individuals remain mitotically quiescent in culture unless a stimulatory agent is added. Phytohemagglutinin (PHA), an extract of the red kidney bean *Phaseolus vulgaris,* is most often used for this purpose. The initiating mechanism is believed to involve mitogen binding to cell surface receptors—a process bearing some resemblance to antigen-induced immune reactions.[30] That metabolic changes are known to accompany this process[30] is further evidenced by transformation—related enhancement of chemical activation to induce SCEs.[38] Primary lymphocyte cultures are short-term, cell division ceasing within 1–2 weeks.[30,37]

In mice, the PHA response appears to be under multifactorial genetic control. The C57 and DBA strains are among the highest and lowest responders, respectively.[39] In certain human disease conditions, impaired levels or deviant patterns of lymphocyte responsiveness to PHA are encountered.[40,41] Normally, however, the number of cells responding depends upon the concentration of PHA.[30,37] The earliest replicators begin their DNA synthesis approximately 24 hr after stimulation; others respond asynchronously up to 4 days or longer after PHA treatment.[30] Thus, while metaphase cells harvested at approximately 42 hr represent mainly first division cells,[37,42] those at considerably later times may represent mixtures of cells in their first, second, third, etc., division. A high proportion of second division cells may be analyzed at 72 hr.[1,37,43] Cell-cycle times of 12–16 hr have been estimated or measured.[37,45] T-Lymphocytes are considered the primary responders to PHA[30,31] although smaller fractions of B-lymphocytes also proliferate.[44,45] Reportedly, the latter cells respond to PHA more slowly,[45] cycle faster,[43] and appear with increasing proportional representation over time.[45] At least one study has determined B cells to have a lower baseline SCE frequency than T cells.[43] However, conflicting information exists concerning differences in SCE frequency for fast- and slow-growing or PHA-responding cells.[43,45–50] The actual extent to which variations in lymphocyte cell type and/or proliferation characteristics may be affecting SCE frequencies is not well understood.

2.2. General Design Considerations

2.2.1. Variable Baseline SCE Levels

Even when technical steps such as culturing conditions and time of cell harvest are held tightly constant, lymphocytes from different individuals, as well as from the same individual over time, may exhibit considerable variability in baseline and inducible SCE levels.[47] Some potential sources of variation are conjectural and may involve subtle differences in metabolism, DNA repair, or lymphocyte history of exposure. Others may pertain to individual characteristics that are routinely describable but as yet insufficiently studied to permit firm conclusions as to their importance. For example, evidence indicates that age and sex are not significant influences upon SCE frequencies in normal human lymphocytes.[25,49] However, experimental studies have shown that cells from older human and animal subjects tend to exhibit a relatively lower SCE response to chemical clastogens than their younger counterparts.[51,52] It has also been reported that male and female benzene-exposed mice experience markedly different levels of SCE induction in bone marrow cells.[53] Several studies are in agreement that smoking can elevate lymphocyte SCE levels.[21,25,54,67] In view of the early stages of SCE monitoring in humans, it seems generally advisable to record all potentially relevant information that is easily obtainable through personal histories, as well as to ascertain basic hematological data from routine blood differential analyses. Time-dependent increases in SCE (from storage)[45] or decreases due to repair or dilution of DNA effects leading to SCE (see Section 3 below) may occur. Thus, the time interval between exposure to a potential SCE-inducing substance and harvest of cells is critical to experimental design and interpretation.

Typical of SCE assays in general is the relatively wide range of individual cell deviations from the mean SCE frequency of a sample. (See Table I.) Whether this is due to cell differences in BrdUrd uptake or past mutagen exposures is uncertain. In any case, experimentally, it is not readily controllable. Wide SCE ranges in control and exposure cell populations are manageable through adjustment of the cohort and/or cell sample size for analysis. Generally, scoring increasing numbers of individuals and cells (i.e., upward from 25/culture) enables detectability of smaller SCE increments. An account of

Table I

In Vitro SCE Frequencies in Human Lymphocytes Treated with Ethyl Carbamate or Vinyl Carbamate

Test chemical	Dose, mg/ml	Number of cells	SCE/cell ranges	SCE frequencies[a]
Control	—[b]	54	3–14	7.4 ± 2.7
Ethyl carbamate[c]	1.0	65	2–15	8.3 ± 3.0
	5.0	54	4–14	7.9 ± 2.7
	10.0	34	3–20	8.2 ± 4.2
Vinyl carbamate[d]	0.01	31	3–17	9.1 ± 3.8
	0.1	27	17–67	41.4 ± 12.4
	0.2	28	17–66	39.3 ± 12.5

[a]Mean value ± standard deviation/sample of cells analyzed.
[b]All control and treatment group cells were grown with 25 μM BrdUrd.
[c]Ethyl carbamate was obtained from Sigma Chemical Co., St. Louis, MO.
[d]Vinyl carbamate was generously provided by Dr. James Miller, McArdle Laboratory for Cancer Research, University of Wisconsin.

outlier cells (with very high numbers of SCEs) through assessment of individual distributions of SCEs is also advised.[23]

2.2.2. BrdUrd Dose

It is well established that BrdUrd induces exchanges.[1,9] However, it is not entirely clear to what extent this may relate to analogue substitution in DNA or to a primary effect at a non-DNA site, i.e., interference with deoxycytidine metabolism.[55] Regardless, the amount of BrdUrd available to the cells can influence baseline SCE levels. Thus, it has been widely recommended that individual laboratories engaged in lymphocyte SCE monitoring standardize the BrdUrd concentration to cell number ratio per culture.[1,23,47] An appropriate ratio may be determined from the establishment of a BrdUrd dose–SCE response curve for constant cell number and culturing conditions. Special attention should be given to maintaining consistency of serum type (and preferably batch) and to eliminating all exposure to light of certain wavelengths, since these are variables that have been clearly shown to influence SCE formation.[1,23] An optimal BrdUrd dose is generally considered to be one that (1) provides high-quality differential staining of sister chromatids, (2) does not markedly inhibit cell replication or cycling rates, and (3) results in an appropriate baseline SCE frequency. The latter may be interpreted in different ways. One line of reasoning holds that an SCE frequency falling in the plateau region of the curve (at higher BrdUrd concentrations) is most suitable, in that the impact of SCE fluctuations stemming from other procedure-related influences will be minimized.[47] Others may contend that the lowest SCE frequency consistent with reliable, high-quality staining results is best, because it provides for maximum assay sensitivity in detecting small SCE increases. Further insight into the potential importance of these and other technical factors is provided in a thorough study by Carrano *et al.*[47]

2.2.3. Combined End Points

SCEs in human lymphocytes are often measured within parallel *in vivo–in vitro* approaches, or in conjunction with other genetic or toxic end points. *In vitro* testing has helped to confirm that negative cytogenetic findings after *in vivo* exposures were due to chemical unreactivity rather than pharmacokinetic factors or repair characteristics of the organism.[56,57] Similarly, chemical exposure trials in culture may help clarify metabolic requirements and activities when positive *in vivo* results are obtained. Correlated incidences of mitomycin C-induced SCEs and gene mutations (HPRT) were recently demonstrated in parallel lymphocyte cultures evaluated for SCE and 8-azaguanine resistance.[18] Cell proliferation and chromosome aberrations may be assessed from the same cultures—and even the same slides—providing SCE information. Since chromosome stain patterns reflect the number of divisions undergone subsequent to BrdUrd exposure, ratios of first, second, and third (or higher) division cells occurring may be determined along with SCE frequencies. Cytotoxicity in the form of increasing proportions of first division cells (corresponding to decreasing incidences of later-division cells) has been noted to accompany SCE induction.[48,53,68] The capability to unequivocally identify and analyze only first division metaphase cells for chromosome aberrations greatly enhances the sensitivity of that assay, since damage that is in cells with inhibited cycling or that is subject to dilution or altered expression by cycling will not be missed.[26] A number of laboratories are presently conducting large-scale studies to determine any disadvantages or potential inaccuracies attached to the analysis of chromosome aberrations in cells substituted with BrdUrd.

2.3. Technical

2.3.1. Human Blood Cultures and Chromosome Preparations

Lymphocyte procedures for SCE analysis follow several common basic steps (Figure 3), although with considerable flexibility in technical detail. This section is summarized from the authors' experience and from several current published works[1,9,23,26,47] that specifically address this topic. In human monitoring studies, blood is obtained by venipuncture, mixed with an anticoagulant such as heparin or acid–citrate–dextrose solution, and set up as sterile replicate cultures of either whole blood or leukocytes obtained after sedimentation or purification on a density gradient such as Ficoll–Hypaque. In our experience, it has proven advantageous to culture blood that was fresh (hours old) as opposed to stored, the latter having exhibited reduced leukocyte recovery. Culture media commonly used include RPMI 1640, Eagle's MEM, or HAM's F 10, with 15–20% fetal bovine serum and antibiotics. Reagent-grade PHA is generally recommended over the purified form, in that it has a wider dose range of effectiveness, has less cytotoxicity, and is more economical.[30] Poor PHA

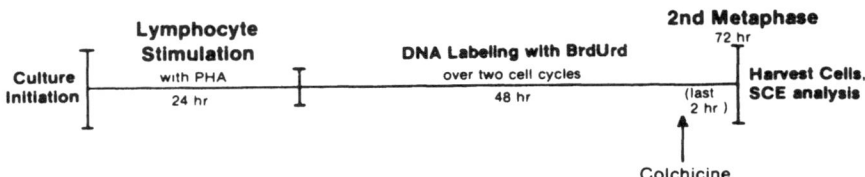

Figure 3. Basic steps involved in culturing human lymphocytes for SCE analysis.

responsiveness often characterizing the lymphocytes of cancer patients has been noted to improve very significantly if cells are washed successively in media prior to culturing with PHA.[58]

Typically, 5- or 10-ml cultures are set up in $\geq$15-ml tubes or flasks (glass or plastic). Cultures should be standardized for the number of cells and for the BrdUrd concentration. White cells, usually counted with a Coulter counter, cytograf, or hemacytometer, are commonly grown in concentrations of 5–8 $\times$ 10^6 cells/culture. BrdUrd, generally used within the range of 10–100 μM concentrations (25 μM is often selected), may be added at the time of culture initiation or after 24 hr, when the first DNA synthesis stage is beginning. Suspension cultures are positioned upright or on a slant in a 37°C, 5% CO_2 incubator. The closely settled cells should be disturbed as little as possible: Continuous agitation inhibits PHA activation.[30] Because light wavelengths $\leq$313 nm can degrade BrdUrd-substituted DNA and induce SCEs,[10] cell cultures should be completely protected from these effects, e.g., by using light-tight incubators and yellow extraneous lighting conditions. Although lymphocyte cycling rates may vary on an individual basis, 72-hr cultures have been found to routinely provide high proportions of second division metaphase cells. A spindle inhibitor such as colchicine or colcemid is added at 68–70 hr in order to halt and collect metaphase stage cells. Standard cytogenetic harvest procedures based upon hypotonic and successive fixative treatments are employed. The most commonly used slide-staining and analysis procedures are those utilizing 33258 Hoechst fluorescence or fluorescence plus Giemsa techniques.[1] A detailed procedure for growing human lymphocytes and for differentially staining chromosomes that has yielded superior results in our laboratory is provided in Appendix A.

Lymphocytes are grown in a similar manner for the purpose of *in vitro* SCE induction tests. A variety of dosing and metabolic activation procedures are effective, the optimal choice depending upon the totality of experimental design and intent considerations. The Gene-Tox Program Report on SCEs[1] has made a number of recommendations concerning *in vitro* chemical testing in human lymphocytes, many of which are enumerated below. It is desirable to obtain information on effects at G_0 and S stages. Exposure might be conducted prior to, at the time of, or at various times (i.e., 24 or 48 hr) after PHA stimulation. The inclusion of S-9 mixture prepared from rat livers[59] has proven effective as a means of adding metabolic activation capabilities; under these conditions, toxicity and optimal serum concentration, exposure times, and exposure durations have been addressed.[1,59] In the absence of exogenous activation, continuous exposure over the last 24 hr of culturing conveniently accomplishes insult during the entirety of the last cell cycle. It is further recommended that at least three doses covering two logs be administered. The highest dose should be at the limits of solubility or produce toxic effects in the form of reduced mitotic indices, chromosome aberrations, or delayed cycling to result in shifts to relatively higher proportions of first metaphase division cells.

Commonly used solvents or carriers have not generally been implicated in SCE induction, although negative control cultures with and without the solvent should always be performed.[1] Effective positive control chemicals include cyclophosphamide with S-9 for chemicals requiring metabolic activation, and ethylmethanesulfonate or mitomycin C as direct-acting agents. Slides should be coded and scored blind (methods of scoring are illustrated in Bloom *et al.* [23]) and SCE frequencies reported on a normalized diploid complement basis. The number of cells analyzed and their statistical treatment depend upon sensitivity requirements and experimental design. A common practice has been the application of T tests for evaluating mean SCE frequency results based upon samples of 25 or more cells/replicate culture (total $= 50+$ cells/group); in some cases the test data are subjected to log or square root transformation to achieve stabilization of variances. Some guidance concerning appropriate interpretations and conclusions in various instances of equivocal results is provided in the Gene-Tox Report on SCEs.[1]

2.3.2. Experimental Animal Blood Cultures

Basically similar protocols have been followed for SCE analysis in peripheral blood lymphocytes from a variety of experimental animals. Specifically, rabbit,[60] cattle, pig, and sheep,[61] mouse[62] and rat[62,63] systems are among those reported. Rabbit and rat systems have been used for *in vivo* and *in vitro* SCE induction analyses. Kligerman *et al.*[63] have thoroughly investigated the conditions for optimal growth and analysis of rat lymphocytes. We have found that their basic procedure provides excellent results: A slightly modified version of it that we routinely employ for *in vivo* and *in vitro* SCE induction trials is given in Appendix B.

3. SELECTED APPLICATIONS

The broad utility of lymphocyte SCE systems is evident in their diverse human monitoring and experimental applications and in their extensive representation within surveys of chemical mutagenesis trials. In addition to their use to signal genetic effects from occupational or medical exposures to various agents, SCE analyses have been used to identify and characterize chromosomal instabilities in cancer-prone individuals. (For review, see Galloway and Tice.[26]) There is also current interest in the prospect that studies of changing SCE frequencies in the blood of cancer chemotherapy patients may prove instructive toward the proper selection of therapeutic agents and treatment regimens.[64] Lymphocyte SCE induction has been used to interpret cell metabolic and DNA repair capabilities[21,22,65–68] and to evaluate the effects of interactions of different agents on modified mutagenic responses.[65] The Gene-Tox Report[1] lists more than 45 different chemicals evaluated for their capabilities to induce SCEs—in some cases relative to efficiencies in the production of other forms of genetic damage. A sample of experimental data from the authors' laboratory, which was obtained with the appendixed protocols, is noted below.

The well-known animal carcinogen ethyl carbamate (urethane) causes extensive SCE induction when injected into mice.[69,70] Yet, in cell culture studies it is considered a "problem" chemical[71] because of its generally weak mutagenicity in such systems.[72] As some other substances thought to require metabolic activation to induce SCEs have proven positive for this effect in human lymphocytes without added activation capabilities,[21,22] we, and others,[73] have examined ethyl carbamate as well as vinyl carbamate for SCE induction under these circumstances. Vinyl carbamate is a suspect metabolite of ethyl carbamate and is considerably more carcinogenic.[74] Although it has recently been reported that ethyl carbamate is more active than vinyl carbamate for SCE induction and can cause a tripling of control-level SCE values in cultured lymphocytes,[73] we have been unable to confirm this (Table I). Over a broad dose range, with inhibited cell replication evident at the highest dose, ethyl carbamate was completely negative for SCE induction. On the other hand, vinyl carbamate caused increases in SCE frequencies that were more than five times that of controls. These findings are consistent with our observations of ethyl carbamate-negative activity in cultured mouse marrow cells[69] and Chinese hamster V-79 cells,[72,75] as well as vinyl carbamate-positive activity in V-79 cells[72,75] and also in rat lymphocytes removed for culturing after *in vivo* exposure (unpublished observations). Despite some seemingly unique metabolic capabilities of human lymphocytes,[21,22] we conclude that ethyl carbamate remains negative for SCE induction although vinyl carbamate is clearly efficient for producing this effect. The discrepancy for these chemicals between our findings and those referenced above is not readily explainable, and it exemplifies the inconsistencies alluded to earlier that may sometimes characterize this assay and may result from any of a number of possible technical reasons. Individual differences in lymphocyte metabolic capabilities may have influenced the conflicting results, although repeat studies in our laboratory using different donors have confirmed our original findings.

The rather small number of human monitoring SCE trials thus far conducted confirm the promise of this approach for detecting genotoxic exposures and also point to important limitations in its application. Some agents that have given positive *in vivo* SCE test results in human blood cells include various cancer chemotherapeutics[1,9,10,26,67] and laboratory chemicals—e.g., solvents,[76] nalidixic acid,[77] vinyl chloride,[78] and ethylene oxide.[25,79] However, in some circumstances, the sensitivity of SCEs was less than that of apparently longer lived chromosome aberrations in revealing genetic effects.[56] In general, it has been found that acute *in vivo* exposures to SCE-active agents give rise to transient induction levels detectable for only days or weeks (an exception is noted below). With repeated dosing, initially high SCE increments tend to fall to more stable intermediate levels of increase before returning to normal frequencies some weeks to months later. These patterns initially reported in experiments with rabbits[60] have been observed in human studies involving different chemicals[64,80]; and reports of negative results are consistent with this as well.[81] Thus, a reasonable conclusion is that the reliability of SCE analysis may be largely limited to instances of high chronic exposure or to assessments immediately (within days) following an acute exposure.[56] Possible explanations for the rapid decline in SCE levels include the death of damaged cells, their dilution by new, undamaged cells, and the repair of damage.[60,64,80]

Although peripheral lymphocytes *in vivo* are considered to be relatively inefficient at excising damaged DNA,[30] some repair ability is suggested by recent observations that methylmethanesulfonate and nitrogen mustard produce significantly more SCEs in cultured human lymphocytes when treatment is at late G_1–S than when it is at early G_1.[67] An unusual SCE induction response has been noted in lymphocytes from cancer patients treated with 1-(2-chloroethyl)-3-cyclohexyl-1-nitrosourea.[67] A single dose of this agent results in a significant elevation of SCEs, which is detectable for 2 months. It is suggested that slow-forming cross-links may be occurring to more than offset repair removal of SCE-related monoadducts.[67,68] Lymphocyte SCE analysis has clearly led to some interesting findings in regard to potential chemical–DNA interactions. The sensitivity of this assay to reveal genetic effects, combined with its versatility within experimental systems and relevance for human monitoring, should assure its continued application in matters of genetic health hazard assessment.

APPENDIX A. A PROCEDURE FOR GROWING AND PREPARING HUMAN LYMPHOCYTES FOR SCE ANALYSIS

1. Blood obtained by venipuncture is collected and gently mixed in 10-cm^3 sterile vacutainer tubes containing 143 units of sodium heparin (Becton-Dickinson).

2. A sample of 0.2 ml is removed for determination of the WBC concentration per milliliter (and optional differential cell count analysis). A Coulter

counter with 100-μm aperture tube and Zap-O-Globin (Coulter Electronics) to lyse red blood cells is conveniently used.

3. Added to replicate, sterile 25-cm^2 culture flasks (Corning) are 5×10^{-6} WBC (typically in 0.7–0.9 ml of blood), along with culture medium PHA, and BrdUrd, to give a total of 10 ml. The medium consists of RPMI 1640 with 15% fetal bovine serum and 100 units/ml of penicillin G + 100 μg/ml streptomycin (GIBCO). Reagent-grade PHA (Burroughs-Wellcome, HA-15) at 0.15 ml/culture and 25 μM BrdUrd (Sigma) are used.

4. Flasks are incubated upright for 72 hr under the conditions of 37°C, 5% CO_2, and complete absence of light. Cells are not disturbed except for the addition of 2.5 μg colcemid (Sigma) to each flask at 70 hr or for the introduction of a mutagen at one of several optional times (see text) for *in vitro* testing. These latter steps are carried out under yellow room lighting. (See text.)

5. Cells are transferred into centrifuge tubes and spun at 400g for 5 min, and the cell pellet is resuspended in several milliliters of 0.075 M KCl hypotonic solution for 10 min. Cells are then repeatedly fixed (three times) in three parts methanol–one part acetic acid (freshly prepared).

6. Drops of cell suspension are applied to cold, wet slides and allowed to air-dry. After staining with 50 μg/ml of Hoechst 33258 dye (Behring Diagnostics, American Hoechst Corp.) in distilled H_2O (pH 7) for 10 min, slides are H_2O-rinsed and layered with McIlvanies buffer at pH 7, coverslipped, and subjected to black light (General Electric, F40B1) photolysis at a distance of 2 inches for 20 min. During this time, slides are on a warmer tray at 50°C. Following a rinse in distilled H_2O, slides are immersed in 4% Giemsa dye prepared with one part McIlvanies buffer–four parts H_2O, pH 7; the slides are rinsed in H_2O again and allowed to dry for subsequent light microscope analysis.

APPENDIX B. A PROCEDURE FOR GROWING AND PREPARING RAT LYMPHOCYTES FOR SCE ANALYSIS*

1. Blood is obtained from the heart or tail vein[82] of CD-1 rats (Charles River). Heart punctures are performed with sterile 5–10-ml heparinized ($\sim$10 units/ml) syringes (Becton-Dickinson) + 23G needles in etherized animals. Approximately 5 ml of blood is routinely obtained. Alternatively, the animal is warmed under a heat lamp to achieve vasodilation and a small razor-cut made in the underside of the tail (after alcohol swabbing) approximately 1 inch from the base; or the distal 0.5 inches of the tail may be snipped. After dis-

*Adapted from Kligerman *et al.*[63]

carding the first 2–3 drops of blood, 10–12 drops are collected in a small sterile tube containing 50 units of sodium heparin (Sigma). Blood and heparin are gently mixed.

2. Heart blood is transferred to a 15-ml centrifuge tube, where it is spun at 500g for 5 min. Washing three times with phosphate-buffered saline (GIBCO), pH 7.4, is advised, as this reportedly provides improved results.[63] Cells are resuspended in medium to a total volume of 5 ml. (Tail vein blood, 0.2 ml, optionally washed, is combined with 1.8 ml medium.) Culture media consists of RPMI 1640 with 25 mM HEPES buffer and 2 × L-glutamine, 10% heat-inactivated fetal bovine serum (GIBCO), and 50 μg/ml gentamicin sulfate (Schering Corp.). Ten units per milliliter of preservative-free sodium heparin (Sigma) is also added. Purified PHA (Burroughs-Wellcome, HA-16; 8 μg/ml culture) or reagent-grade (0.1 ml/culture) PHA (Burroughs-Wellcome, HA-15) has provided excellent mitotic stimulation results. The PHA reactivity may be checked, since it is known to vary among lots.[82]

3. Samples of 0.6-ml heart-blood cell suspension (in media) are transferred to 15-ml sterile culture tubes (Falcon) and combined with additional complete medium to give 5.4 ml culture. (The 2.0-ml tail blood cultures are not diluted.) After incubation for 6 hr at 37°C, 5% CO_2, the cell culture is gently mixed, and cells are returned to the incubator for an additional 18 hr. The complete medium is changed and BrdUrd added to give a final concentration of 10 μM. Cultures are reincubated for an additional 28–30 hr in the complete absence of light. Colcemid (Sigma) at 0.05 μg/ml is introduced for the last 3 hr. These lymphocyte-culturing and BrdUrd-substitution conditions are suitable for *in vivo* or *in vitro* mutagen-exposure experimentation. Cytogenetic techniques for cell harvest, and slide preparation and staining are as described in steps 5 and 6 of Appendix A.

REFERENCES

1. S. A. Latt, J. Allen, S. Bloom, A. Carrano, E. Falke, D. Kram, E. Schneider, R. Schreck, R. Tice, B. Whitfield, and S. Wolff, Sister-chromatid exchanges: A report of the Gene-Tox Program, *Mutat. Res. 87*, 17–62 (1981).
2. G. Marin and D. M. Prescott, The frequency of sister chromatid exchanges following exposure to varying doses of ^{3}H-thymidine or X-rays, *J. Cell Biol. 21*, 159–167 (1964).
3. J. H. Taylor, Distribution of tritium-labeled DNA among chromosomes during meiosis, *J. Cell Biol. 25*, 57–67 (1965).
4. S. A. Latt, Microfluorometric detection of DNA replication in human metaphase chromosomes, *Proc. Natl. Acad. Sci. USA 70*, 3395–3399 (1973).
5. S. A. Latt, Sister chromatid exchanges, indices of human chromosome damage and repair: Detection by fluorescence and induction by mitomycin C, *Proc. Natl. Acad. Sci. USA 71*, 3162–3166 (1974).
6. P. Perry and H. J. Evans, Cytological detection of mutagen–carcinogen exposure by sister chromatid exchange, *Nature 258*, 121–124 (1975).

7. S. Wolff, J. Bodycote, and R. B. Painter, Sister chromatid exchanges induced in Chinese hamster cells by UV irradiation of different stages of the cell cycle: The necessity for cells to pass through S, *Mutat. Res. 25*, 73–81 (1974).

8. H. Kato, Induction of sister chromatid exchanges by chemical mutagens and its possible relevance to DNA repair, *Exp. Cell Res. 85*, 239–247 (1974).

9. P. E. Perry, in: *Chemical Mutagens—Principles and Methods for Their Detection* (F. J. de Serres and A. Hollaender, eds.), Vol. 6, pp. 1–39, Plenum Press, New York (1980).

10. S. A. Latt, R. R. Schreck, K. S. Loveday, C. P. Dougherty, and C. F. Shuler, in: *Advances in Human Genetics* (H. Harris and K. Hirschhorn, eds.), Vol. 10, pp. 267–331, Plenum Press, New York (1980).

11. J. W. Allen, in: *Progress and Topics in Cytogenetics* (A. A. Sandberg, ed.), pp. 297–311, Alan R. Liss, New York (1982).

12. D. G. Stetka, in: *Progress and Topics in Cytogenetics* (A. A. Sandberg, ed.), pp. 99–114, Alan R. Liss, New York (1982).

13. R. J. Reynolds, A. T. Natarajan, and P. H. M. Lohman, *Micrococcus luteus* UV-endonuclease sensitive sites and sister-chromatid exchanges in Chinese hamster ovary cells, *Mutat. Res. 64*, 353–356 (1979).

14. R. B. Painter, A replication model for sister-chromatid exchange, *Mutat. Res. 70*, 337–341 (1980).

15. J. E. Cleaver, Correlations between sister chromatid exchange frequencies and replicon sizes. A model for the mechanism of SCE production, *Exp. Cell Res. 136*, 27–30 (1981).

16. A. V. Carrano, L. H. Thompson, P. A. Lindl, and J. L. Minkler, Sister chromatid exchange as an indicator of mutagenesis, *Nature 271*, 551–553 (1978).

17. D. Turnbull, N. C. Popescu, J. A. DiPaolo, and B. C. Myhr, cis-Platinum (II) diamine dichloride causes mutation, transformation, and sister chromatid exchanges in cultured mammalian cells, *Mutat. Res. 66*, 267–275 (1979).

18. H. J. Evans, and Vijayalaxmi, Induction of 8-azaguanine resistance and sister chromatid exchange in human lymphocytes exposed to mitomycin C and X rays *in vitro, Nature 292*, 601–604 (1981).

19. M. O. Bradley, I. C. Hsu, and C. C. Harris, Relationships between sister chromatid exchange and mutagenicity, toxicity, and DNA damage, *Nature 282*, 318–320 (1979).

20. H. W. Rudiger, F. Kohl, W. Mangels, P. von Wichert, C. R. Bartram, W. Wohler, and E. Passarge, Benzpyrene induces sister chromatid exchanges in cultured human lymphocytes, *Nature 262*, 290–292 (1976).

21. J. M. Hopkin and P. E. Perry, Benzo[a]pyrene does not contribute to the SCEs induced by cigarette smoke condensate, *Mutat. Res. 77*, 377–381 (1980).

22. H. Norppa, M. Sorsa, P. Pfaffli, and H. Vainio, Styrene and styrene oxide induce SCEs and are metabolized in human lymphocyte cultures, *Carcinogenesis 1*, 357–361 (1980).

23. A. D. Bloom, A. V. Carrano, P. G. Archer, M. Bender, J. G. Brewen, and R. J. Preston, in: *Guidelines for Studies of Human Populations Exposed to Mutagenic and Reproductive Hazards* (A. D. Bloom, ed.), pp. 3–35, March of Dimes Birth Defects Foundation, White Plains, New York (1981).

24. J. G. Brewen, Cytogenetic monitoring in the workplace: Is it scientifically sound and practical? *Hazardous Materials Management J. 1*, 28–33 (1980).

25. B. Lambert, in: *Lymphocyte Stimulation* (A. Castellani, ed.), pp. 119–130, Plenum Press, New York (1980).

26. S. M. Galloway and R. R. Tice, in: *The Genotoxic Effects of Airborne Agents* (R. R. Tice, D. L. Costa, and K. M. Schaich, eds.), pp. 463–488, Plenum Press, New York (1982).

27. J. H. Taylor, P. S. Woods, and W. L. Hughes, The organization and duplication of chromosomes as revealed by autoradiographic studies using tritium-labeled thymidine, *Proc. Natl. Acad. Sci. USA 43*, 122–128 (1957).

28. P. Perry and S. Wolff, New Giemsa method for the differential staining of sister chromatids, *Nature 251*, 156–158 (1974).
29. K. Goto, S. Maeda, Y. Kano, and T. Sugiyama, Factors involved in differential Giemsa-staining of sister chromatids, *Chromosoma 66*, 351–359 (1978).
30. N. R. Ling and J. E. Kay, *Lymphocyte Stimulation*, American Elsevier, New York (1975).
31. M. F. Greaves, J. J. T. Owen, and M. C. Raff, *T and B Lymphocytes*, American Elsevier, New York (1974).
32. J. W. Allen, C. F. Shuler, and S. A. Latt, Bromodeoxyuridine tablet methodology for *in vivo* studies of DNA synthesis, *Somatic Cell Genet. 4*, 393–405 (1978).
33. C. C. Huang and M. Furukawa, Sister chromatid exchanges in human lymphoid cell lines cultured in diffusion chambers in mice, *Exp. Cell Res. 111*, 458–461 (1978).
34. Y. Shiraishi and A. A. Sandberg, Effects of various chemical agents on sister chromatid exchanges, chromosome aberrations, and DNA repair in normal and abnormal human lymphoid cell lines, *J. Natl. Cancer Inst. 62*, 27–33 (1979).
35. C. Fonatsch, M. Schaadt, and V. Diehl, Sister chromatid exchange in cell lines from malignant lymphomas (lymphoma lines), *Hum. Genet. 52*, 107–118 (1979).
36. H. Tohda, A. Oikawa, T. Kawachi, and T. Sugimura, Induction of sister-chromatid exchanges by mutagens from amino acid and protein pyrolysates, *Mutat. Res. 77*, 65–69 (1980).
37. R. Tice, P. Thorne, and E. L. Schneider, Bisack analysis of the phytohaemagglutinin-induced proliferation of human peripheral lymphocytes, *Cell Tiss. Kinet. 12*, 1–9 (1979).
38. S. Takehisa and S. Wolff, Sister-chromatid exchanges induced in rabbit lymphocytes by 2-aminofluorene and 2-acetylaminofluorene after *in vitro* and *in vivo* metabolic activation, *Mutat. Res. 58*, 321–329 (1978).
39. H.-J. Heiniger, B. Taylor, E. Hards, and H. Meier, Heritability of the phytohemagglutinin responsiveness of lymphocytes and its relationship to leukemogenesis, *Cancer Res. 35*, 825–831 (1975).
40. B. G. Leventhal, D. S. Waldorf, and N. Talal, Impaired lymphocyte transformation and delayed hypersensitivity in Sjogren's Syndrome, *J. Clin. Invest. 46*, 1338–1345 (1967)
41. P. E. Crossen and W. F. Morgan, Lymphocyte proliferation in Down's Syndrome measured by sister chromatid differential staining, *Hum. Genet. 53*, 311–313 (1980).
42. P. E. Crossen and W. F. Morgan, Occurrence of 1st division metaphases in human lymphocyte cultures, *Hum. Genet. 41*, 97–100 (1978).
43. B. Santesson, K. Lindahl-Kiessling, and A. Mattsson, SCE in B and T lymphocytes. Possible implications for Bloom's syndrome, *Clin. Genet. 16*, 133–135 (1979).
44. J. L. Schwartz and M. E. Gaulden, The relative contributions of B and T lymphocytes in the human peripheral blood mutagen test system as determined by cell survival, mutagenic stimulation, and induction of chromosome aberrations by radiation, *Environ. Mutagen. 2*, 473–485 (1980).
45. H. J. Evans and Vijayalaxmi, Storage enhances chromosome damage after exposure of human leukocytes to mitomycin C, *Nature 284*, 370–372 (1980).
46. E. Giulotto, A. Mottura, R. Giorgi, L. deCarli, and F. Nuzzo, Frequencies of sister chromatid exchanges in relation to cell kinetics in lymphocyte cultures, *Mutat. Res. 70*, 343–350 (1980).
47. A. V. Carrano. J. L. Minkler, D. G. Stetka, and D. H. Moore, II, Variation in the baseline sister chromatid exchange frequency in human lymphocytes, *Environ. Mutagen. 2*, 325–337 (1980).
48. B. Beek and G. Obe, Sister chromatid exchanges in human leukocyte chromosomes: Spontaneous and induced frequencies in early and late-proliferating cells *in vitro*, *Hum. Genet. 49*, 51–61 (1979).

49. W. F. Morgan and P. E. Crossen, The incidence of sister chromatid exchanges in cultured human lymphocytes, *Mutat. Res. 42*, 305–312 (1977).
50. A. J. Snope and J. M. Rary, Cell-cycle duration and sister chromatid exchange frequency in cultured human lymphocytes, *Mutat. Res. 63*, 345–349 (1979).
51. E. L. Schneider and B. Gilman, Sister chromatid exchanges and aging III. The effect of donor age on mutagen-induced sister chromatid exchange in human diploid fibroblasts, *Hum. Genet. 46*, 57–63 (1979).
52. Y. Nakanishi, D. Kram, and E. L. Schneider, Aging and sister chromatid exchange. IV. Reduced frequencies of mutagen-induced sister chromatid exchanges *in vivo* in mouse bone marrow cells with aging, *Cytogenet. Cell Genet. 24*, 6167 (1979).
53. R. R. Tice, D. L. Costa, and R. T. Drew, Cytogenetic effects of inhaled benzene in murine bone marrow: Induction of sister chromatid exchanges, chromosomal aberrations and cellular proliferation inhibition in DBA/2 mice, *Proc. Natl. Acad. Sci. USA 77*, 2148–2152 (1979).
54. J. M. Hopkin and H. J. Evans, Cigarette smoke condensates damage DNA in human lymphocytes, *Nature 279*, 241–232 (1979).
55. R. L. Davidson, E. R. Kaufman, C. P. Dougherty, A. M. Ouellette, C. M. Difolco, and S. A. Latt, Induction of sister chromatid exchanges by BudR is largely independent of the BudR content of DNA, *Nature 284*, 74–76 (1980).
56. D. Anderson, C. R. Richardson, I. F. H. Purchase, H. J. Evans, and M. L. O'Riordan, Chromosomal analysis in vinyl chloride exposed workers: Comparison of the standard technique with the sister chromatid exchange technique, *Mutat. Res. 83*, 137–144 (1981).
57. F. Apelt, J. Kolin-Gerresheim, and M. Bauchinger, Azathioprine, a clastogen in human cells? Analysis of chromosome damage and SCE in lymphocytes after exposure *in vivo* and *in vitro, Mutat. Res. 88*, 61–72 (1981).
58. J. A. Mannick, M. Constantian, D. Pardridge, I. Saporoschetz, and A. Badger, Improvement of phytohemagglutinin reponsiveness of lymphocytes from cancer patients after washing *in vitro, Cancer Res. 37*, 3066–3070 (1977).
59. A. D. White and L. C. Hasketh, A method utilizing human lymphocytes with *in vitro* metabolic activation for assessing chemical mutagenicity by sister-chromatid exchange analysis, *Mutat. Res. 68*, 283–291 (1980).
60. D. G. Stetka, J. Minkler, and A. V. Carrano, Induction of long-lived chromosome damage, as manifested by sister-chromatid exchange, in lymphocytes of animals exposed to mitomycin-C, *Mutat. Res. 51*, 383–396 (1978).
61. A. F. McFee and M. N. Sherrill, Species variation in BrdUrd-induced sister-chromatid exchanges, *Mutat. Res. 62*, 131–138 (1979).
62. G. L. Erexson, J. L. Wilmer, and A. D. Kligerman, Analysis of sister chromatid exchange and cell-cycle kinetics in mouse T- and B-lymphocytes from peripheral blood cultures, *Mutat. Res. 109*, 271–281 (1983).
63. A. D. Kligerman, J. L. Wilmer, and G. L. Erexson, Characterization of a rat lymphocyte culture system for assessing sister chromatid exchange after *in vivo* exposure to genotoxic agents, *Environ. Mutagen. 3*, 531–543 (1981).
64. M. Ohtsuru, Y. Ishii, S. Takai, H. Higashi, and G. Kosaki, Sister chromatid exchanges in lymphocytes of cancer patients receiving mitomycin C treatment, *Cancer Res. 40*, 477–480 (1980).
65. Y. Ishii and M. A. Bender, Caffeine inhibition of prereplication repair of mitomycin C-induced DNA damage in human peripheral lymphocytes, *Mutat. Res. 51*, 419–425 (1978).
66. G. L. Littlefield, S. P. Colyer, A. M. Sayer, and R. J. Dufrain, Sister-chromatid exchanges in human lymphocytes exposed during G_0 to four classes of DNA-damaging chemicals, *Mutat. Res. 67*, 259–269 (1979).

67. B. Lambert, A. Bredberg, W. McKenzie, and M. Sten, Sister-chromatid exchange in human populations: The effect of smoking, drug treatment and occupational exposure, *Cytogen. Cell Genet.* *33*, 62–67 (1982).
68. W. McKenzie and B. Lambert, Induction and reduction of sister chromatid exchange by CCNU in human lymphocytes *in vitro, Cancer Genet. Cytogenet.* *9*, 261–271 (1983).
69. G. T. Roberts and J. W. Allen, Tissue-specific induction of sister-chromatid exchanges by ethyl carbamate in mice, *Environ. Mutagen.* *2*, 17–26 (1980).
70. M. Cheng, M. K. Conner, and Y. Alarie, Multicellular *in vivo* sister-chromatid exchanges induced by urethane, *Mutat. Res.* *88*, 223–231 (1981).
71. J. Ashby, in: *Evaluation of Short-Term Tests for Carcinogens* (F. J. deSerres and J. Ashby, eds.), pp. 112–171, Elseivier/North-Holland, New York (1981).
72. J. W. Allen, Y. Sharief, and R. J. Langenbach, in: *The Genotoxic Effects of Airborne Agents* (R. R. Tice, ed.), pp. 443–460, Plenum Press, New York (1982).
73. I. Csukas, E. Gungl, F. Antoni, G. Vida, and F. Solymosy, Role of of metabolic activation in the sister chromatid exchange-inducing activity of ethyl carbamate (urethane) and vinyl carbamate, *Mutat. Res.* *89*, 75–82 (1981).
74. G. A. Dahl, J. A. Miller, and E. C. Miller, Vinyl carbamate as a promutagen and a more carcinogenic analog of ethyl carbamate, *Cancer Res.* *38*, 3793–3804 (1978).
75. J. W. Allen, R. Langenbach, S. Nesnow, K. Sasseville, S. Leavitt, J. Campbell, K. Brock, and Y. Sharief, Comparative genotoxicity studies of ethyl carbamate and related chemicals: further support for vinyl-carbamate as a proximate carcinogenic metabolite, *Carcinogenesis* *3*, 1437–1441 (1982).
76. F. Fumes-Cravioto, C. Zapata-Gayon, B. Kolmodin-Hedman, B. Lambert, J. Lindsten, E. Norberg, M. Nordenskjold, R. Olin, and A. Swensson, in: *Mutagen-Induced Chromosome Damage in Man* (H. J. Evans and D. C. Lloyd, eds), Edinburgh University Press, Edinburgh, Scotland (1978).
77. J. Kowalczyk, Sister-chromatid exchanges in children treated with nalidixic acid, *Mutat. Res.* *77*, 371–375 (1980).
78. M. Kucerova, Z. Polivkova, and J. Batora, Comparative evaluation of the frequency of chromosomal aberrations and the SCE numbers in peripheral lymphocytes of workers occupationally exposed to vinyl chloride monomer, *Mutat. Res.* *67*, 97–100 (1979).
79. V. F. Garry, J. Hozier, D. Jacobs, R. L. Wade, and D. G. Gray, Ethylene oxide: Evidence of human chromosomal effects, *Environ. Mutagen.* *1*, 375–382 (1979).
80. T. Raposa, Sister-chromatid exchange studies for monitoring DNA damage and repair capacity after cytostatics *in vitro* and in lymphocytes of leukemic patients under cytostatic therapy, *Mutat. Res.* *57*, 241–251 (1978).
81. U. Haglund, S. Hayder, and L. Zech, Sister-chromatid exchanges and chromosome aberrations in children after treatment for malignant lymphoma, *Cancer Res.* *40*, 4786–4790 (1980).
82. K. L. Triman, M. T. Davisson, and T. H. Roderick, A method for preparing chromosomes from peripheral blood in the mouse, *Cytogenet. Cell Genet.* *15*, 166–176 (1975).

8

Unscheduled DNA Synthesis as an Indicator of Genotoxic Exposure

ANN D. MITCHELL AND JON C. MIRSALIS

1. INTRODUCTION

Unscheduled DNA synthesis (UDS),[1] nonsemiconservative repair of damage to DNA, has been shown to occur over the entire genome.[2–4] The process was first revealed by autoradiography when UV irradiation was shown to induce the uptake of labeled thymidine into non-S-phase cells.[5,6] At least three steps are required: adduct formation; excision of the adducts; and DNA-strand polymerization and ligation (Figure 1).[7]

The misrepair or incomplete repair of DNA damage may be initial steps leading to many types of genetic alterations and, indeed, many known chemical mutagens and/or carcinogens have been shown to induce UDS.[8] However, perfect correlations between UDS-inducing chemicals and known mutagens and carcinogens are neither expected nor observed.[8] Although other mechanisms can lead to mutagenesis and carcinogenesis, only those chemicals (or their metabolites) that are electrophilic, and thus capable of reacting with nucleophilic proteins and nucleic acids[9] to induce repairable damage, and that do not inhibit the repair of DNA damage can be detected by UDS. Thus, UDS is, more precisely, an indicator of genotoxic exposure rather than of carcinogenic or mutagenic exposure.

The utility of UDS testing for screening potentially hazardous chemicals was recently evaluated under the auspices of the U.S. Environmental Protection Agency Gene-Tox Program.[8] It was concluded that UDS detection is a

ANN D. MITCHELL AND JON C. MIRSALIS • Cellular and Genetic Toxicology Department, SRI International, Menlo Park, California 94025.

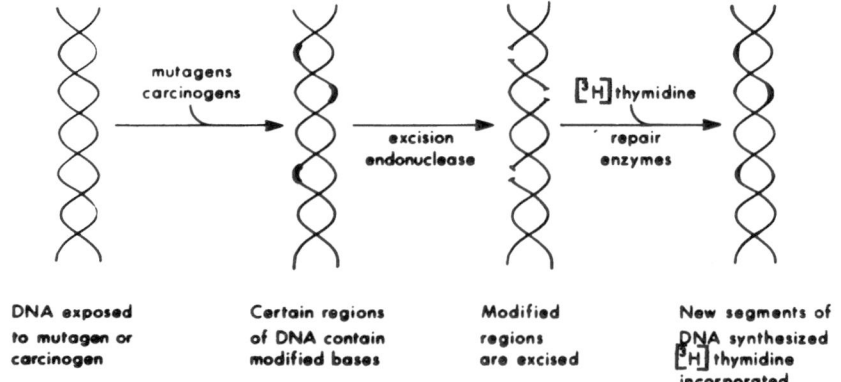

Figure 1. Induction of unscheduled DNA synthesis by genotoxic agents. Electrophilic chemicals or metabolites react with DNA to form some type of alteration in DNA structure. Excision endonucleases cleave these altered regions, and repair enzymes resynthesize the DNA, thereby filling in the gaps. In UDS assays, incorporation of [³H]thymidine can be measured, giving an indication of the amount of DNA repair.

suitable approach for inclusion in mutagenicity and carcinogenicity testing programs because it measures the repair of DNA damage induced by many classes of chemicals, UDS measurements can provide valuable information for evaluating genotoxic mechanisms that may lead to mutagenesis and/or carcinogenesis, and because UDS tests are relatively easy and inexpensive to perform.

A variety of assays have been developed for the measurement of UDS in several cell lines, including HeLa cells,[10,11] transformed human amnion (AV3) cells,[12] Syrian golden hamster embryos,[13] human fibroblasts,[14,15] and a variety of repair-deficient human cells, such as fibroblasts from patients with xeroderma pigmentosum[16] or Cockayne's syndrome.[17] These assays offer rapid and relatively inexpensive systems for measuring DNA damage and its subsequent repair in readily available cell lines, although there are disadvantages to using many of these cell lines for routine screening, as was discussed by the Gene-Tox panel.[8]

More recently, attention has been focused on the use of primary cell cultures from various tissues for UDS assays. These systems may provide more relevant information on the genotoxicity of chemicals to selected target cells. UDS assays have been reported in primary cultures of prespermiogenic cells,[18] salivary gland,[13] rat tracheal epithelium,[19] hamster brain,[20] lymphocytes and spleen,[21] rat pancreas,[22] human lymphocytes,[23] and human intestinal mucosal cells.[24]

The principal drawback of these various systems is that most of the cell lines, as well as primary cultures, are unable to metabolize many classes of procarcinogens to a genotoxic form. Although this problem can be partly resolved by addition of an exogenous metabolic activation system (e.g., containing rat liver microsomes), a more promising solution to this problem was the development of an assay that measures UDS in primary cultures of rat hepatocytes.[25] Such an assay eliminates the need for exogenous activation systems such as S-9 and offers the advantage of having the same cell serve as both the source of metabolic activation and the target for genotoxicity. In this assay, autoradiography is used to measure incorporation of tritiated thymidine ([^{3}H]-dThd) into hepatocyte DNA following excision repair. The *in vitro* hepatocyte DNA repair assay is widely used and has been shown to be an excellent predictor of carcinogenic potential for a wide variety of chemical classes.[26] Similar assays that employ liquid scintillation counting (LSC) for measurement of UDS have been reported[27,28]; however, the high cytoplasmic incorporation of [^{3}H]-dThd by the hepatocytes and the inability to distinguish incorporation due to DNA replication have made these nonautoradiographic methods impractical.

Even *in vitro* UDS assays in hepatocytes do not always reflect the true genotoxic effects present in the whole animal. Such factors as chronic exposure, sex differences, metabolism involving more than one tissue or cell type, and activation by intestinal flora may contribute to genotoxicity in the intact animal, but could obviously not be considered in an *in vitro* assay. The use of *in vivo* assays for the detection and study of genotoxic chemicals results in a more accurate profile of the effects of compounds in the whole animal because uptake, distribution, activation, detoxification, and elimination are all considered. In addition, *in vivo* systems allow the examination of genotoxicity in individual target organs. Several *in vivo* UDS assays have been described. In mice, measurement of DNA repair following *in vivo* treatment has been reported in lung, liver, and kidney,[29,30] spermatogenic cells,[18] and spermatozoa.[31] In rats, UDS assays have been developed for peripheral lymphocytes,[32,33] liver,[34] and kidney.[35]

Comparison of the response observed in hepatocytes following *in vivo* and *in vitro* treatment underscores some basic differences in these two methodologies. Treatment of the whole animal generally provides a more accurate measure of the response in a particular target tissue than *in vitro* assays; however, these tissue-specific assays may frequently miss genotoxic compounds that produce tumors in other target tissues. For example, the *in vitro* hepatocyte UDS assay does not detect the potent hepatocarcinogens 2,6-dinitrotoluene (2,6-DNT) and 1,2-dimethylhydrazine (1,2-DMH) (Table I). 2,6-DNT is metabolized to an active form by the intestinal bacteria[36]; therefore, detection of genotoxicity would not be expected in an *in vitro* assay. Conversely, the potent mutagen benzo(*a*)pyrene is not detected in the *in vivo* UDS assay because it is not a hepatocarcinogen and therefore no genotoxicity occurs in the liver; how-

Table I

Comparison of the Responses of Genotoxic Agents in Hepatocytes following Either *in Vivo* or *in Vitro* Treatment

Chemical	Target organ	*In vitro*	*In vivo*
Methylmethanesulfonate (MMS)	Brain	+	+
Dimethylnitrosamine (DMN)	Liver, kidney	+	+
2-Acetylaminofluorene (2-AAF)	Liver	+	+
Aflatoxin B_1 (AFB_1)	Liver	+	+
Benzidine	Liver, bladder	+	+
Benzo(*a*)pyrene [B(*a*)P]	Mammary, lung	+	−
2,6-Dinitrotoluene (2,6-DNT)	Liver	−	+
1,2-Dimethylhydrazine (1,2-DMH)	Liver, colon	−	+
Safrole	Liver	−	−

ever, this compound is readily detected in the less tissue-specific *in vitro* assay. Neither assay detects the weak hepatocarcinogen safrole, which may be acting as a tumor-promotor in the liver.

Both *in vivo* and *in vitro* UDS assays have obvious advantages and disadvantages. The system chosen will depend on the specific chemical to be tested, the type of information desired, the available funding and expertise, and many other factors. In order to make a rational decision as to which system is appropriate for a testing program requires a working knowledge of the methodology and type of data analysis for each assay. The authors of the Gene-Tox review found no published papers devoted to detailed methodology for UDS testing or detailed criteria for evaluating the results. To meet this need, in subsequent sections of this chapter we will provide more detailed protocols, as used in our laboratory, for the following assays: (1) measurement of UDS by LSC of DNA extracted from diploid human fibroblasts and (2) autoradiographic measurement of UDS in primary rat hepatocytes for both *in vivo* and *in vitro* assays. The use of autoradiography to measure UDS in diploid human fibroblasts will be described briefly.

2. FOUR LABORATORY APPROACHES TO MEASURING UNSCHEDULED DNA SYNTHESIS

2.1. Liquid Scintillation Counting Measurements of UDS in Human Fibroblast DNA

Although the first extensive UDS testing was performed in human fibroblasts by the autoradiography approach,[37,38] we and other investigators experienced difficulties when attempting to use this technique for screening large numbers of chemicals. The method was labor-intensive and the metabolic activation system[37] in use at that time was less than optimal. Subsequently, two different approaches to UDS testing evolved independently—the use of computer-assisted automated autoradiography grain counting (described in subsequent sections) and liquid scintillation counting (LSC) measurements of UDS in DNA extracted from cells exposed to the various chemicals.[39] Features of the LSC approach that we developed include the use of human diploid

Table II

Measurement of UDS by Liquid Scintillation Counting in WI-38 Cells

Compound	Carcinogenicity[a]	Metabolic activation[b]	Concentration range, M	UDS results[c]
Aromatic amines				
2-AAF	UC	−	10^{-6}–10^{-4}	+
2-Aminobiphenyl	NC	−	10^{-7}–10^{-3}	0^d
5-Hydroxy-N-2-fluorenylacetamide	NC	−	10^{-6}–10^{-2}	0
N-Hydroxy-N-2-fluorenylacetamide	PC	−	10^{-7}–10^{-2}	+
		+	10^{-6}–10^{-2}	+
1-Naphthylamine	NC	−	10^{-7}–10^{-3}	0
Alkyl halide				
Benzyl chloride	UC	−	10^{-6}–10^{-2}	+
Polycyclic aromatics				
Benz(a)anthracene	PC	−	10^{-7}–10^{-3}	0^d
		+	10^{-6}–10^{-2}	+
B(a)P	PC	−	10^{-7}–10^{-3}	0^d
		+	10^{-6}–10^{-2}	+
7-Bromomethyl-12-methylbenz(a)anthracene	UC	−	10^{-8}–10^{-4}	+
7,12-Dimethylbenz(a)anthracene	PC	−	10^{-8}–10^{-3}	0
		+	10^{-7}–10^{-2}	+
Phenanthrene	NC	−	10^{-7}–10^{-2}	0
Esters, epoxides, carbamates, etc.				
ϵ-Caprolactone	NC	−	10^{-6}–10^{-2}	0^d
Ethylmethanesulfonate.	UC	−	10^{-6}–10^{-2}	+
Ethyl-p-toluene sulfonate	UC	−	10^{-7}–10^{-3}	+
Glycidaldehyde	UC	−	10^{-7}–10^{-2}	+
Glycidol[e]	NC	−	10^{-6}–10^{-2}	+
MMS	UC	−	10^{-7}–10^{-3}	+
1,3-Propane sultone	UC	−	10^{-7}–10^{-2}	+
β-Propiolactone	UC	−	10^{-6}–10^{-2}	+

(*continued*)

Table II (*Continued*)

Compound	Carcinogenicity[a]	Metabolic activation[b]	Concentration range, M	UDS results[c]
Nitro aromatics and Heterocyclics				
4-Hydroxyaminoquinoline-N-oxide	UC	−	10^{-7}–10^{-3}	+
Methotrexate	NC?	−	10^{-7}–10^{-3}	0^d
4NQO	PC	−	10^{-8}–10^3	+
Nitrosamines				
DMN	PC	−	1.1×10^{-3}–9×10^{-2}	0^d
		+	3×10^{-5}–9×10^{-2}	+
Diphenylnitrosamine	NC	−	10^{-6}–10^{-2}	0^d
N-methyl-N'-nitro-N-nitrosoguanidine	UC	−	10^{-7}–10^{-2}	+
N-Nitrosoethylurea	UC	−	10^{-6}–10^{-2}	+
Fungal toxins				
AFB$_1$	PC	−	10^{-8}–10^{-4}	+
		+	10^{-7}–10^{-3}	+
Miscellaneous heterocyclics				
5-Bromodeoxyuridine	NC	−	10^{-8}–10^{-4}	0
5-Fluorodeoxyuridine	NC	−	10^{-7}–10^{-3}	0
5-Iododeoxyuridine	NC	−	10^{-7}–10^{-3}	0
Miscellaneous nitrogen compounds				
Hydroxylamine hydrochloride	NC	−	10^{-6}–10^{-2}	0
Propyleneimine	UC	−	10^{-6}–10^{-2}	+
Triethyleneimine	UC	−	10^{-7}–10^{-3}	+
Azo dye				
2-Methyl-4-dimethylaminoazobenzene	NC	−	10^{-7}–10^{-3}	0^d
Metallic salts				
Beryllium sulfate	M	−	10^{-7}–10^{-3}	0^d
Lead acetate	M	−	10^{-7}–10^{-3}	0^d
Nickel subsulfide	M	−	8×10^{-7}–8×10^{-3}	+
Platinum sulfate	M	−	3×10^{-7}–3×10^{-3}	+
Platinum tetrachloride	M	−	10^{-6}–10^{-3}	0
Titanocene dichloride	M	−	10^{-7}–10^{-3}	+

[a]UC, ultimate carcinogen; PC, procarcinogen; NC, noncarcinogen; M, metallic salt.
[b](+) Tested with metabolic activation; (−) tested without metabolic activation.
[c](+) Statistically positive UDS results at one or more concentration. These are also presented in Figure 2. (0) No statistically significant response at any concentration tested.
[d]Neither UDS response nor cytotoxic effects were observed.
[e]It has been suggested that, in solution, glycidol is rapidly changed to glycidaldehyde.

fibroblasts (WI-38 cells); inhibition of S-phase synthesis in the fibroblasts by serum depletion and hydroxyurea (HU); exposure of the fibroblasts to the test chemical and [^{3}H]-dThd for 4 hr in the presence and absence of metabolic activation; extraction of cellular DNA following the exposure step; and measurement of the extent of UDS by LSC, expressed per unit of DNA as determined by spectrophotometric measurements of DNA following reaction of the DNA with diphenylamine.

The LSC approach solved some of the problems of the original autoradiography method because grain counting was not required and it was sufficiently rapid so that alternative metabolic activation systems could be examined and a more suitable one could be selected. Moreover, with the LSC approach, the results for each test chemical could be obtained in a shorter time than is normally required for autoradiography.

The LSC system has several obvious drawbacks: (1) larger quantities of cell and test chemicals are required than for autoradiography; (2) frequently, dyes may bind to DNA and prevent accurate spectrophotometric determination of the amount of DNA per sample; (3) because the cells are not visually observed, false positive results might be obtained from agents that reverse the inhibition of S-phase DNA synthesis but do not necessarily induce unscheduled DNA synthesis. With autoradiographic techniques, an increase in DNA replication is easily detected. In spite of these potential concerns, we found that the LSC approach was usually efficient and effective, and we have utilized it to test a large number of chemicals.[39-42] Table II and Figure 2 provide examples of previously unpublished results of assays of chemicals of known carcinogenicity. The distribution of our positive and negative control results is presented in Figure 3.

2.2. Autoradiographic Measurements of UDS in Human Diploid Fibroblasts

The use of autoradiography to measure UDS in human diploid fibroblasts, with and without metabolic activation, was recommended by the Gene-Tox panel. Stich, San, and associates[37,38,43-52] have published the results of testing large numbers of chemicals by this approach, but they seldom used metabolic activation in these studies. It should be possible to couple the cell culture approaches of these researchers or the ones described here for LSC UDS with the metabolic activation system that has been described for LSC UDS and the computer-assisted, automated grain counting to be described for rat hepatocyte UDS (RH-UDS) to conduct autoradiographic measurements of UDS in human diploid fibroblasts in a sensitive and economical manner. Because these techniques are described in detail in association with other sections of this

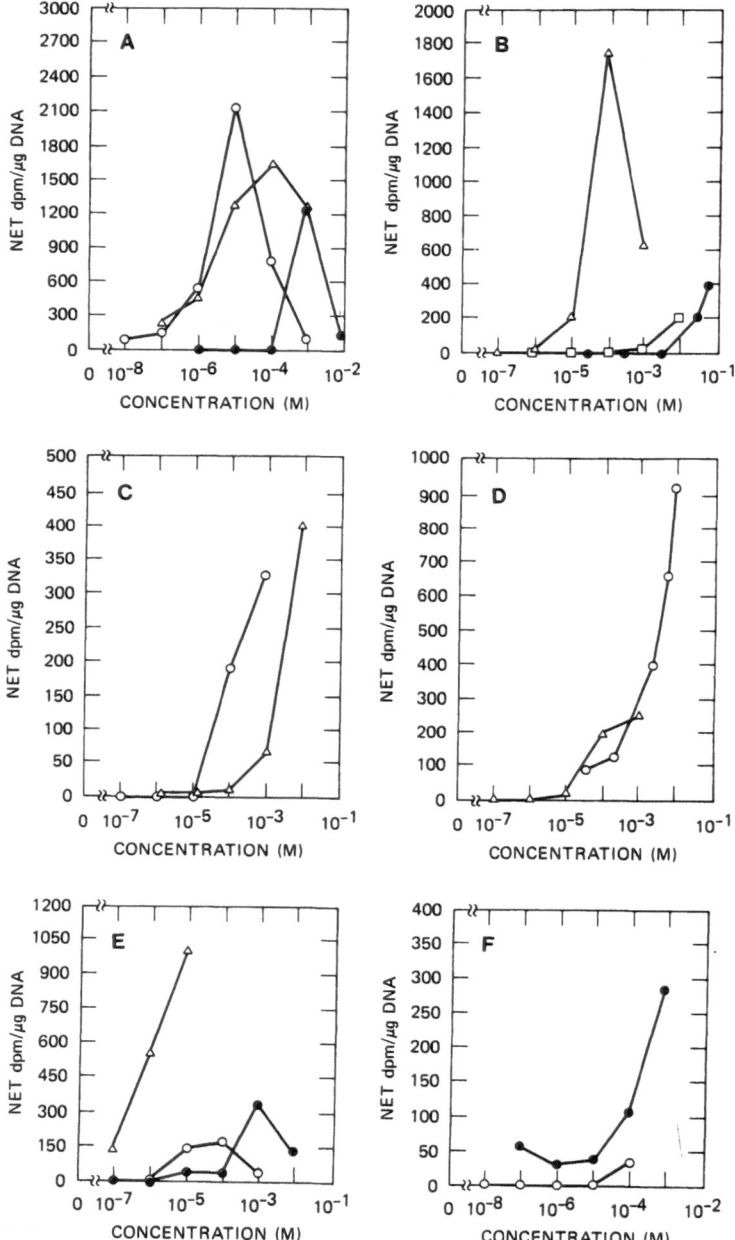

Figure 2. Positive liquid scintillation counting unscheduled DNA synthesis results. (A) 4-Hydroxylaminoquinoline-N-oxide (△) in the absence of metabolic activation and 4-nitroquinoline-N-oxide in the absence of (○) and presence (●) of metabolic activation. (B) N-Methyl-N¹-

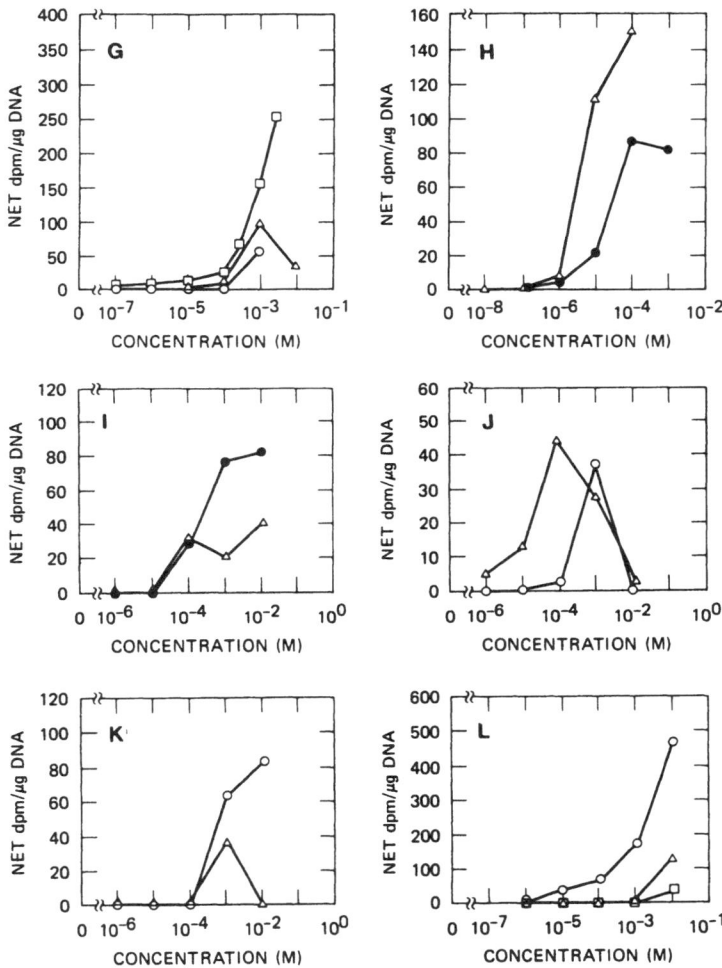

nitro-N-nitrosoguanidine (△) and N-nitrosoethylurea (□) in the absence of metabolic activation and dimethylnitrosamine (●) in the presence of metabolic activation. (C) Ethylmethanesulfonate (△) and methylmethanesulfonate (○) in the absence of metabolic activation. (D) Propyleneimine (○) and triethyleneimine (△) in the absence of metabolic activation. (E) 2-Acetylaminofluorene (△) in the absence of metabolic activation and N-hydroxy-N-2-fluorenylacetamide in the absence (○) and presence (●) of metabolic activation. (F) Aflatoxin B_1 in the absence (○) and presence (●) of metabolic activation. (G) Ethyl-o-toluene sulfonate (○), β-propiolactone (△), and propane sultone (□) in the absence of metabolic activation. (H) 7-Bromomethyl-12-methylbenz(a)anthracene (△) in the absence of metabolic activation and 7,12-dimethylbenz(a)anthracene (●) in the presence of metabolic activation. (I) Benzo(a)pyrene (●) and benz(a)anthracene (△) in the presence of metabolic activation. (J) Benzyl chloride (○) and dimethylcarbamyl chloride (△) in the absence of metabolic activation. (K) Glycidol (○) and glycidaldehyde (△) in the absence of metabolic activation. (L) Platinum sulfate (○), nickel subsulfide (△), and titanocene dichloride (□) in the absence of metabolic activation.

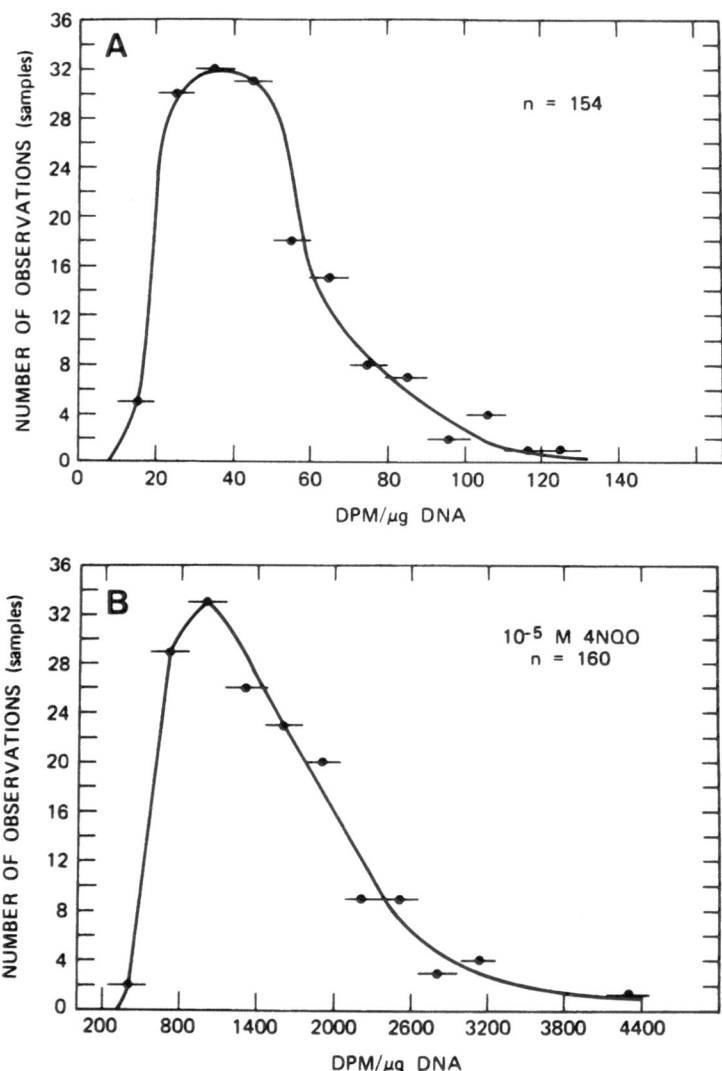

Figure 3. Historical values, dpm/μg DNA, for (A) negative (solvent) and (B) positive (4NQO) controls for the LSC UDS assay.

chapter, and because we have used them only in preliminary studies,[53] we believe further elaboration of this approach is not required.

2.3. Autoradiographic Measurements of UDS in Primary Cultures of Rat Hepatocytes

The use of fibroblast cultures for the detection of genotoxicity is limited by the inability of these cells to metabolize procarcinogens to a genotoxic form. In most early reports on the use of such systems, the investigators were unable to detect carcinogens other than direct-acting agents.[10,12,38] The use of S-9 preparations offered some improvement in terms of approaching the activation profile present in the whole animal; however, many key enzymes required for activation of procarcinogens, including glucuronyltransferase, sulfotransferase, azoreductase, nitroreductase, glutathione transferase, and acetyltransferase, are not functional in S-9.

The development of a UDS assay in primary cultures of rat hepatocytes offered many advantages over these earlier assays: (1) the adult rat liver has a low mitotic index ($\leq 0.1\%$), so inhibitors of DNA replication are not needed; (2) the same cells serve as both activator and target; (3) autoradiographic assessment of UDS offers visual proof of excision repair, simplifies elimination of DNA replication effects, and allows visual examination of cellular morphology; and (4) the intact hepatocytes provide a more accurate profile of metabolism than is obtained with S-9 preparations.

The *in vitro* hepatocyte DNA repair assay has been shown to detect ultimate carcinogens and procarcinogens from a number of different chemical classes, including polycyclic aromatic hydrocarbons, aromatic amines, nitrosamines, direct-acting alkylating agents, and mycotoxins. The assay generally does not detect nitroaromatic and azo compounds, because both nitroreductase and azoreductase are inhibited by oxygen and are not present in appreciable amounts in hepatocytes.

UDS data from hepatocytes treated either *in vitro* or *in vivo* are generally expressed as net grains/nucleus (NG). This value is derived from the nuclear grain count minus the highest number of grains over two to three nuclear-sized areas over the cytoplasm. Some laboratories also express data as the "percentage of cells in repair" (%IR), which is the percentage of cells with ≥ 5 NG. This value is useful in *in vivo* studies because it indicates how many cells in the intact liver were affected. In an *in vitro* assay, however, where a monolayer of cells is uniformly exposed, the %IR is of little value in most situations.

Hepatocytes show significant incorporation of ^3H into the cytoplasm. This may be partly due to mitochondrial DNA synthesis, but probably is also a result of hydrolysis of a $[^3H]\text{-}CH_3$ from thymidine, which can then be incorporated into many different cytoplasmic macromolecules. The use of fresh

Table III
Comparison of Negative and Positive Controls in the *in Vitro*
Hepatocyte DNA Repair Assay

Chemical	Concentration	NG
Solvent controls		
Dimethylsulfoxide (DMSO)	1%	−11.0
Ethanol	1%	−6.2
Williams' medium E	—	−5.7
Positive controls		
DMN	75 μg/ml	45.3
2-AAF	5 μg/ml	58.6

[^{3}H]-dThd reduces this problem, and we recommend using [^{3}H]-dThd that is no more than 2 weeks old. Even under ideal conditions, there are more grains in the cytoplasm than in the nucleus in control cells; therefore, the net grain count is always less than zero for controls, as illustrated in Table III. Negative data must not be reported as 0.0, as this procedure constitutes falsification of data and is a violation of Good Laboratory Practices regulations, and therefore is totally unacceptable for UDS testing of any kind. Some examples of data for negative and positive controls from our laboratory are presented in Table III. For the definitive survey of a large number of chemicals in this assay, we recommend the paper by Probst *et al.*,[26] which presents results of 218 compounds in this test.

2.4. Measurements of UDS in Hepatocytes following *in Vivo* Treatment

In vitro UDS assays in primary cultures of cell lines provide a rapid means of assesing genotoxicity. These assays do not always reflect whole-animal metabolism, however, nor do they identify possible target sites of tumor formation. The *in vivo–in vitro* hepatocyte DNA repair assay[34] measures UDS in hepatocytes following *in vivo* exposure. Treatment of the whole animal offers a true representation of *in vivo* genotoxicity and allows considerable flexibility in experimental protocols. Sex differences,[54] chronic exposure,[54] distribution of responses throughout the liver,[34] the time course of DNA repair,[34] and the effects of gut flora on genotoxicity[36] have all been examined using this assay.

This system has some obvious disadvantages. The major one is that the response is measured in only one potential target tissue, the liver. Although the assay is extremely useful for detection of hepatocarcinogens, it may miss other important classes of nonhepatic carcinogens, such as polycyclic aromatic hydrocarbons.[34] This shortcoming may be partially remedied by the devel-

Table IV

Induction of UDS by Chemicals in the *in Vivo–in Vitro* Hepatocyte DNA Repair Assay[a]

Chemical	Dose, mg/kg	Time, hr	*n*	NG ± SE	%IR ± SE
MMS	20	2	3	9.1 ± 2.2	61 ± 8
	100	2	3	38.0 ± 2.9	98 ± 1
MNNG	50	2	3	1.2 ± 3.5	21 ± 10
DMN	10	2	4	55.8 ± 3.3	91 ± 4
Diethylnitrosamine	50	2	3	30.8 ± 3.4	86 ± 3
2-AAF	50	12	3	45.0 ± 11.3	96 ± 3
Benzidine	200	2	3	6.0 ± 2.1	51 ± 10
		12	3	20.7 ± 9.6	82 ± 9
2,4-Diaminotoluene	150	2	3	15.9 ± 4.8	74 ± 9
		12	3	11.0 ± 9.0	54 ± 22
2,6-Diaminotoluene	150	2	3	−3.5 ± 0.7	5 ± 1
		12	3	−3.3 ± 1.1	6 ± 3
2,6-DNT	5	12	4	1.2 ± 0.9	28 ± 6
	20	12	4	17.9 ± 3.0	82 ± 7
Nitrobenzene	200	12	3	−4.4 ± 1.2	5 ± 2
	500	12	3	−5.6 ± 1.3	6 ± 3
7,12-Dimethylbenz(*a*)-anthracene	150	2	3	−2.5 ± 0.5	6 ± 4
		12	3	−2.6 ± 0.4	7 ± 3
B(*a*)P	100	2	3	−3.4 ± 0.9	6 ± 6
		12	3	−3.6 ± 1.2	3 ± 1
Azaserine	100	12	3	7.4 ± 4.1	47 ± 14
Azoxymethane	10	12	3	36.7 ± 2.9	92 ± 2
Chloroform	400	2	3	−4.4 ± 0.8	1 ± 1
		12	3	−2.7 ± 0.3	4 ± 1
CCl₄	400	2	3	−3.6 ± 0.6	4 ± 4
		12	3	−4.0 ± 1.2	4 ± 4
1,2-DMH	20	12	3	33.9 ± 6.3	90 ± 4
AFB₁	2	2	3	32.3 ± 3.9	95 ± 4
Safrole	200	2	3	−4.6 ± 1.1	3 ± 2
		12	3	−2.3 ± 0.5	6 ± 1
	1000	12	3	−3.1 ± 1.4	7 ± 3
Controls:					
Corn oil		2	7	−5.1 ± 0.5	1 ± 0
		12	13	−4.4 ± 0.5	3 ± 1
Water		2	3	−4.8 ± 0.8	6 ± 2
		12	4	−4.3 ± 0.5	1 ± 1
DMSO		2	3	−3.0 ± 1.7	5 ± 4
		12	3	−3.3 ± 0.6	2 ± 1

[a] *n* is the number of treated animals; NG is the number of grains/nucleus, (standard errors shown represent animal-to-animal variation); and %IR is the percentage of cells with ≥5 NG. (Adapted, with permission, from Ref. 34.)

opment of similar assays in other key target tissues. Another drawback is that liver tumor-promotors or nongenotoxic carcinogens may not be detected.

Despite these limitations, this assay is clearly valuable for the detection and study of genotoxic hepatocarcinogens. A wide variety of chemicals has been examined using this assay; a partial listing is presented in Table IV.

In addition to providing for simple detection of UDS, this assay can be used to study various parameters of genotoxicity. For example, the time course of DNA repair indicates how rapidly DNA damage is produced and how quickly it is repaired. Methylmethanesulfonate (MMS) induces damage to the DNA shortly after treatment, but this damage is rapidly repaired (Figure 4). Conversely, 2-acetylaminofluorene (2-AAF) requires metabolic activation and shows a delay in the peak time of damage as well as a slower rate of repair.

In addition to measuring UDS, the assay may also give an indication of hepatotoxicity, as shown by an increase in cell proliferation. Autoradiographic methods permit identification and quantitation of the heavily labeled S-phase

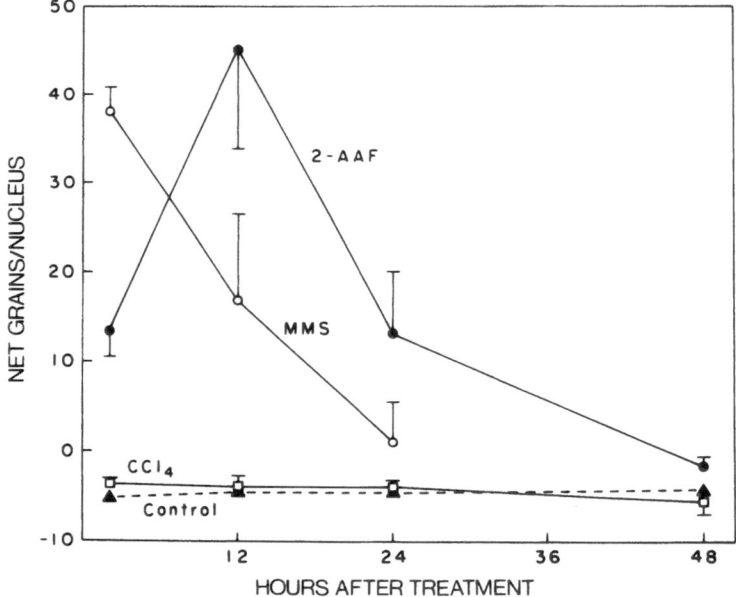

Figure 4. The time course of UDS for 100 mg/kg MMS (o), 50 mg/kg 2-AAF (●), and 400 mg/kg CCl_4 (□). Controls (-▲-) received corn oil. Livers were perfused at the times indicated after treatment by gavage. Standard errors shown represent the variation between animals. (Reprinted, with permission, from Ref. 34.)

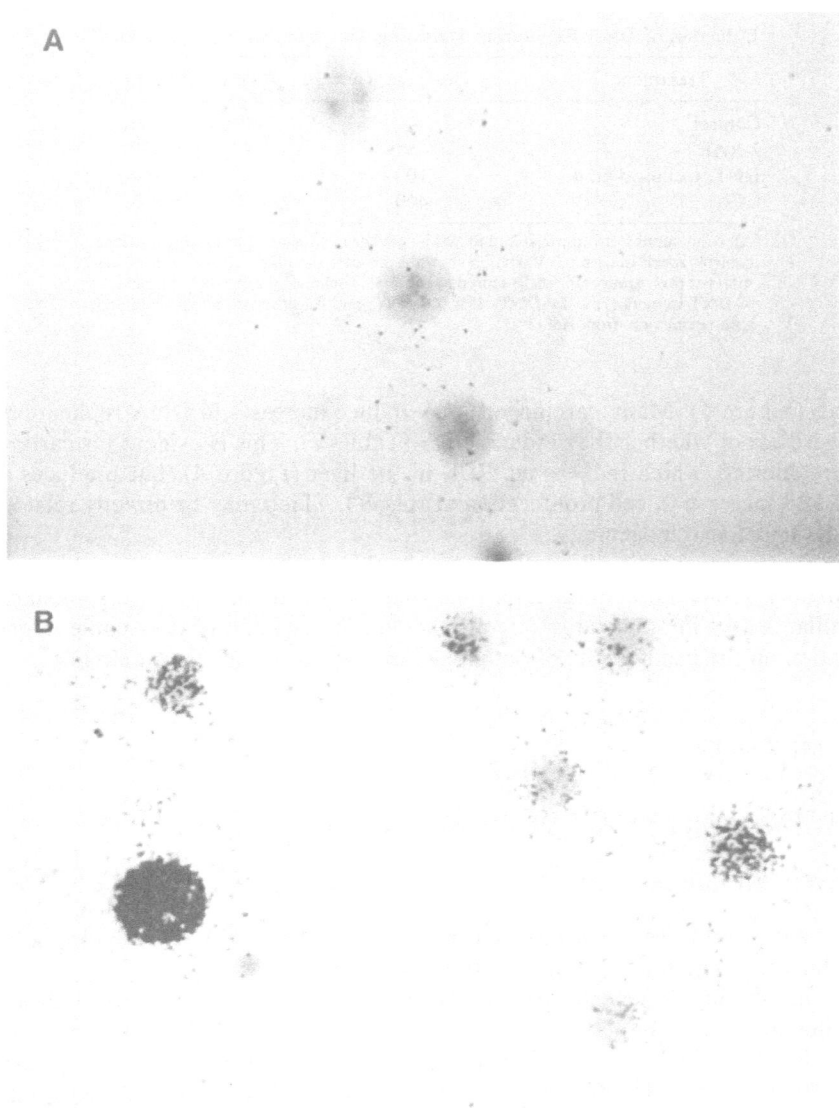

Figure 5. (A) Hepatocytes from a rat treated with a vehicle control show little incorporation of [^{3}H]-dThd into their nuclei. (B) Cells from a rat treated with 50 mg/kg 2-AAF show a significant elevation in incorporation of [^{3}H]-dThd into their nuclei. Cells in S phase are very heavily labeled and are easily distinguished from cells in repair.

Table V

Induction of DNA Replication following Treatment with Hepatotoxins[a]

Treatment	Dose, mg/kg	Percent in S phase
Control	—	0.08 ± 0.01
2-AAF	50	1.8 ± 0.5
DNT, technical grade	100	4.6 ± 0.2
CCl$_4$	400	4.1 ± 1.0

[a]All compounds were administered to rats by gavage in corn oil 48 hr prior to sacrifice; controls received corn oil. Variation shown represents the range of two to three animals for each group; 6000 cells scored per animal. Technical grade DNT is a mixture of DNT isomers (75% 2,4-DNT, 19% 2,6-DNT, and 6% other isomers). (Adapted, with permission, from Ref. 34.)

cells (Figure 5). Many carcinogens may induce increases in DNA replication, regardless of whether they induce UDS (Table V). This is evident for carbon tetrachloride, which induces no UDS in the liver (Figure 4), but produces a 50-fold increase in cell proliferation (Table V), which may be directly related to its hepatocarcinogenicity.

In summary, this assay offers considerable flexibility in assessing the genotoxicity of chemicals in the liver following *in vivo* treatment. Development of similar assays in other target organs should provide additional valuable information on the genotoxicity of potential carcinogens in the whole animal.

3. METHODS

3.1. Procedures for LSC UDS Assays

3.1.1. Cell Culture

All procedures are conducted in a laminar flow hood, with appropriate techniques to maintain sterility of the cell cutures.

a. Obtain WI-38 cells, passage 16–19, from the American Type Culture Collection (ATCC).

b. Thaw the cells according to ATCC directions. Grow them to passage 23 (P23) following Hayflick's procedures[55] for culturing WI-38 cells but using Eagle's basal medium (BME) with Hanks' salts, buffered to pH 7.2 with 15 mM HEPES (N-2-hydroxyethylpiperazine-N′-2′-ethanesulfonic acid), and 10% fetal bovine serum (FBS; growth medium). Periodically check these stock cultures to ensure absence of mycoplasma. Freeze the P23 cells, $\sim 2 \times 10^{-6}$ cells/vial, for later use.

c. Thaw one vial of P23 cells and disperse them into three or four T-75 plastic tissue culture flasks. Subculture them three times in 1 week to maintain a rapid growth rate and $\sim(1-5) \times 10^5$ cells/flask. Between subcultures, replace the growth medium at least once. For subculturing, aspirate medium from the flasks, rinse with ~ 5 ml of Ca^{2+}- and Mg^{2+}-free phosphate-buffered saline (PBS), aspirate the PBS, add ~ 1.5 ml of 0.25% trypsin/flask, and swirl to cover the entire cell monolayer. Incubate the flasks (tightly capped) at 37°C for 3–5 min. Then add 2 ml of growth medium to each flask to neutralize the trypsin. With a Pasteur pipette, break up any clumps and transfer the cells as needed.

d. To initiate samples for an assay, subculture eight T-75 flasks of stock cultures, P25, into 80 T-25 flasks by removing the cells with trypsin and pooling them into 640 ml of growth medium in a 1-liter medium bottle. Maintain the cells in an even suspension (with the aid of a Teflon®-coated magnetic stir bar and a stir plate) while using a Cornwall® syringe to dispense 8 ml of the cell suspension into each T-25 flask (see Figure 6).

Each sample used for a preliminary or definitive UDS assay will consist of a confluent monolayer of P26 cells grown in one plastic T-25 tissue culture flask. For a preliminary assay, which is performed to select concentrations for a definitive assay, four samples will be used for each treatment condition, and 68 T-25 cultures will be required to test five concentrations each of three chemicals, with or without metabolic activation (MA), with positive and negative controls. To achieve statistical confidence in the definitive assay, six samples will be used for each treatment condition. Therefore, to test five concentrations each of two chemicals, with or without MA, with positive and negative controls, 72 T-25 cultures will be required.

e. Observe random cultures from the set of T-25s daily, using an inverted microscope, to determine when the cells reach confluency (this is achieved in approximately 1 week). At that time, replace the medium from each flask with "maintenance medium" (MM)—which is the same as growth medium except that it contains only 0.5% FBS. After approximately 5 or 6 days, cell division will effectively cease, and the cells can be used for a UDS assay.

The measurement of cytotoxicity by methods such as vital stain exclusion is unreliable for selecting an appropriate range of test chemical concentrations for LSC UDS assays. Therefore, concentrations for the definitive UDS assays must be selected based on the results of a preliminary assay, identical to a definitive assay but on a smaller scale. For the UDS assay, the highest concentration selected is the lowest one that produces a "cytotoxic" response, defined as the lowest one in which, because of factors such as cell-killing or repair-enzyme inactivation, the level of UDS is reduced. Usually, the maximum UDS response will be observed at the concentration just below this one. The other

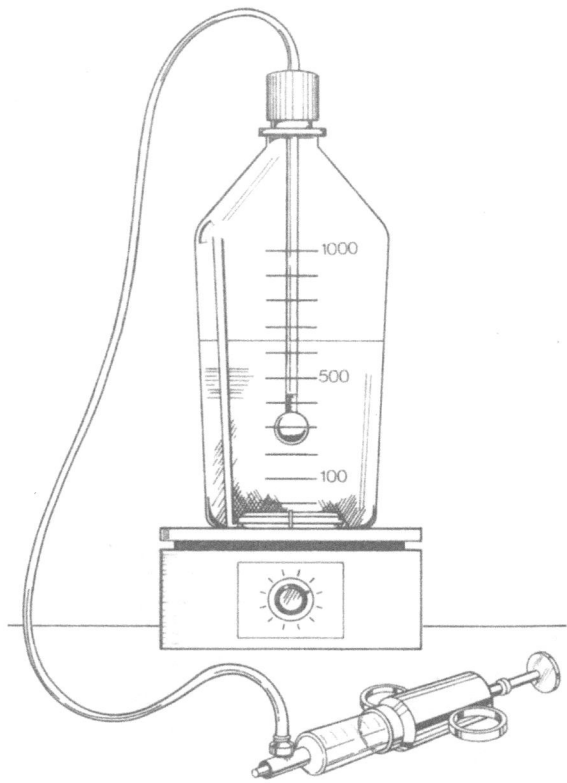

Figure 6. A Cornwall® syringe is attached to a media bottle containing a suspension of WI-38 cells on a stir plate. This allows rapid and even dispensing of the cells into culture flasks.

four concentrations for the UDS assay are selected to cover a range down to the nondetectable UDS-response level in the preliminary assay (see Figure 2).

f. On the day of the assay, check *each* flask to ensure that confluency has been reached and that cell division, as indicated by the presence of mitotic cells, has ceased. Select 72 flasks for use in the UDS assay; discard the other eight. Or, for a preliminary assay, select 68 flasks and discard 12.

3.1.2. Exposures

a. We routinely use as positive controls 10^{-5} M 4-nitroquinoline-N-oxide (4NQO) for testing in the absence of MA and 5×10^{-2} M DMN for testing with MA. The negative control is the test compound solvent, diluted to 0.5% concentration in culture medium.

b. Immediately before use of a test compound in a UDS assay, dissolve it in an appropriate solvent such as water, PBS, ethanol, or dimethylsufoxide (DMSO). This can be accomplished by brief sonication of a capped tube containing the compound and solvent in a sonicating water bath. Dilute this stock concentration of the compound in solvent to form a series of concentrations that, when diluted 200-fold into culture medium, will yield the desired concentrations to be tested. Five concentrations of the chemical will be used for each preliminary or definitive assay.

c. Preincubate the cultures for each assay for 1 hr with 10^{-2} M HU in maintenance medium (MM-HU).

d. For testing without MA, for each flask, replace the MM-HU with 8 ml of MM-HU containing 1 μCi/ml [^{3}H]-dThd (6.7 Ci/mmol) and the appropriate concentration of the test chemical or the positive or negative control.

For testing with MA, replace the MM-HU in each flask with 2 ml of reaction mixture containing the same components as for tests without MA, but with S-9 added (see Section 4.2). Tightly cap the flasks, and place them on a rocker platform in a 37°C incubator so that they can be gently rocked (to enhance oxygenation) during the exposure step.

e. Expose the cells to the reaction mixture, either with or without MA, for 4 hr at 37°C.

f. Remove unincorporated [^{3}H]-dThd by rinsing the cells in each flask twice with 5 ml of PBS containing 100 μg/ml dThd, incubating the cells at 37°C for 30 min in 8 ml of MM-HU containing 100 μg/ml dThd, and rinsing the cells two more times with 5 ml of PBS.

3.1.3. DNA Hydrolysis

DNA is isolated from the treated cultures by a modification of the techniques of Schmidt and Thannhauser.[56]

a. Solubilize the cells in each T-25 flask in 2 ml of 1 N NaOH for 40 min at room temperature. The flasks are on a rocker platform during this step.

b. Transfer the solutions to 15-ml centrifuge tubes and neutralize them with 2 ml of 10% perchloric acid (PCA) at 4°C.

c. Acidify the samples with 1 ml of 5% PCA at 4°C, place the tubes in ice (4°C), and keep them there for at least 15 min while the DNA precipitates.

d. Centrifuge the samples at 725g for 10 min in a Sorvall® GLC-2 centrifuge; discard the supernatants. Usually, after this step, the tubes containing the pellets are stored in a freezer, with subsequent operations being performed at a later time.

e. Break up the pellets with a glass rod, changing glass rods after each treatment group.

f. Twice resuspend the pellets in 2 ml of chilled (4°C) 2% PCA, followed by centrifugation for 10 min at 725g to remove any remaining unbound [³H]-dThd. Remove the supernatant by aspiration and disrupt the pellets by vortexing after each centrifugation.

g. Add room-temperature PCA (15%, 1 ml/tube) to the precipitates, heat the tubes in a 70°C water bath for 30 min, cool them to room temperature, and centrifuge them at 1600g for 15 min.

h. Divide the supernatants of hydrolyzed DNA into two aliquots, 0.6 ml for DNA measurements and 0.2 ml for scintillation counting.

3.1.4. Measurement of DNA Content

DNA content is measured by a modification of the procedures of Richards,[57] i.e., reaction with diphenylamine followed by spectrophotometric reading of optical density at 600 nm.

a. Place an 0.6-ml aliquot from each sample in a 13 × 100 mm culture tube.

b. Add room-temperature PCA (15%, 0.15 ml) to each sample tube. Prepare six blank tubes, each containing 1.50 ml of room-temperature 15% PCA, and duplicate sets of six DNA standards, containing 0.75 ml of 2, 4, 6, 8, 10, or 12 μg calf thymus DNA/ml of 15% PCA.

c. To each of the samples and DNA standards add 0.45 ml of diphenylamine reagent; add 0.9 ml to each blank tube. Cover samples with Parafilm®, shake them vigorously to mix, and store them in a dark place at room temperature for 36–48 hr.

d. Read optical density (OD) at 600 nm with a Beckman model 24 spectrophotometer equipped with a "sipper cell," and record the values. Make readings of blanks interspersed with samples; read the DNA standards last. Correct OD readings for any drift from zero, assuming any drift to be linear, and record the corrected readings.

e. Calculate the slope m for each line formed by the OD reading of each of the 12 DNA standards and the origin from the formula $m = y/x$ (y is the OD reading, x the number of micrograms of DNA). Obtain the average slope $\overline{m}$ by averaging these 12 values. Since $x = y/m$, the number of micrograms of DNA for each sample is calculated by dividing the corrected OD reading by $\overline{m}$.

3.1.5. Measurement of [³H]-dThd Incorporation

LSC measurements of [³H]-dThd incorporation in UDS samples, blanks, and [³H]-dThd standards are made using a Beckman model LS-3145T liquid scintillation counter.

a. Combine a 0.20-ml aliquot of hydrolyzed DNA from each sample with 5 ml of Aquasol® in a scintillation minivial. Prepare blanks by combining 0.20 ml of 15% PCA and 5 ml of Aquasol in each blank minivial. Prepare tritium standards by combining 0.02 ml of a stock solution of [³H]-dThd (1000 μCi/ml) with 9.98 ml of hydrolyzed DNA solution, prepared from untreated cultures of WI-38 cells following the previously described DNA hydrolysis steps. This yields a 2 μCi/ml solution. Then, add 0.20 ml of this standard solution to 5 ml of Aquasol in a minivial. Vortex the sample, blank, and [³H]-dThd standard minivials.

b. Place all minivials in minivial holders. Place the holders in the liquid scintillation counter (interspersing blanks and standards with samples). Place plastic rings around the caps of each minivial.

c. After at least 1 hr, during which time the samples sit idle in the dark, count each sample for 10 min.

d. Calculate adjusted disintegrations per minute (dpm) of [³H]-dThd from the scintillation counts by the following method:

1. Calculate dpm of the standards by the formula

$$\text{dpm/standard} = 2.2 \times 10^6 \text{ dpm/}\mu\text{Ci} \times 0.4 \ \mu\text{Ci} \times \text{decay factor}$$

where 2.2×10^6 dpm $= 1 \ \mu$Ci, by definition; each [³H]-dThd standard contains 0.2 ml of tritiated, hydrolyzed DNA at 2 μCi/ml *or* 0.2 ml $\times$ 2 μCi/ml $= 0.4 \ \mu$Ci; and the decay factor is obtained from the "Half-Life Table of Tritium" provided by Beckman Instruments.

2. Calculate counting efficiency (CE) for each standard:

$$\text{CE} = \frac{\text{cpm}_{std}}{\text{dpm}_{std}}$$

where cpm_{std} is the number of counts per minute from the scintillation counter readout, and dpm_{std} is the known dpm (as calculated above).

3. Calculate and record the mean $\bar{x}$ of the CEs of the standards.

4. Calculate and record the mean blank value (cpm).

5. Calculate dpm for each sample:

$$\frac{\text{dpm}_{sample} - \bar{x} \text{ cpm blank}}{\bar{x} \text{ CE}} = \text{cpm}_{sample}$$

6. Calculate and record adjusted dpm for each sample. Because each sample for scintillation counting contains one-third as much sample as that taken for OD measurement, each dpm sample must be adjusted as follows:

$$\text{Adjusted dpm}_{\text{sample}} = \text{dpm}_{\text{sample}} \times 3$$

e. Calculate adjusted dpm/μg DNA for each sample.

f. Calculate the mean, standard deviation, and standard error of the dpm/μg DNA for each set of (four or six) replicate samples.

g. Statistically analyze the results using either the parametric one-way classification analysis of variance or the nonparametric Kruskal–Wallis one-way analysis of variance.[58] If there is reason to believe that the variances of each of the treatments in a test are equal (i.e., Bartlett's test of variance is negative), use the parametric analysis; if the variances are not equal, use the nonparametric analysis.[59]

h. A chemical is considered to have induced UDS if the control values are within historical ranges from the laboratory (see Figure 3) and incorporation of [^{3}H]-dThd per unit of DNA is significantly elevated, at the 99% confidence level. See Table VI for an example of the manner in which results are presented in reports.

Table VI

LSC UDS Results[a] of Testing 4-Hydroxylaminoquinoline-N-Oxide without Metabolic Activation

	Result at given molar concentration						
	4-Hydroxylaminoquinoline- N-oxide						4NQO[b]
Sample	0	10^{-7}	10^{-6}	10^{-5}	10^{-4}	10^{-3}	10^{-5}
1	43	312	487	1405	1462	1386	1562
2	47	230	473	1087	1495	1121	1888
3	40	276	496	1411	1874	1625	1975
4	51	319	561	1280	1777	1330	1984
5	52	318	577	1389	1675	1280	1845
6	49	298	597	1426	1854	1132	1508
Mean	47	292	532	1333	1690	1312	1794
SD	5	34	53	132	178	186	208
SE	2	14	22	54	73	76	85

[a]Results expressed as dpm/μg DNA.
[b]Positive control.

3.2. Establishment of Primary Cultures of Rat Hepatocytes from Treated or Untreated Animals

3.2.1. Liver Perfusion

Perfusion and culturing of hepatocytes is conducted in a containment hood using sterile solutions and technique. All perfusion solutions should remain in a 37°C bath during perfusion.

a. Sterilize perfusion tubing by circulating a 70% ethanol solution followed by sterile distilled water.

b. Anesthetize an adult Fischer-344 rat with sodium pentobarbital (Nembutal®) (0.20 ml/100 g of body weight) injected intraperitoneally (IP).

c. After anesthesia is complete, place the animal (ventral surface up) on absorbent paper on a cork board. Fold the paper in on each edge to contain perfusate overflow.

d. Wet the abdominal area with 70% ethanol. Open the animal by making a V-shaped incision through the skin and muscle from the center of the lower abdomen to the rib cage. Fold back the skin and muscle over the chest to reveal the abdominal cavity. (See Figure 7).

e. Place a 15-ml centrifuge tube under the back to make the portal vein more accessible. Gently move the intestines out to the right to expose the portal vein.

f. Put a suture in place (but do not tighten it) about two-thirds of the way down the portal vein. Put another around the vena cava just above the right renal branch.

g. Begin the flow of the 37°C [ethylene bis-(oxyethylenenitrilo)] tetraacetic acid (EGTA) solution at 8 ml/min. A Cole-Parmer Masterflex® pump (#7535-10)with a Masterflex® pump head (#7016-10) is used with Cole-Parmer silicon tubing (#6411-01).

h. Cannulate the portal vein with a 23-20GA angiocatheter just below the suture. Remove the inner needle, insert the plastic catheter to about one-third the length of the vein, and tie it in place by the suture. Blood should emerge from the catheter. Then insert the tube containing the EGTA into the catheter (avoid bubbles) and *TAPE IT IN PLACE.*

i. Cut the vena cava below the right renal branch and allow blood to drain from the liver for 1.5 min.

j. Tighten the suture around the vena cava and increase the flow of EGTA to 20 ml/min for 2.5 min. The liver should clear completely of blood and swell. In some cases, gentle massaging of the liver or adjusting the orientation of the angiocatheter may be necessary for complete clearing.

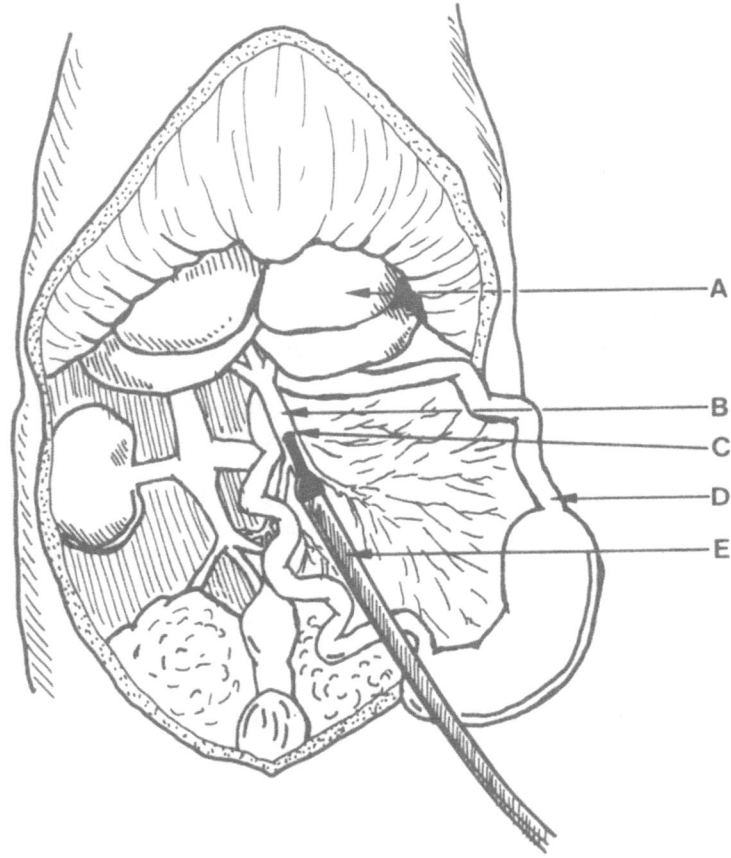

Figure 7. *In situ* perfusion of a rat liver. The liver (A) is perfused by inserting an angiocatheter (C) into the portal vein (B). The intestines and cecum (D) are clamped to one side of the animal. A collagenase solution is pumped through a tube (E) connected to the catheter.

k. Switch the flow to the 37°C collagenase solution for 12 min. During this period the liver is covered with sterile gauze, wetted with sterile saline or media, and a lamp is placed 2 in. above the liver for warming. Allow the perfusate to flow onto the paper and collect it by suction into a vessel connected to a vacuum pump by a trap.

l. After the perfusion is over, remove the catheter and gauze. Remove the liver by cutting away the membranes connecting it to the stomach and lower esophagus, cutting away all but a small piece of the diaphragm, and cutting any remaining attachments to veins or tissue in the abdomen.

m. Using sterile forceps, hold the liver by the small piece of attached diaphragm and rinse it with sterile saline or media. Place it in a sterile petri dish and take it to a sterile hood to prepare the cells.

3.2.2. Preparation of Hepatocyte Cultures

a. Place the perfused liver in a 60-mm petri dish and rinse it in incomplete Williams' medium E (WEI). Remove extraneous tissues (fat, muscle, etc.) with scissors. Place the liver in a clean petri dish and add 40–45 ml of fresh collagenase solution (37°C).

b. Carefully make several small incisions in the capsule of each lobe of the liver. (Large rips in the capsule lead to large unusable clumps of hepatocytes.) Gently comb out the cells with a sterile metal comb (dog-grooming comb), constantly swirling the liver while combing. When only fibrous and connective tissues remain, transfer the cell suspension to a sterile, 50-ml centrifuge tube by a sterile, wide-bore pipette.

c. Centrifuge the cells at 50g for 5 min and discard the supernatant. Gently resuspend the pellet in ice-cold WEI by repeated expulsions from a wide-bore pipette.

d Gently pipette the suspension through a four-ply layer of sterile gauze into a sterile, 50-ml centrifuge tube. While keeping the cells on ice, prepare to perform a cell viability count.

3.2.3. Estimation of Viability and Attachment of Cells

a. Determine viability using the trypan blue exclusion method. Suspend the cells by gently inverting the centrifuge tube a few times.

b. Add 0.5 ml of the cell suspension to 9.5 ml of WEI. Gently mix this suspension and add 0.5 ml to a tube containing 0.1 ml of 0.4% trypan blue solution.

c. Allow to stain for 1 min; then count viable and nonviable (blue) cells in a hemocytometer. Any large clump of cells should be counted as "1."

d. Calculate viability as

$$\text{Viability} = \frac{\text{Number of cells not containing dye}}{\text{Total cells}}$$

e. Calculate cell density as

$$\text{Cells/ml} = \frac{\text{Total cells}}{\text{Hemocytometer fields counted}} \times 2.4 \times 10^5$$

f. Calculate number of viable cells/ml as

$$\text{Viable cells/ml} = (\text{cells/ml}) \times \text{viability}$$

Example: Eight fields counted with 150 viable, 50 nonviable cells:

$$\text{Viability} = 150/(150 + 50) = 0.75 = 75\%$$

$$\text{Cells/ml} = (200/8) \times 2.4 \times 10^5 = 6 \times 10^6 \text{ cells/ml}$$

$$\text{Viable cells/ml} = (6 \times 10^6 \text{ cells/ml}) \times 0.75 = 4.5 \times 10^6$$

g. Place one Thermanox® #5415, 25-mm, round plastic coverslip No. 1½ (Lux Scientific Corp.) into each of six wells of a Linbro® (Flow Labs) tissue culture dish. Add 4 ml of complete Williams' medium E (WEC) to each well.

h. Seed 6×10^5 *viable* cells into each well and distribute over the coverslip by stirring gently with a 1-ml *plastic* pipette in the tissue culture dishes. (Do not use glass pipettes, because they scratch the coverslips.) Gently agitate the hepatocyte–WEC solution in each well so that it covers the entire coverslip.

i. Incubate cultures for 90 min in a 37°C incubator with 5% CO_2, 90% relative humidity, to allow attachment to coverslips.

3.2.4. The *in Vitro* Hepatocyte DNA Repair Assay

A range of five to six concentrations of a test chemical, a solvent control, a media control, and an appropriate positive control are selected for testing.

a. Make appropriate dilutions of chemicals in WEI plus 10 μCi/ml [^{3}H]-dThd (40–60 Ci/mmol).

b. Wash each culture with 4 ml of WEI after the cells are attached. For each concentration, incubate three cultures with 2 ml of the appropriate dilution or control solution. Incubate cultures overnight (16–20 hr) in an incubator (95% air, 5% CO_2) at 37°C, 90% humidity. Incubators should be vented using a negative pressure generator to prevent accumulation of volatile carcinogens or DMSO.

c. After the incubation, aspirate the media and wash each culture three times with 4 ml of WEI (37°C) prior to fixaton.

3.3. The *in Vivo* Rat Hepatocyte UDS Assay

3.3.1. Treatment of Animals

Fischer-344 rats (175–275) of both sexes are used for experiments, though males are used predominantly.

a. Chemicals to be administerd by gavage are dissolved (or suspended) in water or corn oil, depending on solubility. Chemicals to be administered IP are dissolved in saline (0.9% NaCl) or DMSO. Other routes (e.g., inhalation, subcutaneous injection) are also suitable for some compounds.

b. Animals are fasted for at least 6 hr prior to treatment. Each receives 0.1–0.4 ml of test chemical solution per 100 g of body weight. Controls receive the appropriate vehicle solution.

c. Animals treated with volatile biohazardous compounds are maintained in a vented laminar-flow hood or other suitable location to prevent possible human exposure to expired chemicals.

d. Animals are treated at various times prior to sacrifice. For preliminary screening of a compound, 2-hr and 12-hr time points are used.

e. The doses used for a preliminary test should be the LD_{50}, $(0.1-0.25)LD_{50}$ and (optional) $(0.01-0.1)LD_{50}$.

3.3.2. Attachment and Incubation of Cultures

a. Primary hepatocyte cultures are obtained from treated animals and incubated in Linbro® plates with coverslips (in WEC) for 90 min in a 37°C incubator (95% air, 5% CO_2) as is done for *in vitro* cultures.

b. After the 90-min attachment period, aspirate the WEC and wash cultures once with 4 ml of WEI per well.

c. Aspirate off the WEI and add a 2-ml aliquot of a 10 μCi/ml [³H]-dThd–WEI solution to each well.

d. Incubate cultures with [³H]-dThd–WEI solution for 4 hr.

e. After 4 hr, wash the cultures by adding 4 ml of WEI per well.

f. Aspirate the WEI and add 3 ml of unlabeled dThd (0.25 mM)–WEI solution to each well.

g. Incubate cultures overnight (14–16 hr), and wash them two times with 37°C WEI prior to fixation.

3.3.3. Fixation and Washing of Hepatocyte Cultures

a. After washing cultures from *in vivo* and *in vitro* experiments, add 4 ml of 1% sodium citrate (hypotonic solution) to each well in the Linbro® culture plates for 10 min.

b. Aspirate hypotonic solution from each well.

c. Fix cells in three changes (10 min each) of 3 ml of fixative (ethanol–glacial acetic acid, 3:1).

d. Wash out each culture well six times with 3–4 ml of distilled water. In all washes, avoid hitting the cells directly with the stream of liquid from the pipette.

e. Remove the coverslips from the wells with fine-tip, stainless steel forceps and place them on the edge of the labeled dish covers to dry in a dust-free area.

f. When coverslips are dry, use Permount® to mount them cell-side up on a labeled microscope slide, 1–2 cm from the unfrosted end of the slide.

g. After 24 hr, the slides are ready to be prepared for autoradiography.

3.4. Autoradiography

The following procedures are performed in a darkroom. To check for light leaks, the user should remain in darkness for several minutes before beginning the procedures. A safelight may be used (dark red #1 filter) at a distance of 1 ft for short periods of time. It is recommended that as much of the emulsion handling as possible be done in total darkness.

3.4.1. Applying Emulsion Layer

a. Place Kodak NTB-2 emulsion in an incubator (37°C) for several hours to melt. Dilute emulsion 1:1 in distilled deionized water (~40°C) and place in a 37°C incubator for 2–4 hr to allow loss of air bubbles. Diluted emulsion may be used immediately or refrigerated and melted for later use.

b. Pour melted emulsion into a dipping cup in a 40°C water bath and allow it to sit for 5 min.

c. Mount the slides in plastic slide grips (Lipshaw). To dip the slides, lower them into the cup until they touch the bottom and then pull them out of the emulsion with a smooth action, usually over a period of 5–6 sec. Allow the excess emulsion to drain off into the cup and touch the ends of the slides to a paper towel to remove any excess emulsion.

d. Hang the slides/holders in a vertical position in total darkness (light-proof box) for 2–3 hr or until the emulsion dries. After the slides are dry, pack them into slide boxes containing a false bottom packed with desiccant. Seal any seams of the slide box with black electrical tape and wrap the boxes in aluminum foil.

e. Store the slides at −20°C for 12–14 days for *in vivo* experiments or 7 days for *in vitro* experiments.

3.4.2. Developing Autoradiograms

a. After the 7–14 day exposure, remove the slide boxes from the freezer and allow them to thaw for 2 hr. Then unpack the slides and load them into a slide rack that is suitable for slide-staining or development.

b. Place the slides in 15°C Kodak D-19 developer for 3 min. Agitate the rack up and down every 30 sec without lifting it out of the developer.

NOTE: To avoid air bubbles that can result in undeveloped areas of emulsion, tap the rack against the bottom of the developing dish vigorously several times when the slides are first placed in D-19.

c. Place slides in 15°C distilled water for ~30 sec to rinse.

d. Place slides in 15°C Kodak Fixer (*not* Rapid-Fix) for 8 min, with agitation every 60 sec.

e. Remove slides from the fix and place them in running water for ~25 min. Avoid hitting the slides directly with the water stream. (At this time, the lights may be turned on.)

f. Remove slides from water. Slides may be stained while still wet or after drying.

3.4.3. Staining

a. Immerse the developed slides in stain (methyl green pyronin Y solution) at room temperature for 10–30 sec.

b. Rinse the slides two to four times in distilled water for ~30 sec by moving the rack up and down in the staining dish.

NOTE: DO NOT OVERSTAIN CELLS. Overstaining may cause artifacts that will affect the grain counts.

c. Verify staining quality through microscopic evaluation prior to coverslipping. Cells should have light blue-green nuclei and pale pink cytoplasm.

3.4.4. Coverslipping

a. When slides are dry, mount 25-mm square coverslips over the round coverslip, using a thin layer of Permount®.

b. When the slides have dried overnight, they are ready for grain counting.

3.4.5. Grain Counting

Grain counting is accomplished using an Artek model 880 or 980 colony counter interfaced to a Zeiss Universal microscope with an Artek TV camera. The data are fed directly into a Digital Equipment Corp. VAX 11/782 or a similar computer via an Artek BCD-RS232 Omni-Interface. Computer programs may be developed for each particular computer system for data recording and processing.

a. Randomly select a patch of cells on the slide and record the starting coordinates. Focus the cells, using the 10× objective. Align the microscope according to manufacturer specifications. Place a drop of immersion oil on the slide and switch to the 100× oil objective. (The Optovar may be set at 2.0 for higher magnification.) Pull the light-path pushrod all the way out.

b. The following cells should not be counted:

1. Morphologically altered cells, eg., cells with pyknotic nuclei (<10 μm), lysed nuclei, etc.
2. Isolated nuclei not surrounded by a cytoplasm
3. Cells that show unusual staining artifacts or the presence of debris such that an artificially high "grain count" is obtained

c. All other morphologically unaltered cells encountered while moving the stage should be counted.

d. Make all counts with the mode switch set on OBJ. AREA. This allows accurate measurement of large patches of grains or multiple grains that are touching. When using the area mode, a correction must be made for the differences in magnification for each counting system. This can be determined by counting several patches of grains manually and with the OBJ. AREA mode. The correction factor will be the actual (manual) grain count/the area count. This number is usually in the range of 1.0–1.5. All grain counts should be multiplied by this factor.

e. For each cell, use the following procedure:

1. Adjust the aperture so that it is directly over the nucleus and is the same size as the nucleus.
2. Adjust the sensitivity to the highest possible level that does not produce the appearance of spurious "flags" over nonexistent grains.
3. Hit the count button to record the nuclear count. Without changing the aperture size or the sensitivity, count two to three areas over the cytoplasm that are directly adjacent to the nucleus and that show the heaviest labeling of grains.

f. Score 50 cells by moving the x-axis of the microscope stage in a line from the starting point. If 50 cells have not been scored before coming to the edge of the slide, move the stage one to two fields on the y-axis, then resume counting in the opposite direction, parallel to the first line. Make a note of the furthest y-axis coordinate before changing direction.

g. The NG is calculated as the nuclear count minus the highest of the cytoplasmic counts. The percent of cells in repair is defined as the percent of cells with ≥ 5 NG.

h. Specific computer programs can be developed for tabulation of data from slides, pooling animals for given doses, etc. Some sample outputs are shown in Figure 8.

```
40JJ                    ST:110,  21.4    END:107,  21.5
Counter=880             scored by Karen,  18813
TOTAL CELLS       50    Area to grain conversion=   1.26

                              MEAN        S.D.      SUM SQ.        SUM
NUCLEAR COUNTS                55.82      18.70    172910.2777   2790.90
BACKGROUND                    11.87       3.52      7650.6443    593.46
NET GRAINS PER NUCLEUS        43.95      19.27    114770.7794   2197.44

98.0 PERCENT GREATER OR EQUAL TO 5 GRAINS/NUC

 #    NUC       BKG       NET       #     NUC       BKG       NET
 1   65.52     10.08     55.44      2    74.34     10.08     64.26
 3   66.78      8.82     57.96      4    26.46     10.08     16.38
 5   68.04     12.60     55.44      6    60.48      7.56     52.92
 7   73.08     16.38     56.70      8    76.86     10.08     66.78
 9   68.04     12.60     55.44     10    52.92     10.08     42.84
11   36.54      8.82     27.72     12    41.58     11.34     30.24
13   41.58      6.30     35.28     14    35.28      7.56     27.72
15   30.24      5.04     25.20     16    10.08      8.82      1.26
17   30.24     11.34     18.90     18    47.88     11.34     36.54
19   60.48     15.12     45.36     20    74.34     15.12     59.22
21  100.80      8.82     91.98     22    66.78     13.86     52.92
23   37.80     15.12     22.68     24    51.66     16.38     35.28
25   50.40     16.38     34.02     26    54.18     15.12     39.06
27   54.18     20.16     34.02     28    69.30      8.82     60.48
29   37.80     15.12     22.68     30    54.18     17.64     36.54
31   47.88     13.86     34.02     32    81.90     12.60     69.30
33   42.84     15.12     27.72     34    69.30      7.56     61.74
35   84.42      6.30     78.12     36    26.46     15.12     11.34
37   84.42      8.82     75.60     38    71.82      8.82     63.00
39   80.64     17.64     63.00     40    42.84     12.60     30.24
41   54.18      6.30     47.88     42    65.52     10.08     55.44
43   22.68     15.12      7.56     44    46.62     13.86     32.76
45   42.84     11.34     31.50     46    54.18     12.60     41.58
47   74.34      8.82     65.52     48    68.04     12.60     55.44
49   54.18     16.38     37.80     50    57.96     11.34     46.62
A
```

(*continued*)

Figure 8. Grain counting data are input directly into the computer. The slide code, starting and ending coordinates, counter number, and scorer are all input at the terminal. Data are summarized by the computer for individual slides (A) or animals can be pooled together to give totals for a given dose group (B). A frequency distribution (C) is easily constructed from the raw data for subsequent plotting or statistical analysis.

```
SUMMARY FOR 12hr, 50mg/kg    2-Acetylaminofluorene                      pg.  1

SLIDE       NUC +/- S.D.       BKG +/- S.D.       N.G. +/- S.D.      %I.R.
-----       ------------       ------------       ------------      -----
240         38.83   9.10       13.41   4.98       25.43   10.39      98.0
24AA        44.00  10.25        8.97   3.70       35.03   11.79     100.0
24WWW       56.88  18.30       13.05   7.69       43.82   20.90      98.0

29A         33.29  10.04       10.26   5.05       23.03    9.13     100.0
29U         41.03  17.24        9.93   5.22       31.10   17.75      98.0
29U2        52.57  11.39       11.89   5.55       40.67   13.00     100.0

30S         44.50  15.22       18.30   5.72       26.21   15.20      94.0
30SS        42.36   9.59        9.55   3.78       32.81   10.65     100.0
30S2        45.28  10.76       13.58   4.66       31.70   10.43      98.0


DOSE TOTALS
-----------

TOTAL # OF ANIMALS =  3
TOTAL # OF SLIDES  =  9
TOTAL # OF CELLS   = 450

             MEAN         ANIMAL        SLIDE         CELL
                          [S.E.]        [S.E.]        [S.D.]
             ----         ------        ------        ------

NUC          44.30         1.24          2.34         14.37
BKG          12.10         0.91          0.97          5.90
NET          32.20         1.34          7.30         15.12

% REPAIR     98.4          0.6           1.9*          ----

B
                                            * S.D. for % in repair
```

Figure 8 *(continued)*

4. REAGENTS, SOLUTIONS, STAINS, AND MEDIA

The lower case letters that appear in a footnote position in this section have the following meanings:

[a]Store at room temperature.
[b]Store at −20°C.
[c]Store at 4°C.
[d]Store desiccated.
[e]Protect from light.
[f]Store in lead shield.
[g]Store in regulated area.

4.1. Reagents

    1. Acetic acid, glacial (HAc), #2504-5; Mallinckrodt, Inc., St. Louis, MO.[a]

```
SUMMARY FOR 12hr. 50mg/kg    2-Acetylaminofluorene            pg.  2

Frequency Distribution       Median=    31.50
===========================
NET GRAINS        PERCENT              NET GRAINS        PERCENT
  < -20            0.2                    25              4.0
    -20                                   26              2.4
    -19                                   27
    -18                                   28              3.8
    -17                                   29              2.2
    -16                                   30              3.3
    -15                                   31
    -14                                   32              5.1
    -13                                   33              4.0
    -12                                   34              4.7
    -11                                   35              2.7
    -10                                   36
     -9                                   37              2.9
     -8            0.2                    38              2.9
     -7                                   39              4.9
     -6                                   40              2.2
     -5                                   41
     -4            0.2                    42              1.6
     -3            0.2                    43              2.2
     -2                                   44              2.9
     -1                                   45              2.2
      0            0.4                    46
      1            0.2                    47              0.7
      2                                   48              3.1
      3                                   49              1.6
      4                                   50              1.6
      5            0.4                    51
      6            0.4                    52              0.4
      7                                   53              0.9
      8            0.9                    54              0.4
      9            0.2                    55              0.2
     10            0.9                    56
     11            2.0                    57              0.7
     12                                   58              0.9
     13            1.1                    59              0.2
     14            1.6                    60
     15            1.8                    61
     16            3.1                    62              0.4
     17                                   63              0.4
     18            1.6                    64              0.4
     19            2.9                    65
     20            4.0                    66
     21            2.7                    67
     22                                   68              0.2
     23            3.3                    69              0.2
     24            2.7                    70
                                        > 70              2.4
C
```

Figure 8 (*continued*)

2. Albumin from bovine serum (BSA), crystallized and lyophilized, #A-4375; Sigma Chemical Co., St. Louis, MO.[b,d]
3. Aquasol LSC Cocktail, #NEF-934; New England Nuclear Corp., Boston, MA.[a]
4. Aroclor® 1254, #RCS-088B; Analabs, Inc., New Haven, CT.[a]

5. Autoradiography developer, D-19; Eastman Kodak, Rochester, N.Y.[a]

6. Autoradiography emulsion, NTB-2; Eastman Kodak, Rochester, N.Y.[c,e,f]

7. Basal medium (Eagle's) with Hanks' balanced salt solution (BME), #G-12; Grand Island Biological Co., Santa Clara, CA.[c]

8. Chloroform ($CHCl_3$), #4440; Mallinckrodt, Inc., St. Louis, MO.[a]

9. Citric acid; Fisher Scientific Co., Fair Lawn, N.J.[a]

10. Collagenase (Type 1), #C-0130; Sigma Chemical Co., St. Louis, MO. Or #4196; Worthington Biochemical, San Francisco, CA.[b,d,e]

11. "Count-Off"[®] Radioactivity Decontaminant, #NEF-942; New England Nuclear Corp., Boston, MA.[a]

12. Cupric sulfate ($CuSO_4 \cdot H_2O$), #1843; J. T. Baker Chemical Co., Phillipsburg, N.J.[a]

13. Deoxyribonucleic acid (DNA) from calf thymus, Type 1, #D1501; Sigma Chemical Co., St. Louis, MO.[c,d]

14. Dimethylsulfoxide analytical reagent (DMSO), #4948; Mallinckrodt, Inc., St. Louis, MO.[a]

15. Diphenylamine crystals (DI-Φ-NH_2), #D2385; Sigma Chemical Co., St. Louis, MO.[c,d,e]

16. Erythrosin B, #3-446; J. T. Baker Chemical Co., Phillipsburg, N.J.[a]

17. Ethanol, absolute; Industrial Chemical, Los Angeles, CA.[a]

18. [Ethylene bis-(oxyethylenenitrilo)] tetraacetic acid (EGTA), #8276; Eastman Kodak, Rochester, N.Y., or Sigma Chemical Co., St. Louis, MO.[a]

19. Ethylenedinitrilotetraacetic acid (EDTA), #4931; Mallinckrodt, Inc., St. Louis, MO.[a]

20. Fetal bovine serum (FBS), #14-501B; Microbiological Associates, Los Angeles, CA.[b]

21. Fixer, #KP6781313; Eastman Kodak, Rochester, N.Y.[a]

22. Folin and Ciocalteu's phenol reagent, 2 N, #F-9252; Sigma Chemical Co., St. Louis, MO.[c,e]

23. Gentamicin sulfate, #G-7507; Sigma Chemical Co., St. Louis, MO.[c]

24. Glucose-6-phosphate, disodium salt (G-6-P), #G7250; Sigma Chemical Co., St. Louis, MO.[b,d]

25. L-Glutamine, #810-1051; Grand Island Biological Co., Santa Clara, CA.[b]

26. Hanks' balanced salt solution 10× (without Ca^{2+} and Mg^{2+}), #310-4180; Grand Island Biological Co., Santa Clara, CA.[a]

27. HEPES buffer, #845-1344; Grand Island Biological Co., Santa Clara, CA.[c] Or #H3375; Sigma Chemical Co., St. Louis, MO.[a]

28. Hydroxyurea (HU), #H-8627; Sigma Chemical Co., St. Louis, MO.[b,d]

29. D,L-isocitric acid, trisodium salt (isocitrate), #1-1252; Sigma Chemical Co., St. Louis, MO.[b,d]

30. Magnesium chloride ($MgCl_2 \cdot H_2O$), #CB487; Matheson, Coleman, and Bell, Norwood, OH.[a]

31. Methyl alcohol, #3016-8; Mallinckrodt, Inc., St. Louis, MO.[a]

32. Methyl green pyronin, #1A560; Roboz Surgical Inst., Washington, D.C.[a]

33. Niacinamide, #4813; Calbiochem, La Jolla, CA.[b,d]

34. Nicotinamide adenine dinucleotide phosphate (NADP), #N-0505; Sigma Chemical Co., St. Louis, MO.[b,d]

35. Paraldehyde, Eastman #198; Sargent-Welch, Anaheim, CA.[a,e]

36. Penicillin–streptomycin (Pen-strep), #600-5140; Gibco, Santa Clara, CA.[b]

37. Perchloric acid, 70% (PCA), #A-229; Fisher Scientific Co., Fair Lawn, N.J.[a]

38. Permount,® #72856; Fisher Scientific Co., Fair Lawn, N.J.[a]

39. Phenol, liquid, #A-931; Fisher Scientific Co., Fair Lawn, N.J.[a]

40. Potassium chloride (KCl), #1-3040; J. T. Baker Chemical Co., Phillipsburg, N.J.[a]

41. Potassium phosphate monobasic (KH_2PO_4), #7100; Mallinckrodt Inc., St. Louis, MO.[a]

42. Resorcinol; Fisher Scientific Co., Fair Lawn, N.J.[a]

43. Sodium bicarbonate, #7412; Mallinckrodt Inc., St. Louis, MO.[a]

44. Sodium carbonate (Na_2CO_3) #3602; J. T. Baker Chemical Co., Phillipsburg, N.J.[a]

45. Sodium chloride (NaCl), #1-3624; J. T. Baker Chemical Co., Phillipsburg, N.J.[a]

46. Sodium citrate, #0754; Mallinckrodt, Inc., St. Louis, MO.[a]

47. Sodium hydroxide (NaOH) pellets, #7708-1; Mallinckrodt, Inc., St. Louis, MO.[a]

48. Sodium pentobarbital (60 mg/ml), #NDC 14035-1032-4; Trico Pharmaceutical Co., San Carlos, CA.[a]

49. Sodium phosphate dibasic, anhydrous (Na_2HPO_4), #7917-1; Mallinckrodt Inc., St. Louis, MO.[a]

50. Sodium phosphate dibasic, dodecahydrate ($Na_2HPO_4 \cdot 12H_2O$); Mallinckrodt, Inc., St. Louis, MO.[a]

51. Sodium phosphate dibasic, heptahydrate ($Na_2HPO_4 \cdot 7H_2O$) Mallinckrodt, Inc., St. Louis, MO.[a]

52. Sodium phosphate monobasic, anhydrous (NaH_2PO_4), #7892; Mallinckrodt Inc., St. Louis, MO.[a]

53. Sodium potassium tartrate, #S-387; Fisher Scientific Co., Fair Lawn, N.J.[a]

54. Sucrose, #S-5, 79112; Fischer Scientific Co., Fair Lawn, N.J.[a]
55. Thymidine, #T-9250; Sigma Chemical Co., St. Louis, MO.[a,e]
56. Tritiated thymidine ($[^3H]$-dThd), specific activity 40–60 Ci/mmol, TRK.418; Amersham Corp., Arlington Heights, FL. Or specific activity 6.7 Ci/mmol, #NEC-027; New England Nuclear Corp., Boston, MA.[c,g]
57. Trypan blue vital stain (0.4%), #630-5250; Grand Island Biological Co., Santa Clara, CA.[a]
58. Trypsin, #610-5090; Gibco, Santa Clara, CA.[b]
59. Williams' medium E (powdered) formula, #78-5133; Gibco, Santa Clara, CA.[c]
60. Williams medium E without L-glutamine, #12-502-54; Flow Laboratories, Inglewood, CA.[c,e]
61. Xylene, #8668-1; Mallinckrodt, Inc., St. Louis, MO.[a]

4.2. Solutions and Stains

1. Acetic acid (glacial)–15% PCA (5:3).[a] To make 600 ml, combine these ingredients in the following order:

a. 295 ml of deionized H_2O
b. 80 ml of 70% perchloric acid (PCA)
c. 225 ml of glacial acetic acid
   or
a. 375 ml of 15% PCA
b. 225 ml of glacial acetic acid

2. Autoradiography developer.[a,b] Ingredients:

a. Deionized H_2O, 3.8 liter
b. Kodak D-19 developer, one package

Heat water to 38°C, then slowly add the contents of one package of Kodak D-19 developer while stirring. Dissolve completely and store in a brown, 1-gallon jug. Make fresh once a month.

3. Autoradiography fixer.[a,e] Ingredients:

a. Deionized H_2O, 3.8 liters
b. Kodakfixer, one package

Add contents of one package of Kodak fixer (not Rapid-Fix) to the water and stir until dissolved completely. Store in a brown 1-gallon jug.

4. Bovine serum albumin (BSA) standard.[b] Procedure:

a. Using an analytical balance (Mettler Model H51), weigh 50 mg of BSA to five decimal places.
b. Calculate the amount of deionized water needed to make a 500 μg/ml solution ($\sim$100 ml). Dissolve completely.
c. Aliquot $\sim$3.5 ml/tube and store until needed for Lowry assay of protein standards.

5. Calf thymus DNA standard solution.[c] Procedure:

a. Using an analytical balance, weigh 2.5 mg of calf thymus DNA to five decimal plces.
b. Calculate the amount of 1$\times$ SSC (sodium citrate, saline) needed to make a 500 μg/ml DNA solution and add it to the DNA.
c. Add one drop of chloroform and place the solution in a 37°C bath until dissolved (3–5 hr). Store refrigerated and dilute 1:5 to 100 μg/ml as needed, following instructions below.
d. Dilute to 100 μg/ml with 15% PCA (perchloric acid) and hydrolyze in a 70°C bath for 30 min.
e. Cool and store at $\sim$4°C until needed for preparation of DNA diphenylamine standards for UDS assays. Discard after 2 months.

6. Collagenase (100 units/ml).[c] Ingredients:

a. Collagenase, 35,000 units
b. Williams' medium E, 350 ml

Dissolve collagenase in the medium for 20 min, then add:

c. HEPES (2 M), 1.75 ml
d. NaOH (2 N), 0.70 ml

Should be made up no more than 24 hr before each use. Filter-sterilize with 0.45-μm filter (and prefilter) and add 0.1 cm^3 gentamicin sulfate per 100 ml.

7. Diphenylamine reagent (Di-Φ-NH$_2$).[a,e] Ingredients must be added in *the following order*. Work under a fume hood.

a. 500 ml of glacial acetic acid
b. 0.05 ml of 4% paraldehyde
c. 20 g of diphenylamine crystals

Store in black tape-wrapped bottle at room temperature.

8. EDTA.[c] Procedure:

a. Dissolve 1% (by volume) of EDTA in double-deionized H_2O (1 g of EDTA in 100 ml of H_2O).
b. Adjust the pH of the solution to 7.2–7.4 with 1 N NaOH.
c. Filter-sterilize through 0.22-μm Nalgene® filter.

9. Erythrosin B.[a] Procedure: Add 0.4 g to 100 ml of PBS.

10. Giemsa (3%). Ingredients:

a. Giemsa stain (improved R66 solution), 6 ml
b. Sorensen's buffer, pH 6.8, 194 ml

Make fresh just before use.

11. Hank's balanced salt solution (HBSS) with EGTA.[c] Ingredients:
a. HBSS, 100 ml
b. EGTA, 21 mg

Dissolve EGTA in HBSS in water bath for at least 1 hr. Then add the following:

c. HEPES (2 M), 0.5 ml
d. NaOH (2N), 0.2 ml

Filter-sterilize with 0.2-μm filter and add 0.1 cm^3 of gentamicin sulfate/100 ml. Store at 4°C until use.

12. HEPES buffer, (N-2-hydroxyethylpiperazine-N'-2'-ethanesulfonic acid.[c] Ingredients:

a. Powdered HEPES, 240 g
b. H_2O distilled (deionized), 1000 ml

Filter-sterilize with 0.22-μm Nalgene filter.

13. Lowry solutions.
Lowry A solution[c]: Ingredients:

a. Na_2CO_3, 20.0 g
b. NaOH, 4.0 g
c. Na tartrate or K tartrate, 0.2 g
d. H_2O up to 1.0 liter

Lowry B solution[c]: Ingredients:

a. $CuSO_4 \cdot 5H_2O$, 5.0 g
b. H_2O up to 1.0 liter

Phenol stock reagent[a,e]: 2 N Folin and Ciocalteau; dilute 1:2 (to 1 N) just before use.

Lowry AB[a]:

a. 49 ml of A solution
b. 1 ml of B solution

Make up *only* 1 hr before using in Lowry assay.

NOTE: Lowry A and Lowry B solutions can be made up separately and stored indefinitely.

14. Methyl green pyronin solution.[a,e]

Solution A: Mix the following in a graduated cylinder:

a. Na_2HPO_4, 7.45 g
b. Methanol, 66.0 ml

Add distilled water to bring volume to 263 ml.

Solution B: Mix the following in another graduated cylinder:

a. Citric acid, 5.0 g
b. Methanol, 59.0 ml

Add distilled water to bring volume to 240 ml.
Mix both solutions when they are dissolved. Then add to the mixed solutions:

a. Phenol (liquid), 12.5 μl
b. Resorcinol, 125.0 mg
c. Methyl green pyronin Y, 5.0 g

Allow to sit for 2 weeks before use. Keep in dark bottle and filter before each use. Discard after approximately 6 months or when an obvious decrease in staining intensity is observed.

15. Perchloric acid (PCA).[a] Ingredients:

	H_2O, ml	70% PCA, ml
2%	971.4	28.6
5%	928.6	71.4
10%	857.1	142.9
15%	785.7	214.3

Only deionized H_2O should be used. Always add *acid to water*.

16. Phosphate-buffered saline (PBS)[a] Procedure:

a. Combine the following in an Erlenmeyer flask (all quantities/liter H_2O):

   1. NaCl, 8.0 g
   2. KCl, 0.2 g
   3. $Na_2HPO_4 \cdot 12H_2O$, 2.89 g
     or
     $Na_2HPO_4 \cdot 7H_2O$, 2.16 g
     or
     Na_2HPO_4 (anhydrous), 1.15 g
   4. KH_2PO_4, 0.2 g

b. Add deionized H_2O to flask and mix on stir plate until totally dissolved.
c. Transfer contents of flask to Nalgene aspirator bottle. Bring up to final volume with deionized H_2O; mix.
d. Dispense PBS into 500-ml media bottles, filling to approximately 300–400 ml.
e. Cap loosely. Autoclave at 15 lb for 30 min on the same day that the solution is prepared. Alternatively, PBS may be filter-sterilized prior to dispensing into 500-ml bottles. PBS *must* be filter-sterilized for WI-38 culture.

17. Phosphate-buffered KCl.[c] Ingredients (all quantities/liter H_2O):

a. KCl, 11.50 g
b. Na_2HPO_4 (anhydrous), 0.230 g
   or
   $Na_2HPO_4, \cdot 7H_2O$, 0.436 g
   or
   $Na_2HPO_4 \cdot 12H_2O$, 0.580 g
c. NaH_2PO_4 (anhydrous), 0.052 g
   or
   $NaH_2PO_4 \cdot H_2O$, 0.060 g

18. Rat liver homogenate, S-9.[b] The rat S-9 liver homogenate contains approximately 3 mg/ml of protein and is prepared aseptically from the livers of adult male Fischer 344 rats treated 5 days before sacrifice with 500 mg/kg Aroclor®. It is stored in 3-dram vials in liquid nitrogen.

19. Rat S-9 cofactor preparation.[c] To make 144 ml of S-9 liver preparation and complete medium (this is the quantity required for a definitive +MA LSC UDS assay):

a. Cofactors:

    1. NADP, 0.360 g
    2. Isocitrate, 0.675 g

b. Liver, 15.0 ml of rat S-9
c. Maintenance medium, 60.0 ml

Dissolve cofactors in medium, neutralize with 1–2 drops of 10 N NaOH, and add S-9. Dilute 1:2 into medium for UDS exposures without MA.

20. Saline sodium citrate (IX) (SSC).[a] Ingredients:

a. Na citrate, 2.2 g
b. NaCl, 4.3 g
c. Deionized H_2O, 500.0 ml

21. Sodium bicarbonate (7.5%).[c] Ingredients:

a. $NaHCO_3$, 7.5 g
b. Deionized H_2O, 100.0 ml

Autoclave or filter-sterilize and store at 4°C.

22. Sodium citrate (1%).[a] Ingredients:

a. Sodium citrate, 10.0 g
b. Deionized H_2O, 1000.0 ml

23. Sodium hydroxide (NaOH).[c] Ingredients:

	1 N	2 N
a. Anhydrous NaOH pellets	40 g	8 g
b. Deionized H_2O	1 liter	100 ml

NOTE: This is an exothermic reaction; therefore, NaOH pellets should be added to H_2O slowly, with the solution cooling on ice between additions. Filter-sterilize with 0.2-μm filter and store at 4°C.

24. Sorensen's buffer, pH 6.8.[c] Ingredients:

a. KH_2PO_4, 13.26 g
b. $Na_2HPO_4 \cdot 7H_2O$, 5.12 g
c. Deionized H_2O, 2.0 liters

Adjust pH to 6.8 with 1 NaOH.

25. Sucrose–phosphate buffer.[c] Ingredients:

a. Sucrose, 85.6 g
b. Na_2HPO_4, 0.230 g
   or
   $Na_2HPO_4 \cdot 12H_2O$, 0.581 g
   or
   $Na_2HPO_4 \cdot 7H_2O$, 0.435 g
c. NaH_2PO_4, 0.053 g
   or
   $NaH_2PO_4 \cdot H_2O$, 0.061 g
d. Deionized H_2O, 1.0 liter

Adjust pH to 7.4; autoclave; sterilize 20 min. only.

26. Thymidine (100 μg/ml). Ingredients:

a. Thymidine, 6.1 mg
b. WEI, 100.0 ml
c. HEPES (2 M), 0.3 ml

Final concentration is 0.25 mM. Filter-sterilize with 0.2-μm filter. Make up just before using. Make ~20 ml per animal.

27. 0.4 μCi Tritium standard (for LSC UDS assays).[c] See Section 3.1.3 for method of preparing hydrolyzed WI-38 DNA solution (~10 ml). Prepare ~10 ml of a 2-μCi/ml solution of tritiated thymidine ([^{3}H]-dThd)–DNA solution as follows:

a. Stock [^{3}H]-dThd (1000 μCi/ml), 0.02 ml
b. Hydrolyzed WI-38 DNA solution, 9.98 ml

Vortex and store at 4°C until needed.
To make a 0.4-μCi ^{3}H standard for scintillation counting, combine 0.20 ml of above standard with 5 ml of Aquasol® in a minivial and vortex.

28. Trypan blue. A 0.4% solution comes prepared from Gibco.

29. Trypsin.[b] Procedure:

a. As needed, thaw 100 ml (one bottle) and dispense into 5-ml aliquots in sterile, screw-cap test tubes. Keep frozen until use.
b. For "working" trypsin solution, thaw 5 ml of trypsin and add to 45 ml of sterile PBS.
c. *Optional:* 1 ml of sterile 1% EDTA can be added to enhance effectiveness of trypsin for WI-38 cells.

4.3. Media

1. Basal medium (Eagle's) with Hanks' salt (BME).[a] Ingredients:

a. Powdered medium, one packet for 10 liters
b. Distilled, deionized H_2O, 10 liters
c. Sodium bicarbonate, 3.5 g

Sterilize by pressure filtration, filling 500-ml medium bottles in laminar-flow hood.

Growth medium[c] (serum concentration 10%). Ingredients:

a. BME, 450 ml
b. FBS, 50 ml
c. L-Glutamine, 5 ml
d. HEPES, 5 ml

Maintenance medium[c] (serum concentration 0.5%). Ingredients:

a. BME, 450 ml
b. FBS, 2.5 ml
c. L-Glutamine, 5 ml
d. HEPES, 5 ml

Thaw medium[c] (serum concentration 10%). Ingredients:

a. BME, 450 ml
b. FBS, 50 ml
c. L-Glutamine, 5 ml
d. HEPES, 5 ml
e. Pen-strep, 5 ml

Freezing medium[b] (serum concentration ~20%). Ingredients:

a. Thaw medium, 33.5 ml
b. FBS, 6.5 ml
c. DMSO, 10.0 ml

Medium for LSC UDS exposures without MA.[c] Ingredients:

a. BME, 600.0 ml
b. HU, 0.48 g
c. FBS, 3.0 ml
d. HEPES, 12.0 ml

The above solution is 10^{-2} M HU, 0.5% FBS, and 25 mM HEPES in BME. Prepare just before using.

Medium for LSC UDS exposures with MA.[c] See Section 4.2, item 19.

2. Fetal bovine serum (FBS).[b] Thaw 500-ml bottle of FBS that was stored at $-20°C$. Heat-inactivate at $56°C$ for 30 min. Then put 50-ml portions into sterile 120-ml bottles.

3. L-Glutamine (200 mM).[b] Ingredients:

a. L-Glutamine, 2.92 g
b. Distilled H_2O, 100 ml

Heat in $37°C$ bath if needed to dissolve. Filter-sterilize and store in 5-ml aliquots.

4. Pen-strep.[b] Procedure:

a. As needed, thaw 100 ml (one bottle) and dispense 5-ml aliquots into sterile, screw-cap tubes.
b. Thaw and use aliquots as needed.

5. Williams' E complete (WEC).[c] Ingredients

a. Williams' medium E, 500 ml
b. Fetal bovine serum, 50 ml
c. L-Glutamine (200 mM), 5 ml
d. Gentamicin, 0.5 cm³

Add FBS that has been heat-inactivated (30 min at $56°C$) to WEI (item 6 below).

6. Williams' E incomplete (WEI).[c] Ingredients:

a. Williams' medium E, 500 ml
b. L-Glutamine, 5 ml
c. Gentamicin sulfate, 0.5 cm³

5. EQUIPMENT AND SUPPLIES

5.1. Balances

Mettler analytical balances, models H34, P3N, and P163; Mettler Instruments Co., Princeton, NJ

5.2. Calculators

1. #HP-11C, Hewlett-Packard calculator; Hewlett-Packard Corp., Palo Alto, CA
2. TI-5010 printing calculator; Texas Instruments, Dallas, TX

5.3. Centrifuges

1. IEC Model CU-5000 centrifuge; International Equipment Co., Needham Heights, MA
2. Sorvall GLC-2B centrifuge; Dupont Company, Newton, CT

5.4. Computer Equipment

1. VAX 11/782 computer; Digital Equipment Corp., Maynard, MD
2. VT/100 terminal; Digital Equipment Corp.
   or
   Zenith Data Systems Z-19 terminal; Zenith Radio Corp., Glenview, IL

5.5. Filters

1. Filter units, 0.2 μm, 115-ml capacity, #09-740; Fisher Scientific, Pittsburgh, PA
2. Stainless steel filter holder, 142 mm, #4422-142-30; Millipore Corp., Bedford, MA
3. Dispensing pressure vessel, 20-liter capacity, #XX67-00P-20; Millipore Corp.
4. Prefilter, #AP25-142-50; Millipore Corp.
5. Filter unit, 0.45 μm, 500-ml capacity, #F3200-6; American Scientific Products, Evanston, IL
6. Filters for media preparations, 0.2 μm, 142-mm diameter, Gelman Cat. #60305; Gelman Sciences, Ann Arbor, MI

5.6. Grain Counters

1. Colony counter, Model 880 or 980; Artek Systems Corp., Farmingdale, NY
2. Omni-Interface, BCD-RS232; Artek Systems Corp.
3. Auxiliary TV camera model #73307; Artek Systems Corp.

5.7. Incubators and Related Apparatus

1. Forma Scientific CO_2 incubator, model 3209; Forma Scientific, Marietta, OH
2. Forma negative-pressure generator, model #3044; Forma Scientific
3. CO_2 analyzer, Bacharach 105000, Cat. #G-1725; American Scientific Products
4. Precision Scientific incubator, #31032; GCA Precision Scientific, Chicago, IL

5.8. Laminar-Flow Hoods

1. Bioguard hood, model NCB-6, class II, type II; Baker Co., Sanford, ME
2. Sterilgard hood, model VBM-600; Baker Co.

5.9. Microscopes

1. Zeiss universal microscope, #47-16-90; Carl Zeiss, New York, NY
2. Wild Heerbrugg inverted microscope, model M40; Max Erb Instruments, Los Angeles, CA

5.10. Mixer

Vortex-genie mixer, #12-812; Fisher Scientific

5.11. Pipetting Apparatus

1. Pipet-Aid with filter, #13-681-16; Fischer Scientific
2. Cornwall pipetter, 10 ml, #P5173-10; American Scientific Products
3. Oxford sampler micropipette, continuously adjustable, 2–1000 μl, #3001-3004; Oxford Laboratories, Foster City, CA
4. Oxford sampler tips, #910 and 911; Oxford Laboratories
5. Miscellaneous disposable glass pipettes; Various scientific vendors

5.12. Pump Apparatus

1. Barnett Masterflex pump, #7520-10; Cole Parmer Instruments, Chicago, IL
2. Barnett Masterflex pump-head, #7016-21; Cole Parmer Instruments

3. Barnett Masterflex two-head kit, #7013-05; Cole Parmer Instruments
4. Gast pressure vacuum pump, #P8401-2; American Scientific Products

5.13. Rocker Platform

Bellco rocker platform, #7740; Bellco Glass, Vineland, NJ

5.14. Scintillation Counter

Beckman liquid scintillation counter, model LS-3145T; Beckman Instruments, Fullerton, CA

5.15. Spectrophotometer

Beckman model 24 spectrophotometer (with sipper system); Beckman Instruments

5.16. Tissue Culture Supplies

1. Culture dishes, 100 × 20, #3003; Falcon Plastic Division, Becton-Dickinson Corp., Oxnard, CA
2. Culture plates, six-well Linbro®, #76-058-05; Flow Laboratories, Inglewood, CA
3. Centrifuge tubes, 15 ml (Corning), #5-538-51; Fisher Scientific
4. Centrifuge tubes, 50 ml, #2098; Falcon
5. Thermanox® coverslips #5451-2 mm, #1.5, Cat. #62-415-07; Flow Laboratories
6. Culture tubes, 16 × 125 mm, #2025; Falcon
7. Culture tubes, 13 × 100 mm, #2027; Falcon
8. Culture flasks, T-75, Corning #25110; American Scientific Products
9. Culture flasks, T-25, Corning #25100; American Scientific Products
10. Ampules for freezing cells, NUNC Inter Med, 2 cm³; Vangard International, Neptune, NJ

5.17. Water Baths

1. Thelco models 184 and 186; Precision Scientific
2. Ultrasonicating water bath; Untrasonics, Plainview, NY

5.18. Water System

Super Q water system; Millipore Corp.

5.19. Miscellaneous Equipment

1. Freezers; Various appliance dealers
2. Hand counter with two units, #02-67-012; Fisher Scientific
3. Hemocytometer, Bright Line, #02-671-5; Fisher Scientific
4. Kodak Adjustable Safelite, Model B, #141-2212; Eastman Kodak, Rochester, NY
5. Kwick-Set Lab Chron Timer, #C65525-2; American Scientific Products
6. Lead donuts, #LD-5C; Instruments for Research & Industry, Chelterham, PA
7. Liquid nitrogen refrigerator, Linde #LR-40; Union Carbide Corp. New York, NY
8. Magnetic stir plate, Tekstir, #S8250-1; American Scientific Products
9. Metal dog-grooming comb; Various pet suppliers
10. Pharmaseal needle destruction device, #9655; American Scientific Products
11. Pilot box, six-outlet, #91-437; Fisher Scientific
12. Polypropylene centrifuge tube holder, #14-8091; Fisher Scientific
13. Refrigerators; Various appliance dealers
14. Stirring bar, ⅜ in × 1½ in, #58949; VWR Scientific
15. Stopcock, Pharmaseal, three-way, #S8965-1; American Scientific Products
16. Tensor lamp, 25 W, #11-990-15; Fisher Scientific
17. Tissue grinder, Con-Torque power unit, Eberbach #2360, SP #T4029; American Scientific Products
18. Tissue grinder (Potter Elvehjem), Wheaton, SP #T4028-30; American Scientific Products

5.20. Miscellaneous Supplies

1. Cover glass, 25 × 25, Corning Cat. #M6020-3; American Scientific Products
2. Catheters, Deseret Angiocath 20G, 1.25 in., #2878; Bischoff's Surgical Supples, Oakand, CA
3. Mini LSC vials, #NEF-943; New England Nuclear, Boston MA

4. Permount® mounting medium, #SO-P-15; American Scientific Products
5. Scintillation vial holders; American Scientific Products
6. Silk sutures, Ethicon 4-0, #LA-53G; Bischoff's Surgical Supplies
7. Silicon tubing, #6411-02; Cole-Parmer Instruments
8. Slides, 75 × 25, frosted end, Corning Cat. #M6171; American Scientific Products
9. Syringes, tuberculin, one ml, with needle, #14-823-220; Fisher Scientific
10. Vials, 3 dram, for storage of S-9, #B7807-3; American Scientific Products

ACKNOWLEDGMENTS. The authors gratefully acknowledge the assistance of Cathy Contreras, Erica Loh, Michelle Mack, Patricia McAfee, Douglas Robinson, Karen Steinmetz, Kim Tyson, and Adeline Will in the preparation of this manuscript. Development of the LSC UDS system was partially supported by NCI Contract N01/CP-33394, NIEHS Grant ES01281, and EPA Contract 68-01-2458.

REFERENCES

1. B. Djordevic and L. J. Tolmach, Responses of synchronous populations of HeLa Cells to ultraviolet irradiation at selected stages of the generation cycle, *Radiat. Res. 32*, 327–346 (1967).
2. L. Meltz, N. J. Whittam, and W. H. Thornburg, Random distribution of highly repetitive and intermediate frequency mouse L-929 cell DNA sequences synthesized after UV light exposure, *Photochem. Photobiol. 27*, 545–550 (1978).
3. M. J. Smerdon and M. W. Lieberman, Nucleosome rearrangement in human chromatin during UV-induced DNA repair synthesis, *Proc. Natl. Acad. Sci. USA 75*, 4238–4241 (1978).
4. W. J. Bodell and M. R. Banerjee, The influence of chromatin structure on the distribution of DNA repair synthesis studied by nuclease digestion, *Nucl. Acids Res. 6*, 359–370 (1979).
5. R. E. Rasmussen and R. B. Painter, Radiation-stimulated DNA synthesis in cultured mammalian cells, *J. Cell Biol. 9*, 11–19 (1966).
6. R. B. Painter and J. E. Cleaver, Repair replication in HeLa cells after large doses of X-irradiation, *Nature (London) 216*, 369–370 (1967).
7. J. J. Roberts, the repair of DNA modified by cytotoxic, mutagenic and carcinogenic chemicals, *Adv. Radiat. Biol. 7*, 211–436 (1978).
8. A. D. Mitchell, D. A. Casciano, M. L. Meltz, D. E. Robinson, R. H. C. San, G. M. Williams, and E. S. von Halle, Unscheduled DNA synthesis tests: A report of the "Gene-Tox" Program, *Mutat. Res. 123*, 363–410 (1983).
9. E. C. Miller and J. A. Miller, The metabolism of chemical carcinogens to reactive electrophiles and their possible mechanisms of action in carcinogenesis, *Chemical Carcinogens*, ACS

Monograph 173 (C. E. Searle, ed.), pp. 737–762 American Chemical Society, Washington, D.C. (1976).

10. R. E. Rasmussen and R. B. Painter, Evidence for repair of ultraviolet damaged deoxyribonucleic acid in cultured mammalian cells, *Nature (London) 203,* 1360–1362 (1964).

11. C. N. Martin, A. C. McDermid, and R. C. Garner, Testing of known carcinogens and noncarcinogens for their ability to induce unscheduled DNA synthesis in HeLa cells, *Cancer Res. 38,* 2621–2627 (1978).

12. J. E. Trosko and J. D. Yager, A sensitive method to measure physical and chemical carcinogen-induced "unscheduled DNA synthesis" in rapidly dividing eukaryotic cells, *Exp. Cell Res. 88,* 47–55 (1974).

13. F. Ide, T. Ishikawa, S. Takayama, and S. Umemura, Autoradiographic demonstration of unscheduled DNA synthesis in oral tissues treated with chemical carcinogens in short-term organ cultures, *J. Oral Pathol., 10,* 113–123 (1981).

14. R. H. C. San and H. F. Stich, DNA repair synthesis of cultured human cells as a rapid bioassay for chemical carcinogens, *Int. J. Cancer 16,* 284–291 (1975).

15. P. K. Gupta and M. A. Sirover, Sequential stimulation of DNA repair and DNA replication in normal human cells, *Mutat. Res. 72,* 273–284 (1980).

16. R. D. Snyder and J. D. Regan, DNA repair in normal human and xeroderma pigmentosum group A fibroblasts following treatment with various methanesulfonates and the demonstration of a long-patch (U.V.-like) repair component, *Carcinogenesis 3,* 7–14 (1982).

17. A. J. Rainbow and M. Howes, A deficiency in the repair of UV and gamma-ray damaged DNA in fibroblasts from Cockayne's Syndrome, *Mutat. Res. 93,* 235–247 (1982).

18. I. P. Lee and K. Suzuki, Induction of unscheduled DNA synthesis in mouse germ cells following 1,2-dibromo-3-chloropropane (DBCP) exposure, *Mutat. Res. 68,* 169–173 (1979).

19. T. Ishikawa, S. Takayama, and F. Ide, Autoradiographic demonstration of DNA repair synthesis in rat tracheal epithelium treated with chemical carcinogens *in vitro, Cancer Res. 40,* 2898–2903 (1980).

20. H. L. Gensler, Low level of U.V.-induced unscheduled DNA synthesis in postmitotic brain cells of hamsters: Possible relevance to aging, *Exp. Gerontol. 16,* 199–207 (1981).

21. H. Tuschl and H. Altmann, Unscheduled DNA synthesis in lymphocytes of rheumatoid arthritis patients and spleen cells of rats with experimentally induced arthritis, *Med. Biol. 54,* 327–333 (1976).

22. K. L. Steinmetz and J. C. Mirsalis, Measurement of DNA repair in primary cultures of rat pancreas cells treated with genotoxic agents, *Environ. Mutagen. 5,* 481 (1983).

23. K. Tatsumi, T. Sakane, H. Sawada, S. Shirakawa, T. Nakamura, and G. Wakisaka, Unscheduled DNA synthesis in human lymphocytes treated with neocarzinostatin, *Gann 66,* 441–444 (1975).

24. H. J. Freeman and R. H. C. San, Use of unscheduled DNA synthesis in freshly isolated human intestinal mucosal cells for carcinogen detection, *Cancer Res. 40,* 3155–3157 (1980).

25. G. M. Williams, Carcinogen induced DNA repair in primary rat liver cell cultures; a possible screen for chemical carcinogens, *Cancer Lett. 1,* 231–236 (1976).

26. G. S. Probst, R. E. McMahon, L. E. Hill, C. Z. Thompson, J. K. Epp, and S. B. Neal, Chemically-induced unscheduled DNA synthesis in primary rat hepatocyte cultures: A comparison with bacterial mutagenicity using 218 compounds, *Environ. Mutagen. 3,* 11–32 (1981).

27. G. Michalopoulos, G. L. Sattler, L. O'Connor, and H. C. Pitot, Unscheduled DNA synthesis induced by procarcinogens in suspensions and primary cultures of hepatocytes on collagen membranes, *Cancer Res. 38,* 1866–1871 (1978).

28. J. D. Yager and J. A. Miller, DNA synthesis in primary cultures of rat hepatocytes, *Cancer Res. 38,* 4385–4394 (1978).

29. H. F. Stich and D. Kieser, Use of DNA repair synthesis in detecting organotropic actions of chemical carcinogens, *Proc. Soc. Exp. Biol. Med. 145*, 1339–1342 (1974).
30. G. Brambilla, M. Cavanna, P. Carlo, R. Finollo, and S. Parodi, DNA repair synthesis in primary cultures of kidneys from BALB/c and C3H mice treated with dimethylnitrosamine, *Cancer Lett. 5*, 153–159 (1978).
31. N. Tanaka and M. Katoh, Unscheduled DNA synthesis in the germ cells of male mice *in vivo*, *Jpn. J. Genet. 54*, 405–414 (1979).
32. T. M. Michel and M. S. Legator, DNA repair synthesis and chromosomal aberrations induced *in vivo* by triethylenemelamine, *Mutat. Res. 24*, 41–45 (1974).
33. M. J. Skinner, B. DeCastro, and J. F. Eyre, Detection of unscheduled DNA synthesis in rat lymphocytes treated *in vivo* with cyclophosphamide and triethylenemelamine, *Environ. Mutagen. 2*, 277–278 (1980).
34. J. C. Mirsalis, C. K. Tyson, and B. E. Butterworth, Detection of genotoxic carcinogens in the *in vivo–in vitro* hepatocyte DNA repair assay, *Environ. Mutagen. 4*, 553–562 (1982).
35. C. K. Tyson and J. C. Mirsalis, Measurement of chemically induced DNA repair in rat kidney following *in vivo* treatment, *Environ. Mutagen. 5*, 482 (1983).
36. J. C. Mirsalis, T. E. Hamm, J. M. Sherrill, and B. E. Butterworth, Role of gut flora in the genotoxicity of dinitrotoluene, *Nature (London) 295*, 322–323 (1982).
37. H. F. Stich and B. A. Laishes, DNA repair and chemical carcinogens, in: *Pathobiology Annual* (H. L. Ioachim, ed.), pp. 341–376, Appleton-Century Crofts, New York (1973).
38. R. H. C. San and H. F. Stich, DNA repair synthesis of cultured human cells as a rapid bioassay for chemical carcinogens, *Int. J. Cancer 16*, 284–291 (1975).
39. D. E. Robinson and A. D. Mitchell, The unscheduled DNA synthesis response of human fibroblasts, WI-38 cells, to 20 coded chemicals, in: *Evaluation of Short-Term Tests for Carcinogens* (F. J. deSerres and J. Ashby, eds.), pp. 517–527, Elsevier/North-Holland, New York (1981).
40. V. F. Simmon, A. D. Mitchell, and T. A. Jorgenson, Evaluation of Selected Pesticides As Chemical Mutagens, *in Vitro* and *in Vivo* Studies, U.S. Environmental Protection Agency Environmental Health Effects Research Series, #EPA-600/1-177-028 (May 1977), pp. 1–5, 12–16, 25–27, and 78–117.
41. V. F. Simmon, D. C. Poole, A. D. Mitchell, and D. E. Robinson, *In Vitro* Microbiological Mutagnicity and Unscheduled DNA Synthesis Studies of Eighteen Pesticides, SRI International, Menlo Park, CA, Project LSU-3447, Report for the U.S. Environmental Protection Agency (August 1978), pp. 1–4, 11–16, 24–39, and 112–164.
42. V. F. Simmon, E. S. Riccio, D. E. Robinson, and A. D. Mitchell, *In Vitro* Microbiological Mutagenicity and Unscheduled DNA Synthesis Studies of Fifteen Pesticides, SRI International, Menlo Park, CA, Project LSU-3447, Report for the U.S. Environmental Protection Agency (August 1979), pp. 1–4, 11–16, 25–27, and 103–171.
43. R. H. C. San, W. Stich, and H. F. Stich, Differential sensitivity of xeroderma pigmentosum cells of different repair capacities towards the chromosome breaking action of carcinogens and mutagens, *Int. J. Cancer 20*, 181–187 (1977).
44. H. F. Stich, O. Hammerberg, and B. Casto, The combined effect of chemical mutagen and virus on DNA repair, chromosome aberrations, and neoplastic transformation, *Can. J. Genet. Cytol. 14*, 911–917 (1972).
45. H. F. Stich and B. A. Laishes, The response of xeroderma pigmentosum cells and controls to the activated mycotoxins aflatoxin and sterigmatocystin, *Int. J. Cancer 16*, 266–274 (1975).
46. H. F. Stich and R. H. C. San, DNA repair and chromatid anomalies in mammalian cells exposed to 4-nitroquinoline-1-oxide, *Mutat. Res. 10*, 389–404 (1970).

47. H. F. Stich and R. H. C. San, DNA repair and chromatid anomalies in mammalian cells exposed to 4-nitroquinoline-1-oxide, *Mutat. Res. 13*, 279–282 (1971).

48. H. F. Stich and R. H. C. San, DNA repair synthesis and cell survival of repair-deficient cells exposed to the K-region epoxide of benz(*a*)anthracene, *Proc. Soc. Exp. Biol. Med. 142*, 155–158 (1973).

49. H. F. Stich, R. H. C. San, and Y. Kawazoe, DNA repair synthesis in mammalian cells exposed to a series of oncogenic and non-oncogenic derivatives of 4-nitroquinoline-1-oxide, *Nature (London) 229*, 416–419 (1971).

50. H. F. Stich, R. H. C. San, and Y. Kawazoe, Increased sensitivity of xeroderma pigmentosum cells to some chemical carcinogens and mutagens, *Mutat. Res. 17*, 127–137 (1973).

51. H. F. Stich, R. H. C. San, J. A. Miller, and E. C. Miller, Various levels of DNA repair synthesis in xeroderma pigmentosum cells exposed to the carcinogens N-hydroxy and N-acetoxy-2-acetylaminofluorene, *Nature New Biol. 238*, 9–10 (1972).

52. H. F. Stich, L. Wei, and P. Lam, The need for a mammalian test system for mutagens: Action of some reducing agents, *Cancer Lett. 5*, 199–204 (1978).

53. J. C. Beck, G. P. Sterling, M. L. Hay-Kaufman, and A. D. Mitchell, Unscheduled DNA synthesis testing of six promutagens using an autoradiography approach, *Environ. Mutagen. 3*, 315 (1981).

54. J. C. Mirsalis and B. E. Butterworth, Induction of unscheduled DNA synthesis in rat hepatocytes following *in vivo* treatment with dinitrotoluene, *Carcinogenesis 3*, 241–245 (1982).

55. Leonard Hayflick, Subculturing human diploid fibroblast cultures, in: *Tissue Culture Methods and Applications* (P. F. Kruse and M. K. Patterson, Jr., eds.), pp. 220–223, Academic Press, New York (1973).

56. G. Schmidt and S. J. Thannhauser, A method for the determination of desoxyribonucleic acid, ribonucleic acid and phosphoproteins in animal tissues, *J. Biol. Chem. 161*, 83–89 (1945).

57. G. M. Richards, Modification of the diphenylamine reaction giving increased sensitivity and simplicity in the estimation of DNA, *Anal. Biochem. 57*, 369–374 (1974).

58. W. C. Guenther, *Analysis of Variance*, pp. 20–43, Prentice-Hall, Englewood Cliffs, NJ (1964).

59. J. H. Zar, *Statistical Analysis*, pp. 109–111, Prentice-Hall, Englewood Cliffs, NJ (1974).

9

The Micronucleus Test as an Indicator of Mutagenic Exposure

Robert R. Racine and Bernhard E. Matter

1. HISTORICAL BACKGROUND

The widespread demand for protection against chemical substances in the environment that may damage genetic material emphasizes the need for reliable and comprehensive assay systems for the detection of genotoxic effects. Such effects can be classified in three broad categories, namely (1) gene and point mutations, (2) chromosome mutations, and (3) genome mutations. It is well known that in humans these effects may lead to severe clinical disorders that may be transmissible to future generations if they occur in the germ line. A number of chemical substances that could cause such adverse effects in humans have already been identified by means of experimental work with biological assay systems.

The classical assays for the identification of categories (2) and (3) are mostly cytogenetic methods, i.e., metaphase preparations of meiotic/mitotic cells. These metaphase preparations, derived either from cells of animals treated *in vivo* or from cell cultures treated *in vitro,* are studied for the presence of chromosome aberrations.[1,2] These assays not only make it possible to identify compounds that cause such aberrations, but they also make it possible to distinguish among various types of chromosome aberrations and to indicate possible modes of action of the mutagens. Nevertheless, these methods have severe drawbacks. First, the scarcity of mitosis, and the resulting lack of suitable metaphase spreads, often does not permit satisfactory evaluation. Second, microscopic evaluation is quite time-consuming; it is a deplorable situation for

Robert R. Racine and Bernhard E. Matter • Sandoz Ltd., Preclinical Research, Toxicology, CH-4002 Basle, Switzerland.

a cytogeneticist to have to study a high number of compounds in a limited period of time. It is not surprising, therefore, that cytogeneticists began to look for short-term tests that might serve as indicators of cytogenetic effects. One of these attempts led to the development of the micronucleus test.

Micronuclei have long been known in the field of medicine under the name of "Howell–Jolly bodies." They are cytoplasmic chromatin masses that look like very small nuclei. They arise from chromosomes lagging at anaphase or from acentric chromosomal fragments resulting from mitotic/meiotic disturbances. The production of micronuclei as a result of chromosome damage caused by ionizing radiation has been known for many years.[3-7] Evans et al.[8] used the incidence of micronuclei in plant root-tips to quantitatively monitor cytogenetic damage caused by ionizing radiation.

In the late 1960s and early 1970s Schmid and coworkers initiated an extensive research program in order to determine the parameters that might serve as the most useful indicators of cytogenetic damage in bone-marrow cells of rodents treated in vivo with chemical mutagens.[9-15] Independently of this development, other researchers were also active in this field.[16-19]

From a historical point of view, the initial work of Schmid and coworkers and Heddle is of particular interest because it led directly to the development of the "bone-marrow micronucleus test," which today is widely used as a screening system for the identification of compounds that cause chromosome/genome mutations.[20-24]

2. RATIONALE OF THE TEST SYSTEM

The micronucleus test is based on several unusual features of maturing red blood cells of the bone marrow. During the anaphase of mitosis, centric elements move, or are moved by, the spindle fibers toward the spindle poles. Acentric chromatid/chromosome fragments produced by a clastogen lag behind during this process but are included in the cytoplasm of the daughter cells. These lagging elements are then transformed into one or several secondary nuclei. Since they are smaller than the parent nucleus, they are called micronuclei. Similar events occur as a consequence of partial impairment of

Figure 1. Bone marrow smears of a CD-1 mouse treated twice (24 hr apart) with 0.5 mg/kg triethylenemelamine. The slide was prepared according to the method described in Section 3.5. An Ilford HP5 (400 ASA/27 DIN) film was used. (A) Overview. (B) Enlargement. Several cell types can be identified: (1) Polychromatic erythrocytes (the population of cells to be scored for micronuclei); (a) with micronucleus; (b) without micronucleus. (2) Normochromatic erythrocytes. (3) Lymphocytes. (4) Immature granulocytes; (a) with micronucleus; (b) without micronucleus. (5) Crushed cells (not considered in the micronucleus test).

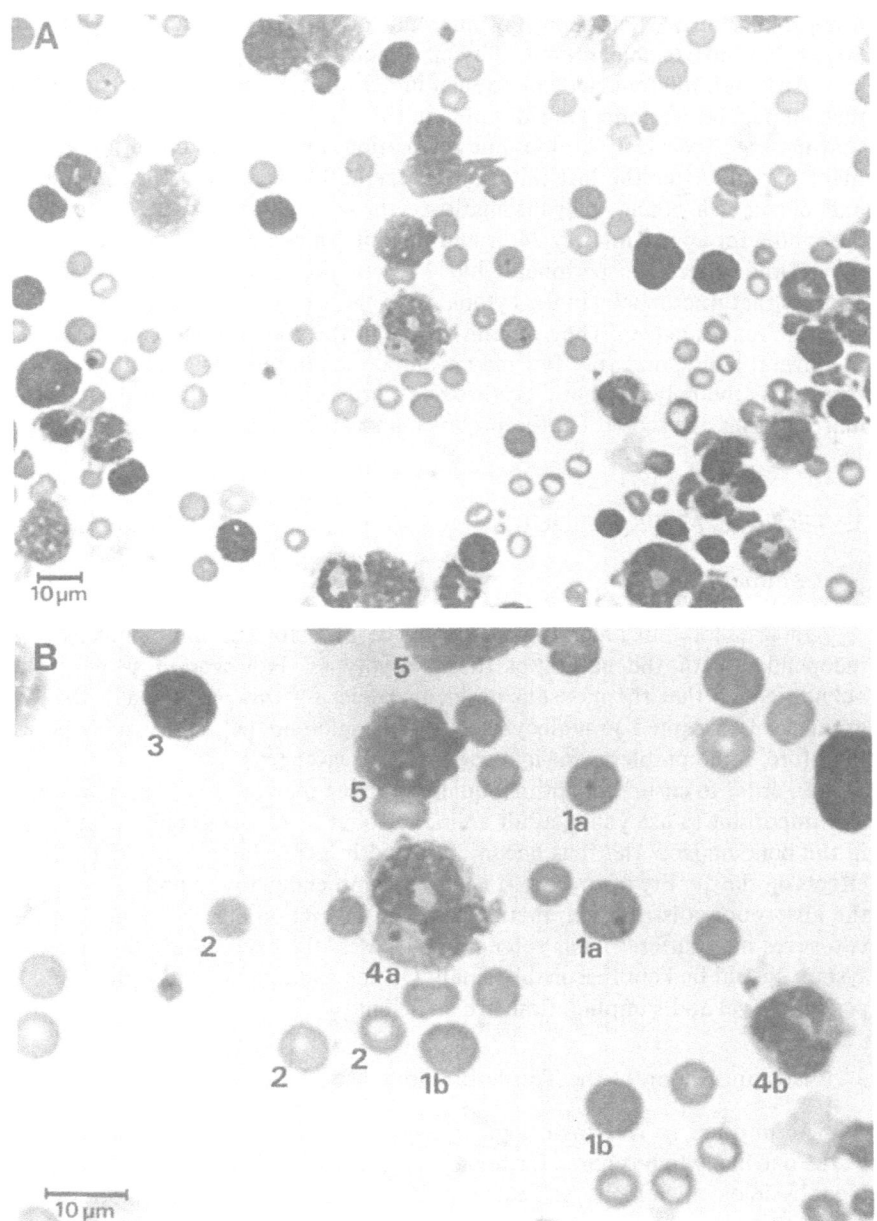

the spindle apparatus by spindle poisons. In such cases the main nucleus is often replaced by whole groups of micronuclei. Such micronuclei may also be larger than micronuclei produced by clastogens.

Although micronuclei can be seen in various types of bone marrow cells, the cell population under consideration in this chapter consists of erythroblasts that undergo their last chromosome replications and mitoses during the treatment period. After the last mitosis, the erythroblast expels its main nucleus and becomes a young, polychromatic erythrocyte. It retains its cytoplasmic basophilia for approximately 24 hr and then becomes a normochromatic erythrocyte and enters the peripheral blood circulation. For unknown reasons it appears that micronuclei in the cytoplasm of these cells are not always expelled with the main nucleus. They remain visible in the polychromatic erythrocytes for several hours, and very few may even be seen in normochromatic erythrocytes. It is the polychromatic erythrocytes, present in large quantities in bone marrow, that are scored for the presence and absence of micronuclei (Figure 1).

3. TECHNICAL PROCEDURE

3.1. Animals

In principle, all animal species may be used for the micronucleus test, independently of the nature of their karyotypes. However, it is generally acknowledged that the mouse is an ideal species for this purpose. (In the rat, granula of disrupted granulocytes resemble micronuclei; this species poses, therefore, some problems for inexperienced researchers.)

In order to ensure an optimal quality of bone-marrow smear preparations, it is important to use young adult animals, about 8–15 weeks old, as fat tissue in the bone marrow that has accumulated with increasing age has deleterious effects on the quality of smears. It is also recommended to use both sexes, since the absorption, distribution, metabolism, and excretion of a compound in the two sexes may differ.[25] For screening purposes, the expenditure of the assay system should be kept reasonably small. On the average, four to eight animals per dose level and sampling time are sufficient.

3.2. Administration of the Test Substance

As in other *in vivo* toxicological assays, the administration route should be the one likely to be chosen for humans, usually the oral one for medicines.[26] Nonphysiological vehicles/solvents must be avoided since quite often they are more toxic than the test compound in question. If a test agent is insoluble in physiological saline, it is suspended in 2% gelatin or a similar vehicle. Mice receive a single or double administration by stomach tube at a volume of 25 ml/kg body weight. It is no handicap to suspend a compound instead of dissolving it as long as resorption can be demonstrated either by measuring its toxicity or its simple kinetics. In order to enhance the yield of effects in test systems that utilize proliferating tissues such as bone marrow, two types of experiments can be used with about equal success.

One is to apply the test agent twice or several times in order to ensure that the mitoses are attacked in different phases. Bone marrow smears are then usually prepared at one particular sampling time, e.g., 6 or 24 hr after the last application. The other method is to use a single or double application; the bone marrow is then sampled at various times (see Section 3.4).

3.3. Determination of Dosage

Positive findings in a micronucleus test are not relevant when animals die of a too high dosage. The procedure described below to determine the dosage has been proven useful and it is also widely accepted. Dose levels can best be selected on the basis of toxicity tests. For this purpose the researcher can choose between either a LD_{50}/LD_5 determination or a simple determination of the lowest lethal dose. Therefore an LD_5 or a dose near the lowest lethal dose may be selected as the highest dose level for a micronucleus test, while one-tenth of this dose and the logarithmic middle point between the two may serve as the low and mid doses, respectively. Thus, in each experiment, three dose levels are used, as well as a negative control in which animals receive only the plain vehicle. Since the reproducibility of results within a given laboratory is usually excellent, it may not always be necessary to use a positive control (mutagen) in each experiment. Studies also using mutagens should, however, be done at regular time intervals.

3.4. Sampling Times

The yield of micronucleated erythrocytes produced by a mutagen depends on various features of the test compound and test system. Its maximum frequency may occur at various time intervals after treatment, depending on the following, among other factors:

1. Metabolic activation/detoxification
2. Mode of action of the test compound or metabolites on chromosomes or spindle apparatus
3. Cytotoxicity/toxicity versus mutagenicity
4. Dose levels and number of applications

5. Maturation of the polychromatic erythrocytes into normocytes
6. Enucleation of the erythroblast and disappearance of the micronuclei in the polychromatic erythrocytes or normocytes

It has been amply demonstrated by Schmid and coworkers,[9-11,13-15] and Salamone et al.,[27] that the maximum frequency of micronucleated polychromatic erythrocytes can be reached anywhere between about 12 and 72 hr after a single application, or 6–48 hr after the last of a series of applications, depending on the substance. Researchers have, consequently, used different types of test protocols. It must be remembered, however, that their development was based on retrospective screening, that is, the researchers used known mutagens. It is obvious that, ideally, test protocols should be adapted to the particular features of a test compound and, finally, each chemical substance should have its specific test protocol. However, for prospective testing of chemical substances for which no information is yet available, except perhaps their acute toxicity, the only way to deal with this problem is to standardize the test protocol and use the simplest one, especially if the researcher is faced with large numbers of test substances (see Section 3.9).

One should also remember that in the field of prospective testing using short-term tests the primary interest lies in qualitative answers, i.e., the identification of a substance as a mutagen (yes/no). Quantitative aspects are almost impossible to study by means of test systems that involve proliferating tissues since the slightest deviation from a given test protocol will have an influence on the yield of effects, i.e., the shape of the dose–response curve.

3.5. Preparation of the Bone Marrow Smears

The animals are killed by cervical dislocation under CO_2 anesthesia. Both femora are removed by cutting through the pelvic bones and tibia below the knee. The femora are freed of muscle tissues and cut with scissors at both ends until a small opening to the marrow canal becomes visible. A needle fitted to a 1-ml plastic syringe containing 1 ml of fetal calf serum (FCS) is then inserted a few millimeters from the distal end of the femur into the bone marrow canal. The marrow is flushed into a small centrifuge tube containing 2 ml of FCS. Bone marrow of both femora of one animal are pooled. The tube is then centrifuged at 1000 rpm for 5 min and the supernatant removed with a Pasteur pipette. Cells in the sediment are gently stirred with a Pasteur pipette. A small drop of the viscous suspension thus obtained is put on a microscope slide and a smear made according to the conventional hematological method.[13] The quality of the staining must make it possible to differentiate between polychromatic and normochromatic erythrocytes. It is mandatory that the erythrocytes preserve their original morphology. This is the reason the processing of the bone marrow is done in FCS.

The bone marrow smears are air-dried. If drying is too slow, especially with thickly spread slides, the morphology of the erythrocytes can be altered. These drying artifacts can make scoring more difficult. The staining is done in conventional staining glass jars as follows:

- 5 min in pure ethanol
- 3 min in 5% May–Grünwald stain diluted with pure ethanol
- 2 min in 50% May–Grünwald stain diluted with Sorensen's phosphate buffer pH 6.8
- 10 min in 14% Giemsa stain diluted with Sorensen's phosphate buffer pH 6.7
- 10 sec in Sorensen's phosphate buffer pH 6.7
- 10 sec in Sorensen's phosphate buffer pH 6.8
- 10 sec in distilled water
- As before, the preparations are air-dried for at least 1 day and then mounted with coverslips.

3.6. Scoring of Micronuclei

The slides are prescreened using 10 × 16 magnification for regions where cells are well spread and optimally stained. Such regions are often located in a zone near the end of the smear. The morphology of the nucleated cells can serve as a criterion for a good-quality slide.

The erythrocytes should be visible separately, be well spread, and not have fuzzy contours. Their staining should be brilliant, yellowish-red for mature erythrocytes and with a strong bluish tint in the young, immature forms, the polychromatic erythrocytes.

We recommend using coded slides to count the micronucleated polychromatic erythrocytes among the polychromatic erythrocytes. About 1000 polychromatic erythrocytes should be scored per animal. At the same time the number of mature erythrocytes should be scored as well (see Section 3.8). The scored element is the number of micronucleated, polychromatic erythrocytes and not the number or micronuclei (Figure 1).

Due to the obvious variability of the cytogenetic parameters from animal to animal, and therefore from experiment to experiment, even within the same laboratory, the use of adequate negative controls cannot be overemphasized. In our laboratory data from negative control animals were therefore collected for several years in order to determine the mean frequencies of spontaneously occurring micronuclei and the variability of these frequencies among single animals. Some of the results of these studies, which show minimal variability, have been published.[28]

The recognition of artifacts is usually not a problem.[13,15] Difficulties can sometimes occur with stain residues. In order not to confuse micronuclei with artifacts, we recommend always registering the micronucleated normochromatic erythrocytes. This is a safeguard, since it can be assumed that artifacts are evenly distributed between polychromatic and normochromatic erythrocytes. An almost equal ratio of micronuclei in these two types of cells is, therefore, an indication of the presence of artifacts.

3.7. Data Evaluation

In our laboratory we evaluate data, after decoding the slides, according to three criteria:

1. The accumulated negative control ranges (normal ranges) found in individual animals and groups
2. Statistical evaluation
3. The presence of a dose–effect relationship

1. One of the negative control studies performed in our laboratory consisted of 144 CD-1 mice (equal numbers of females and males). The range of micronucleated polychromatic erythrocytes in single animals lay between 0% and 0.5% (mean 0.10%). A total of 143 (out of 144) animals had micronucleated polychromatic erythrocytes ranging between 0% and 0.4%. Furthermore, the ranges of the mean values among negative control groups of 36 individual experiments were 0.08–0.3%. Hence, micronucleated polychromatic erythrocytes at the frequencies of 0.4% for single animals and 0.3% for individual groups were taken as the upper limits of the normal values.

2. When the values obtained are above the normal range, they are evaluated statistically using the standard tables of Kastenbaum and Bowman[29] for comparing the negative control group with each of the other treated groups.

3. Data also suggest a drug effect when there is an indication of a dose–effect relationship. However, even if the values obtained show a trend toward dose dependence, they are interpreted as being negative insofar as they lie within the normal range.

It has to be emphasized that these criteria are based on our practical experience and have proved useful. Other evaluation criteria may be used if felt necessary.

A search in the micronucleus test literature reveals that there are a few papers in which the authors could not clearly decide whether the test agent in question was able to induce micronuclei or not. The compound was called "weak," "borderline," "questionably effective," or having "minimal activity." In most of these cases, to our knowledge, a data base on negative historical controls seems to be nonexistent. The authors, therefore, are not aware of the normal fluctuation of results among untreated animals or groups, and thus have difficulties when faced with making a decision.

3.8. Other Useful Information on the Micronucleus Test

Certain substances such as antimetabolites may severely inhibit DNA replication and consequently cause a pronounced reduction in the proportion of polychromatic erythrocytes and nucleated bone-marrow cells. Such a finding may not be paralleled by an increase in micronucleated erythrocytes. Potential chromosome damage may reveal itself only after the release of the blocked cells.

This means that the compound in question, although judged negative in the standard micronucleus test, may be able to damage chromosomes.[13] By initiating a new experiment using different sampling times or lower dose levels one could expect to find micronuclei.

This example demonstrates that the experienced researcher should keep his or her eyes open and carefully study the general appearance of the bone marrow smear, the ratio of polychromatic/normochromatic erythrocytes, etc. In this way a researcher will gain important additional information on the proliferative state of the tissue, the relative cytotoxicity of the compound in question, and perhaps even the cell-cycle specific time of action of the mutagen.[13]

3.9. Manpower and Costs

One of the most widely used test protocols for screening purposes consists of the use of four animals per dose level and sampling time, four dose levels including the negative control, two applications 24 hr apart, bone marrow preparation about 6–48 hr (see Section 3.4) after the second application, and scoring of 1000 polychromatic erythrocytes per animal for the presence of micronuclei.[28] Such an experiment can start on a Monday and the report can be written on Friday of the same week, and involve approximately 40–50 manhours per test substance. The total costs will amount to about $2000–$3000. The experiment can be performed by one or two well-trained technicians working under the close supervision of a scientist.

4. RESULTS AND COMPARATIVE STUDIES

Most of the micronucleus test results obtained so far are summarized in several review articles.[20,22,24,30] They show that clastogens and spindle poisons are clearly detectable in this assay.

The micronucleus test compares favorably with the classical cytogenetic methods or the SCE (sister chromatid exchange) *in vivo* assay.[13,28,31−34] It is noteworthy that some anticancer chemotherapeutics cause micronuclei at therapeutic dose levels. This indicates that a positive found in this test is, indeed, a serious concern, especially if it occurs at a similar or low multiple of the human exposure level.

Scientists frequently raise the question of whether bone marrow behaves the same way as germ cells do when treated with a mutagen. They fear that a substance causing no effect in the micronucleus test could still cause chromosome aberrations or spindle damage in germ cells or vice versa. No such substance is known, according to the published evidence. However, since chemical substances are hardly ever evenly distributed among all organs, it is to be expected that the yield of effects from the bone marrow and germ cells would differ quantitatively.

It is self-evident that the micronucleus test does not compare favorably with test systems that measure end points other than chromosome aberrations or genome mutations. Several known carcinogens and Ames-positive substances cannot be detected by the micronucleus test (for review see de Serres and Ashby[35]). Furthermore, not all substances that produce sperm abnormalities in mice can be detected by the micronucleus test.[20]

These findings clearly emphasize the need to use other test systems in conjunction with the micronucleus test in order to detect as many mutagens as possible.

5. RELATED ASSAY SYSTEMS

This chapter has so far dealt with the bone marrow micronucleus test. The "nucleus anomaly test" as developed by Müller et al.[17] may be regarded as an extension of the micronucleus test in that bone marrow smears are also scored for other types of nuclear damage in various types of bone marrow cells. This assay system has not found wide application because it is more time-consuming than the micronucleus test and requires extensive knowledge of bone marrow pathology. It is exactly these difficulties, recognized earlier by Schmid and co-workers,[9−11] that triggered the development of the more practical micronucleus test.

A further application of the micronucleus test is in animal embryos. Cole et al.[36,37] have demonstrated the possibility of utilizing livers and peripheral blood for the determination of micronuclei in embryos of mothers who have been treated with clastogens and spindle poisons. Thus, the effects produced in embryos can be compared with those found in the bone marrow of mothers in order to gain information on transplacental effects of clastogens and spindle poisons.

Although peripheral blood in embryos can be monitored easily due to its peculiar hemopoietic system, attempts to use peripheral blood instead of bone marrow in adult animals have not produced clear-cut results. MacGregor et al.[38] claim that this system works, while other researchers have so far failed in these attempts (B. E. Matter and W. Schmid, unpublished). Therefore, more work is required to clarify the situation.

The bone-marrow micronucleus test can also be applied to humans.[39-41] For this purpose, bone marrow aspirates from patients receiving chemotherapeutic treatment with cytostatic drugs for life-threatening diseases are studied for the presence of micronuclei. A considerable drawback of this method is that for ethical reasons it is not possible to obtain bone-marrow aspirates from untreated persons to be used as negative controls.

As mentioned in the introduction, the micronucleus test can, in principle, be applied to all tissues and cells, in vivo or in vitro, that undergo natural or artificial (by means of a mitogen) mitosis. The test also seems to work in various systems, as shown in reports describing the effects of chemical substances in plants,[8,42,43] lymphocytes,[23,44] spermatids,[45] and hepatocytes.[46]

6. ADVANTAGES

1. The micronucleus test is simpler and more practical than conventional cytogenetic (metaphase) methods. The results of both methods correlate well.
2. It can be done in all laboratory mammalian species independently of the nature of the karyotype.
3. It is an in vivo test that takes metabolism into account.
4. It detects chromosome-breaking agents (clastogens) and spindle poisons and is thus able to detect more types of genotoxic effects than metaphase methods. If the micronucleus test is used in this context, the false positive and false negative ratio is very low.
5. It is highly predictive for humans. Anticancer cytostatic drugs induce micronuclei in mammals and humans at therapeutic dose levels. Positive results, therefore, suggest direct mutagenic hazards to humans.
6. Virtually unlimited numbers of scorable cells are available, and the background level of micronuclei is low. From a statistical point of view the test therefore has advantages over classical cytogenetic methods.
7. It is an established method used in many laboratories worldwide. Approximately 70 publications on more than 200 chemical substances can be found in the literature.

7. LIMITATIONS

1. The micronucleus test does not necessarily detect mutagens that (a) act tissue/cell-specifically, (b) do not reach the target cells in sufficient con-

centrations to damage chromosomes or spindle fibers, (c) induce point/ gene mutations only, (d) are strongly cytotoxic, or (e) are toxic to the animals themselves, thereby masking mutagenic effects. Therefore the test system may not be the first choice for the screening of carcinogens.

2. The micronucleus test does not readily distinguish among different types of chromosomal aberrations or modes of action of the test agent (clastogens versus spindle poisons).

3. It is based on a proliferating tissue, which means that quantitative aspects (e.g., shapes of dose–response curves) are difficult to interpret.

It is noteworthy that most of these limitations apply also to other *in vivo* tests for chromosome aberrations (SCE, etc.).

8. APPLICATION OF THE MICRONUCLEUS TEST

As already discussed, the micronucleus test was developed in order to facilitate the work of cytogeneticists confronted (1) with inherent problems of conventional metaphase methods and (2) with high numbers of substances to be tested within a given time period. Research work over the past 12 years has shown that the micronucleus test fulfills these prerequisites; it is a very useful method for prospective screening and identification of compounds that damage the chromosome complement. Results may thus serve as a basis for decision-making as to whether or not further tests with more laborious techniques, e.g., metaphase methods, the dominant lethal test, or the heritable translocation test, are necessary. In other words, the micronucleus test can indeed substitute for some of these classical, more time-consuming *in vivo* mammalian methods to identify substances with potential to damage chromosomes or the genome as a whole.

This test method should not be used in isolation to fulfill objectives other than those mentioned above. It must be used in conjunction with other tests for the identification of mutagens or carcinogens in general (battery or tier approach). Scientists should always keep in mind that the test methods should be selected according to the objectives, and not vice versa.

Researchers interested in this test system may obtain further information from a recently published illustrated course.[47]

REFERENCES

1. H. J. Evans, in: *Chemical Mutagens: Principles and Methods for Their Detection* (A. Hollaender, ed.), Vol. 4, pp. 1–29, Plenum Press, New York (1976).
2. M. M. Cohen and K. Hirschhorn, in: *Chemical Mutagens: Principles and Methods for Their Detection* (A. Hollaender, ed.), Vol. 2, pp. 515–534, Plenum Press, New York (1971).

3. H. Brenneke, Strahlenschädigung von Mäuse- und Rattensperma, beobachtet an der Frühentwicklung der Eier, *Strahlentherapie 60*, 214–238 (1937).

4. K. Mather, The experimental determination of the time of chromosome doubling, *Proc. R. Soc. Lond. B 124*, 97–106 (1937).

5. J. M. Thoday, The effect of ionizing radiations on the broad bean root. Part IX. Chromosome breakage and the lethality of ionizing radiations to the root meristem, *Br. J. Radiol. 24*, 572–576 (1951).

6. J. M. Thoday, The effect of ionizing radiations on the broad bean root. Part IX. (Concluded), *Br. J. Radiol. 24*, 622–628 (1951).

7. L. B. Russell and W. E. Russell, Pathways of radiation effects in the mother and the embryo, *Cold Spring Harbor Symp. Quant. Biol. 19*, 50–59 (1954).

8. H. J. Evans, G. J. Neary, and F. S. Williamson, The relative biological efficiency of single doses of fast neutrons and gamma-rays on vicia faba roots and the effect of oxygen. Part II. Chromosome damage: The production of micronuclei, *Int. J. Radiat. Biol. 1*, 216–229 (1959).

9. K. Boller and W. Schmid, Chemische Mutagenese beim Säuger. Das Knochenmark des Chinesischen Hamsters als *in vivo*-Testsystem. Hämatologische Befunde nach Behandlung mit Trenimon, *Humangenetik 11*, 35–54 (1970).

10. B. E. Matter and W. Schmid, Trenimon-induced chromosomal damage in bone marrow cells of six mammalian species, evaluated by the micronucleus test, *Mutat. Res. 12*, 417–425 (1971).

11. M. Von Ledebur and W. Schmid, The micronucleus test. Methodological aspects, *Mutat. Res. 19*, 109–117 (1973).

12. B. E. Matter, I. Jaeger, and J. Grauwiler, The relationship between the doses of various chemical mutagens required to induce micronuclei in mouse bone marrow and their lethal doses, *Proc. Eur. Soc. Study Drug Toxic. 15*, 275–279 (1973).

13. W. Schmid, Chemical mutagen testing on *in vivo* somatic mammalian cells, *Agents Actions 3/2*, 77–85 (1973).

14. W. Schmid, The micronucleus test, *Mutat. Res. 31*, 9–15 (1975).

15. W. Schmid, in: *Chemical Mutagens: Principles and Methods for Their Detection* (A. Hollaender, ed.), Vol. 4, pp. 31–53, Plenum Press, New York (1976).

16. V. Smoliar, Cinétique des micronoyaux du rein après irradiation et néphrectomie unilatérale. Effet de la cystamine, *Int. J. Radiat. Biol. 16*, 227–231 (1969).

17. D. Müller, M. Langauer, R. Rathenberg, F. F. Strasser, and R. Hess, 40. Mikrokerntest sowie Chromosomenuntersuchungen an somatischen und gonosomalen Zellen des Chinesischen Hamsters nach Cyclophosphamidgabe, *Verh. Dtsch. Ges. Pathol. 56*, 381–384 (1972).

18. J. A. Heddle, A rapid *in vivo* test for chromosomal damage, *Mutat. Res. 18*, 187–190 (1973).

19. J. J. Roberts and J. E. Sturrock, Enhancement by caffeine of N-methyl-N-nitrosourea-induced mutations and chromosome abberations in Chinese hamster cells, *Mutat. Res. 20*, 243–255 (1973).

20. W. R. Bruce and J. A. Heddle, The mutagenic activity of 61 agents as determined by the micronucleus, *Salmonella*, and sperm abnormality assays, *Can. J. Genet. Cytol. 21*, 319–334 (1979).

21. D. Jenssen and C. Ramel, The micronucleus test as part of a short-term mutagenicity program for the prediction of carcinogenicity evaluated by 143 agents tested, *Mutat. Res. 75*, 191–202 (1980).

22. B. E. Matter and D. Wild, in: *Comparative chemical mutagenesis* (F. J. de Serres and M. D. Shelby, eds.), pp. 657–679, Plenum Press, New York (1981).

23. J. A. Heddle, A. S. Raj, and A. B. Krepinsky, in: *Short-Term Tests for Chemical Carcinogens* (H. F. Stich and R. H. C. San, eds.), pp. 250–254, Springer, New York (1981).

24. J. A. Heddle, M. Hite, B. Kirkhart, K. Mavournin, J. T. MacGregor, G. W. Newell, and M. F. Salamone, The induction of micronuclei as a measure of genotoxicity, *Mutat. Res. 123*, 61–118 (1983).

25. M. Henry, S. Lupo, and K. T. Szabo, Sex difference in sensitivity to the cytogenetic effects of ethyl methanesulfonate in mice demonstrated by the micronucleus test, *Mutat. Res. 69*, 385–387 (1980).

26. Committee on Toxicology, in: *Principles and Procedures for Evaluating the Toxicity of Household Substances*, Publication 1138, p. 2, National Academy of Sciences, Washington, D.C. (1978).

27. M. Salamone, J. Heddle, E. Stuart, and M. Katz, Towards an improved micronucleus test. Studies on 3 model agents, mitomycin C, cyclophosphamide and dimethylbenzanthracene, *Mutat. Res. 74*, 347–356 (1980).

28. B. E. Matter, Failure to detect chromosome damage in bone-marrow cells of mice and Chinese hamsters exposed *in vivo* to some ergot derivates, *J. Int. Med. Res. 4*, 382–392 (1976).

29. M. A. Kastenbaum and K. O. Bowman, Tables for determining the statistical significance of mutation frequencies, *Mutat. Res. 9*, 527–549 (1970).

30. D. Jenssen and C. Ramel, Factors affecting the induction of micronuclei at low doses of X-rays, MMS and dimethylnitrosamine in mouse erythroblasts, *Mutat. Res. 58*, 51–65 (1978).

31. T. Tsuchimoto and B. E. Matter, Comparison of micronucleus test and chromosome examination in detecting potential chromosome mutagens, *Mutat. Res. 46*, 240 (1977).

32. T. Tsuchimoto and B. E. Matter, *In vivo* cytogenetic screening methods for mutagens, with special reference to the micronucleus test, *Arch. Toxicol. 42*, 239–248 (1979).

33. B. E. Matter and T. Tsuchimoto, Mutagenicity test systems for the detection of chromosome aberrations *in vivo*, *Arch. Toxicol. 46*, 89–98 (1980).

34. A. S. Raj and J. A. Heddle, Simultaneous detection of chromosomal aberrations and sister-chromatid exchanges. Experience with DNA intercalating agents, *Mutat. Res. 78*, 253–260 (1980).

35. J. F. de Serres and J. Ashby, *Evaluation of Short-Term Tests for Carcinogens* (Report of the international collaborative program), Elsevier/North-Holland, Amsterdam (1981).

36. R. J. Cole, N. A. Taylor, J. Cole, and C. F. Arlett, Transplacental effects of chemical mutagens detected by the micronucleus test, *Nature 277*, 317–318 (1979).

37. R. J. Cole, N. A. Taylor, J. Cole, and C. F. Arlett, Short-term tests for transplacentally active carcinogens. I. Micronucleus formation in fetal and maternal mouse erythroblasts, *Mutat. Res. 80*, 141–157 (1981).

38. J. T. MacGregor, C. M. Wehr, and D. H. Gould, Clastogen-induced micronuclei in peripheral blood erythrocytes: The basis of an improved micronucleus test, *Environ. Mutagen. 2*, 509–514 (1980).

39. M. Krogh Jensen and M. S. Hüttel, Assessment of the effect of azathioprine on human bone marrow cells *in vivo*, combining chromosome studies and the micronucleus test, *Dan. Med. Bull. 23*, 152–154 (1976).

40. M. Krogh Jensen, Cytogenetic findings in pernicious anaemia. Comparison between results obtained with chromosome studies and the micronucleus test, *Mutat. Res. 45*, 249–252 (1977).

41. M. Krogh Jensen, G. G. Rasmussen, and S. Ingeberg, Cytogenetic studies in patients treated with penicillamine, *Mutat. Res. 67*, 357–359 (1979).

42. K. Linnainmaa, T. Meretoja, M. Sorsa, and H. Vainio, Cytogenetic effects of styrene and styrene oxide, *Mutat. Res. 58*, 277–286 (1978).

43. T. Ma, A. H. Sparrow, L. A. Schairer, and A. F. Nauman, Effect of 1,2-dibromoethane on meiotic chromosomes of *Tradescantia*, *Mutat. Res. 53*, 112–113 (1978).
44. P. Countryman and J. Heddle, A true microculture technique for human lymphocytes, *Hum. Genet. 35*, 197–200 (1977).
45. J. Lähdetie and M. Parvinen, Meiotic micronuclei induced by X-rays in early spermatids of the rat, *Mutat. Res. 81*, 103–115 (1981).
46. A. D. Tates, I. Neuteboom, M. Hofker, and L. den Engelse, A micronucleus technique for detecting clastogenic effects of mutagens/carcinogens (DEN, DMN) in hepatocytes of rat liver *in vivo, Mutat. Res. 74*, 11–20 (1980).
47. B. E. Matter, Test systems in mutagenicity: the micronucleus test; in: *Lectures in Toxicology*, number 10 (G. Zbinden, ed.), pp. 1–5, Pergamon Press, Oxford (1981).

10

The Identification of Somatic Mutations in Immunoglobulin Expression and Structure

DONALD J. ZACK AND MATTHEW D. SCHARFF

1. INTRODUCTION

Naturally occurring and induced mutations have played a major role in molecular biology. In bacteria, mutants provided the crucial insights into the regulation of gene expression and have been used to define the biosynthetic pathways of macromolecules. Mutants in both bacterial and animal viruses have made it possible to define their interactions with host cells and to identify and map the functions that they perform. Naturally occurring mutations and polymorphisms have made it possible to map many of the genes in higher organisms. While the genetic and structural complexity and long division time of animal cells has made it more difficult to establish useful genetic systems, the very complexity of such cells demands that molecular genetics be used if we are ever to fully understand how they function.

In recent years, a number of somatic-cell genetic systems have been established with animal cells. Among these, cultured cells producing large amounts of immunoglobulin have several unique characteristics. Cultured mouse myeloma and hybridoma cells are neoplastic cells that synthesize large amounts of antibody and secrete it into the medium. This means that 20–100 μg of mutant protein can be obtained from 1 ml of medium. If more is needed, mutant cells can be injected into animals and hundreds of milligrams of mutant gene prod-

DONALD J. ZACK AND MATTHEW D. SCHARFF • Department of Cell Biology, Albert Einstein College of Medicine, Bronx, New York 10461.

ucts can be obtained from the serum or ascites fluid of tumor-bearing animals.[1] Since the complete structure and function of many antibody molecules have been determined,[2] mutant gene products can be easily identified and their phenotype established. Spontaneous variants occur at rates of 10^{-3}–10^{-4}/cell per generation and in some instances the frequency of mutation can be increased 10- to 20-fold with mutagenesis.[3–5] With such frequent mutations, it is not absolutely necessary to have selective techniques. Since the immunoglobulin molecule itself is not required for cell viability or proliferation, many different types of mutants are tolerated by the cell. The immunoglobulin genes have been extensively studied and the molecular mechanisms of mutation can be determined. Finally, this is one of the few somatic-cell genetic systems based on a differentiated or luxury function, and it could provide insights into the regulation of differentiation not otherwise available.

In addition to their usefulness in studying the molecular genetics of antibody production, the identification of mutants with changes in antibody structure provides an opportunity to extend our knowledge of the structural basis of antigen binding and of effector functions such as the fixation of complement and the binding to Fc receptors on phagocytic and other cells. With the increasing use of monoclonal antibodies, the generation of mutants may make it possible to improve the usefulness of monoclonal antibodies both as diagnostic reagents and in passive immunization and drug targeting.[6] The quantitative analysis of immunoglobulin mutants may also prove suitable for the screening of potentially mutagenic and carcinogenic agents.

In the sections that follow, we will briefly review the essential features of the structure of antibodies and the organization of the genes that code for them. We will then review some of the methods that have been used to induce and identify mutants in mouse myeloma and hybridoma cells. Finally, the phenotypes of the mutants that have been identified will be summarized and a few of the better-characterized mutants will be described.

2. IMMUNOGLOBULIN PROTEIN AND GENE STRUCTURE

A typical antibody molecule is composed of two identical light (L) and two identical heavy (H) chains joined together by disulfide bonds (Figure 1). Amino acid sequence analysis of numerous H and L chains produced by myeloma, hybridoma, and normal cells reveals extensive sequence variability in the amino-terminal 110–115 amino acids (open area, Figure 1) and even greater variability in the hypervariable regions.[7] In contrast, the carboxy-terminal (cross-hatched area, Figure 1) parts of the heavy and light chains are highly conserved. These findings led to the suggestion that the variable (V) regions

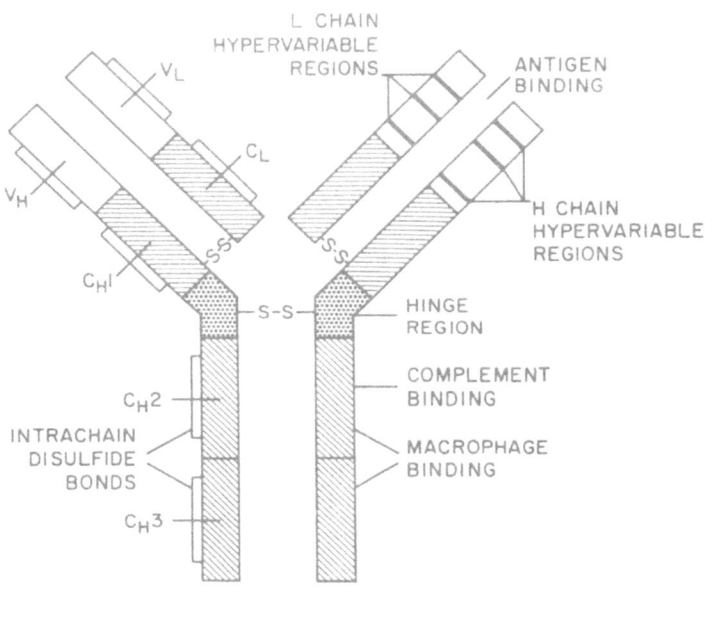

Figure 1. Schematic representation of a typical antibody molecule. The cross-hatched and dotted areas represent the constant regions; the clear areas represent the variable regions. V_L, C_L, V_H, C_H1, C_H2, and C_H3, designate the light-chain variable region, light-chain constant region, heavy-chain variable region, and first, second, and third heavy-chain constant regions, respectively. (Reprinted with permission from *CRC Critical Reviews in Immunology*.[78])

are coded for by hundreds to thousands of genes, while constant (C) regions are coded for by only about 10 different genes.

These differences in sequence variability are associated with different functions. The V regions react with antigen, with the hypervariable regions forming the actual antigen binding site.[8] The H-chain C region determines the class and subclass (IgM, IgA, IgG, etc.) of the antibody and is responsible for the various effector functions, such as complement fixation and binding to the Fc receptors on phagocytic cells. Most species produce two classes of L chains, κ and λ, which have distinctly different C and V regions.

The genetic and evolutionary difficulties in generating and maintaining sequence diversity in one part of a polypeptide chain while maintaining constancy in the other part led Dreyer and Bennett to suggest that the immunoglobulin V and C regions are separately encoded in the germ-line DNA.[9] Molecular genetic studies during the last several years have amply confirmed and extended the Dreyer–Bennett hypothesis. The κ, λ, and H chains are each encoded by a separate multigene family. In the germ line, the L chain consists of four noncontiguous gene elements—signal sequence (S), variable (V_L), joining (J_L), and constant (C_L) (see Figure 2, but note that for simplicity the signal sequence element is not shown).[10] During lymphocyte differentiation a DNA rearrangement occurs that brings together a particular V_L exon and a particular J_L exon (for instance, V_κ and J_2 in Figure 2).[10,11] The remaining intervening sequences between S and $V_L J_L$ and between $V_L J_L$ and C_L are not removed at the DNA level but rather by RNA splicing. The DNA rearrangement mechanism permits both great diversity and constancy by allowing the combinatorial joining of hundreds of V_κ genes with one of four J_κ genes (in the mouse) and one C_κ gene. Furthermore, the DNA joining mechanism is flexible, thus providing for further sequence diversity at the V_κ–J_κ junction.[12] There is also evidence for a somatic mutational process that can introduce point mutations within the V region.[13–16] The mechanism for formation of an active H-

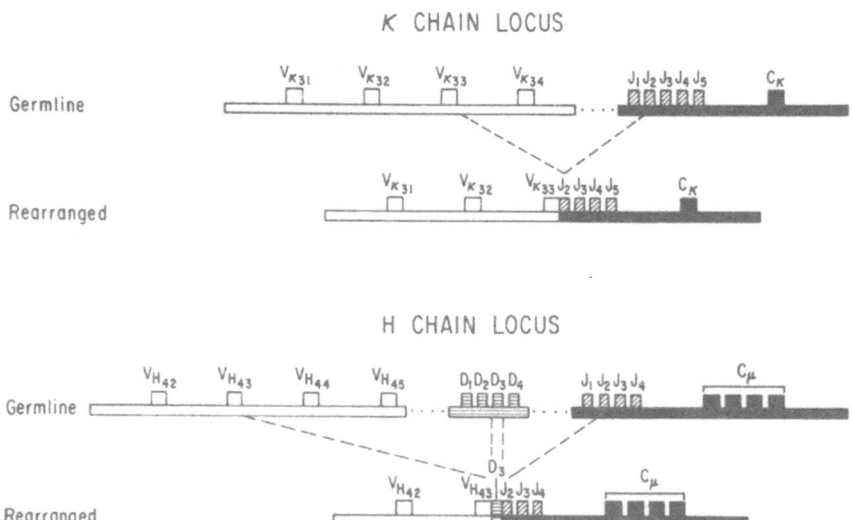

Figure 2. Somatic rearrangement of germ-line immunoglobulin genes leading to the formation of an active complex. The numbering of the V regions and D_H segments is for illustrative purposes only because the actual numbers are unknown. (Modified from Adams.[105])

chain gene is similar except that it involves an extra gene element, the diversity (D) segment (see Figure 2).[17] The V_L-J_L and $V_H-D_H-J_H$ joining are thought to be mediated by DNA deletions guided by complementary sequences on the 3' side of V, the 5' side of J, and both sides of D.[18,19]

In general, at any one time an individual B-lymphocyte makes only one species of antibody, with a single L-chain V region and a single H-chain V region. During differentiation, the first H-chain C region expressed is μ (IgM). Subsequently, a "class switch" can occur in which the same V region is expressed with a new H-chain constant region.[20] For instance, switching from a μ gene to a γ_3 gene would result in synthesis of an IgG_3 molecule instead of an IgM. Cloning studies have shown that the H-chain C-region genes are arranged tandemly on an approximately 100-kb region of DNA in the order μ, δ, γ_3, γ_1, γ_{2b}, γ_{2a}, ϵ, and α,[10,21,22] Evidence suggests that, except for μ and δ double expression, which may be mediated by a splicing mechanism,[23,24] switching involves DNA deletion between so-called switch sequences, which results in moving the new C region closer to the expressed V region.[25,26]

3. METHODS FOR THE ISOLATION OF MUTANTS

3.1. Mutagenesis

Methods for the mutagenesis of myeloma and hybridoma cells are similar to those that have been used for other cultured mammalian cells. Since different cell lines vary in their sensitivity to mutagenic agents, killing curves have to be carried out with each cell line. Although the number of mutants analyzed is still small and only high-frequency events have been analyzed, mutagenesis does not appear to increase the spectrum of phenotypes. The frequency of mutants is increased by the acridine half-mustard ICR-191 (0.0625–4.0 g/ml),[4,5] the phenylanine mustard Melphalan (0.2–0.8 μg/ml),[27] and nitrosoguanidine (0.025–2.0 μg/ml).[4] It is particularly interesting that Melphalan is mutagenic in this system since it is also one of the primary therapeutic agents used in the treatment of multiple myeloma in humans. Ethylmethanesulfonate (EMS) (50–300 μg/ml) did not increase the frequency of mutants in one cell line[4] but did in another that had a lower frequency of spontaneous mutants. (See Table I.) In most of the studies reported, cells were incubated with mutagen in complete growth medium for 24 hr, washed, and resuspended in mutagen-free medium for at least 24 hr before being analyzed for mutants. Recent studies with other somatic-cell genetic systems suggest that longer expression times may be desirable.[28] In addition, since nitrosoguanidine is unstable in serum-containing medium, more reproducible mutagenesis can be achieved by treating for 2–4 hr in serum-free medium.[29]

Table I
Effect of Mutagens on the Incidence of Heavy-Chain Nonsecreting Mutants.[a]

Cell line	Mutagen	Dose (μg/ml)	Percentage of cell survival	Incidence of variants[b]	Percentage	Ref.
MPC-11	ICR-191	0	100	18/2104	0.86	4
		1	60	25/3635	1.54	
		2	25	110/3404	3.24	
		4	<1	15/229	6.55	
MPC-11	Melphalan	0	100	17/3777	0.45	27
		0.2	32	31/2336	1.33	
		0.4	28	100/5926	1.69	
		0.6	16	55/2961	1.86	
		0.8	9	31/1298	2.39	
MPC-11	Nitrosoguanidine	0	100	29/4993	0.58	4
		0.25	90	46/3828	1.21	
		0.5	68	33/4332	0.76	
		1.0	33	14/2404	0.58	
		2.0	8	10/1977	0.51	
MPC-11	Ethylmethanesulfonate	0	100	13/2168	0.60	4
		50	85	13/1594	0.81	
		100	45	10/1288	0.80	
		200	13	4/721	0.55	
Y5606	Ethylmethanesulfonate	0	100	15/4167	0.36	5
		100	69	35/4124	0.82	
		200	19	24/2806	0.86	
		300	5	40/3598	1.14	

[a]Frequencies were measured by the immunoplate assay (see Section 3.2.1).
[b]Number of unstained per total.

Some of the mutagens are difficult to dissolve. Melphalan [p-di-(2-chloroethyl)amino-lL-phenylalanine from Burroughs Wellcome] is prepared as a stock solution of 0.2–1.0 μg/ml in polyethylene glycol.[27] Nitrosoguanidine (N-methyl-N'-nitro-N-nitrosoguanidine from K and K Laboratories, Plainview, NY) is made up as a stock solution of 100–200 μg/ml in 0.1 M sodium acetate, pH 5, and sterilized by filtration through a Millex filter. It can be stored for at least several months at −70°C.[30] Aliquots are thawed and used immediately.

One of the major problems in studying quantitative mutagenesis is the high spontaneous rate of mutation of the immunoglobulin genes in many mouse myeloma and hybridoma cell lines (see Section 4). The only solution currently available is to use a relatively stable cell line, to screen fresh subclones for ones that have not accumulated many spontaneous mutants, and then to use those subclones quickly. Since many of the assays used involve negative identification rather than positive selection (see Section 3.2), the high background and the need to characterize all of the putative mutants makes this a difficult system for quantitative mutagenesis. Some of the newer approaches that will be described below may overcome these difficulties and make this a more useful system for evaluating mutagenic agents in animal cells.

3.2. Screening Techniques

Due to the frequency with which mutants arise in cultured mouse myeloma and hybridoma cells, it is possible to isolate mutants by brute force screening. In one such tour de force, Milstein and his colleagues uncovered four mutants producing structurally altered immunoglobulins by isoelectric focusing the radiolabeled secretions of 7000 subclones of the IgG_1-producing P_3 cell line.[31,32] However, several approaches have been devised that make it possible to screen for mutants more easily and a few investigators have begun to use selective methods. Those techniques that are used in our own laboratory will be described in somewhat more detail but we will only include methodological details when these have not been published elsewhere.

3.2.1. Immunoplate Assay

The immunoplate assay was one of the first methods used to detect mouse myeloma mutants.[3,4,33,34] In essence, cells are cloned in soft agarose over feeder layers. Antibody against the immunoglobulin that is secreted by the cells is added to the plate and diffuses through the agarose. The immunoglobulin secreted by the clone of myeloma cells precipitates with the antibody and the clone is surrounded by an antigen–antibody precipitate, which is seen as a collection of dark granules and specks under low or medium power with an inverted microscope (Figure 3). Clones that are not surrounded by precipitate are putative variants. If the myeloma or hybridoma is secreting an antibody that reacts with a known antigen, the clones can be overlayed with antigen, which will then react with the secreted antibody.[35] However, antigen precipitate is smaller and more difficult to see than antibody precipitate.

We and others continue to use these assays not only to look for mutants of myeloma and hybridoma cells, but also to clone hybridomas and identify the subclones that are still producing the desired antibody. While this technique has been described previously,[3,33,34] there have been sufficient modifications in the intervening years so that we will describe it in some detail here.

In order to obtain a high efficiency of cloning, rat embryo or other feeder layers are used. The feeder cells should contact-inhibit when they reach confluence so that they do not deplete the nutrients in the medium or produce large amounts of lactic or other acids. They must also provide growth-promoting factors to the hybridoma or myeloma cell line. In our hands, primary rat

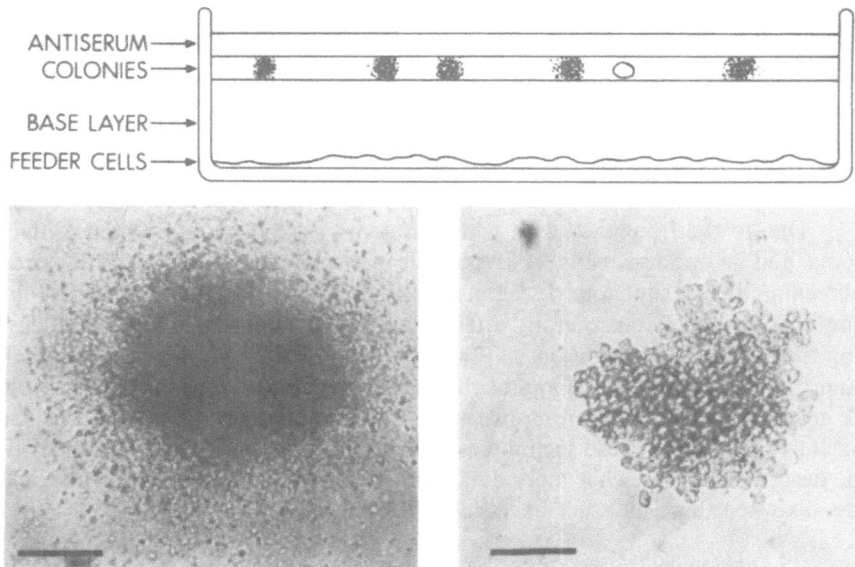

Figure 3. Immunoplate assay with antibody overlay. The left insert shows a stained clone, while that on the right shows an unstained one.

embryo fibroblasts have been effective, although others have used continuous cell lines such as 3T3 or human fibroblasts. The feeders are plated out in 60-mm plastic tissue culture dishes and when they have reached half confluence they are overlayed with 5 ml of growth medium containing approximately 0.4–0.6% of Sea Plaque agarose (Marine Colloids Division, FMC Corp.). While many different types of agarose have been used successfully, Sea Plaque agarose has the benefit of remaining in solution till the temperature is lowered to 19°C. This means that the agarose solution can be maintained at 37°C rather than at 42°C, reducing the chance of killing the cells when they are suspended in the agarose. Once the underlayer of agarose-containing medium has gelled in the cold, the plates are ready to be overlayed with cells.

It is preferable to use myeloma or hybridoma cells when they are in the logarithmic growth phase. The optimum number of clones per plate is between 500 and 1000. Most cell lines that have been in culture for some time clone at efficiencies of 50–100%. However, hybridomas that are only a few weeks old often have lower cloning efficiencies. The myeloma or hybridoma cells are counted and diluted, and one volume of cells is mixed with four volumes of agarose-containing growth medium. One milliter of cells in agarose-containing growth medium is gently distributed over the underlayer on each dish. This means that the cell layer contains a 20% lower concentration of agarose than the underlayer.

The looser the agarose, the better the cloning efficiency. We empirically determine the concentrations to be used for each batch of agarose by making up a stock solution of 5–7% agarose in water, dissolving the agarose by autoclaving, and then determining whether a final solution containing 7, 8, 9, or 10 ml of agarose per 100 ml of growth medium will produce a gel that is so loose that is is almost sloppy but still firm enough to suspend the clones. If the clones do not "vibrate" in the agarose when gently jarred, the agarose is too concentrated. The agarose stock solution (5–7%) should not be autoclaved and reused more than three times.

We clone cells in the type of medium in which they are growing and often provide certain additives to increase cloning efficiency. For example, we routinely use Dulbecco's modified Eagle's medium (DMEM) containing high glucose (H-21, Grand Island Biological Co., GIBCO) supplemented with glutamine, penicillin, and streptomycin (if it is not already present), nonessential amino acids (all 1×, from GIBCO), 10% NCTC 109 (Microbiological Associates), and 10–20% heat-inactivated (56°C for 30 min) fetal calf or horse serum. We screen batches of serum by limiting dilution cloning for ones that will produce the highest cloning efficiency. In some laboratories, perhaps related to the water supply, higher cloning efficiencies can be achieved with commercially available liquid medium than with medium reconstituted from commercial powder. Medium sterilized through a Triton-containing filter will inhibit clones. For example, we use Millex rather than regular millipore filters to sterilize our media. There have been reports that medium exposed to normal fluorescent light is toxic[36] and we have confirmed that shielded medium will sometimes give higher cloning efficiencies. For hardy cell lines, many of these precautions are not necessary.

Once the dishes have been overlayed, they are placed at 4°C on a level surface for a few minutes to solidify and then placed in a CO_2 incubator that is as humid as possible and is equilibrated with 7–8% CO_2. Since it is difficult to prevent some drying of the plates in incubators that are heated by blown air, we use water-jacketed incubators.

Although antibody against the secreted immunoglobulin can be added when the cells are plated, we usually wait 2–3 days until the clones contain 8–16 cells. This allows one to be certain that each dish contains the desired number of clones and that the plates are not contaminated. In addition, the growth of some cells is inhibited by antibody (even in the absence of complement) if the antibody is present at the time of plating. Clones are overlayed with heat-inactivated (56°C for 30 min) antiserum or antigen in 1 ml of agarose-containing medium. The optimum amount of antigen or antibody must be determined empirically for each reagent. However, we make a preliminary estimate of the amount of antiserum needed by lysing 1×10^7 myeloma or hybridoma cells in 50λ of 0.5% NP-40 in isotonic buffer, removing the nuclei by centifugation, and placing the cytoplasmic lysate in the center well of an Ouchterlony plate. Twofold dilutions of the antiserum are then added to the surrounding wells. If the one-fourth dilution of the antiserum still reacts with the lysate, then we add 0.1 ml of antiserum to each plate. If the titer of the antiserum is higher, then proportionately less is added. It is worth noting that antiserum should be filtered before heat inactivation since some antisera either aggregate or are trapped on the filter after being treated at 56°C for 30 min.

If the clones are to be overlayed with antigen, a polyvalent form of the antigen must be used. When antibody is used to detect mutants, each secreted immunoglobulin will precipitate with approximately five antibody molecules. When antigen is used, it will require a number of secreted immunoglobulin molecules to precipitate each antigen molecule. The antigen-induced precipitates are therefore smaller and often difficult to see. We have increased the size of such precipitates by adding a small or subliminal amount of antiimmunoglobulin to the cells when they are plated.[35] The antigen is added 3 days later. While we are not certain why this helps, we think that the antibody slows the diffusion of the secreted immunoglobulin away from the clones, thereby increasing the local concentration of antibody that will react with antigen. It also increases the amount of protein in the precipitate. The amount of sublimal anti-immunoglobulin must be adjusted so that it alone will not produce a visible precipitate with the secreted immunoglobulin when the clones are scored 5–6 days after plating. Obviously, a control with subliminal antibody alone must be included and the antiimmunoglobulin should not contain antibody against the antigen-binding site of the secreted immunoglobulin.

The plates are usually examined for clones that are not surrounded by a visible antigen–antibody precipitate between 6 and 10 days after plating, which is 3–7 days after overlaying with antibody or antigen. In plates that have been overlayed with antibody, as the clones get larger the precipitate surrounding the clones may be solubilized (in antigen excess) by immunoglobulin being secreted by the clone. Since clones continue to grow for 10–14 days, and the larger the clone the more certain one is that it can be recovered, presumptive variants sometimes need to be marked. Marking the dish is useless because the agarose can rotate. We use a technique developed by Dr. Sherie Morrison when she was in this laboratory. Spangles are purchased in a notion store, autoclaved, and gently laid on the agarose next to the presumptive mutants using a fine tweezer.

Desired clones are removed from the agarose using a finely drawn, benttipped Pasteur pipette and gentle mouth-controlled suction. The cells are then deposited in a well of a 96-well tissue culture microtiter dish containing 0.1 ml of medium. If clones from a particular cell line are difficult to recover, we use conditioned medium. In our experience, the best-conditioned medium is identical to the medium in which the clone has been growing. When cloning cells, we therefore prepare some dishes with feeder layers, overlay with agarose, and then overlay the agarose with 5 ml of the medium we are using for cloning. This "conditioned" medium is removed after 24–72 hr, stored at 4°C, and, when the clones are to be recovered, diluted 1:2 or 1:4 with fresh medium. While it would be logical to make conditioned medium from the fibroblasts directly, we have found such medium to inhibit growth. This type of conditioned medium is stable for at least a few weeks at 4°C but not when frozen and thawed.

While this procedure has been used to generate many mutants,[3-5,33-35,37-41] it has some serious drawbacks. First, it is a tedious screening assay, which requires that many wild-type clones be visualized in the microscope for each mutant that is detected. Since no more than 10,000–20,000 clones can be examined in each experiment, only mutants that occur frequently will be identified. Second, in most cases, it is a negative assay, in which a particular clone that is not surrounded by a visible precipitate may have lost the ability to synthesize or secrete either or both of the immunoglobulin polypeptide chains, may be secreting decreased amounts of wild-type immunoglobulin, or may be producing a structurally altered immunoglobulin molecule. This means that every presumptive mutant must be recovered from the agarose and its phenotype determined. In some situations, the assay can be used as a positive method of detecting certain types of mutants. For example, when we were looking for subclones that had switched from producing IgG_{2b} immunoglobulin to IgG_{2a}, we overlayed the clones with antisera specific for the $\gamma2a$ heavy chain and looked for clones that were surrounded by a precipitate. Similarly, when we were looking for revertants of a myeloma that had lost its ability to bind antigen,[35] we overlayed with antigen and found clones that contained an antigen–antibody precipitate around them. We have also made the assay more discriminating by overlaying first with an antiserum that reacts with only one part of the immunoglobulin molecule and then with a more broadly reactive antiserum. For example, if mutants with deletions in the C_H3 domain (see Figure 1) were being sought, we overlayed the clones with an antiserum that was specific for that domain. Clones that were not surrounded by a visible precipitate were marked, and then the plates were overlayed again with an antiserum that reacted with other parts of the immunoglobulin molecule. Previously unstained clones that were now surrounded by a visible precipitate were variants that had lost antigenic determinants in their C_H3 domains but were still synthesizing and secreting detectable amounts of immunoglobulin.

Finally, the immunoplate assay when done with conventional antiserum detects mutants that have undergone gross changes in gene expression or in the structure of the immunoglobulin molecule. This is because even highly absorbed conventional antisera almost always react with multiple antigenic determinants on the immunoglobulin molecule. If a single antigenic determinant is lost through a point mutation, the conventional antiserum will still react with the mutant immunoglobulin molecule and the mutation will be undetected. This explains why the antibody overlay assay has provided us with mutants containing large deletions, frameshifts, and class switches. In order to find mutants with more subtle changes, we have overlayed clones with monoclonal antibodies. We did not expect a single monoclonal to give a visible precipitate since at best it might react with one determinant on each heavy chain and would not cross-link enough molecules to form a visible precipitate. However, mixtures of monoclonals that did give a visible precipitate by Ouchterlony analysis still did not give such precipitates when layered over clones. This may be due to the relatively low affinity of the monoclonals we were using. We believe that further work will allow us to use monoclonal antibodies to detect point mutations.

When the S107 myeloma, which produces a phosphocholine-binding antibody, was overlayed with antigen, mutant molecules with single amino acid substitutions associated with changes in antigen binding were detected (see Section 4.2).[35,42,43] Presumably, this is because small changes in structure can lead to significant changes in antigen binding.

3.2.2. Plaque Assays

Because the immunoplate assay described above is both tedious and has many limitations, we have adapted the Jerne hemolytic plaque assay[44] so that it can be used to detect mutant clones in soft agarose. This assay is also a useful way to detect hybridoma clones or subclones that are producing particular antibodies and in fact was used by Kohler and Milstein[45] to detect some of the first hybridomas.

The Jerne hemolytic plaque method was originally developed in order to identify and count individual antibody-secreting cells in a mixture of lymphocytes.[44] In its simplest form, lymphocytes making anti-sheep red blood cell antibodies are mixed with sheep red blood cells (SRBC) in a thin layer of agar. After a period of incubation, complement is added. Areas of lysis (plaques) form around the anti-SRBC secreting cells because the secreted antibody binds to the surrounding SRBC and causes their lysis by activating the complement cascade. IgM-producing cells are most easily detected because the IgM molecule fixes complement most effectively. For plaquing IgG- or IgA-secreting cells, an antiserum against IgG or IgA, respectively, is added in order to facilitate complement fixation. The generality of the technique can be increased by chemically attaching an antigen of choice to SRBC. This allows one to screen for cells producing almost any antibody rather than just ones against SRBC.

For plaquing to be useful in the isolation of variant myeloma and hybridoma cells, it obviously must be possible to recover the cells of interest. Since this is difficult to do with single cells, the method has been adapted for clones. Although the SRBC layer can be added after the clones have grown to a reasonable size (as was done for the screening of some of the first hybridoma fusions), we have found that more discrete and reproducible plaques are obtained if the SRBC are included in the myeloma/hybridoma cell layer.

Our current protocol is in fact very similar to that described in Section 4.1.1 for the antibody/antigen overlay. The feeders and 5-ml agarose underlayer are prepared in the same manner. The 1-ml cell layer, in addition to 0.8 ml of the agarose-cloning medium mix, contains 0.15 ml of cloning medium containing sufficient myeloma or hybridoma cells to produce 500 clones, 0.05 ml of a 20% suspension of antigen-coated SRBC (in DME), and several microliters of a rabbit facilitating antiserum. The exact amount of antiserum must be determined for each batch (for IgA plaques, we use 2 μl of a Bionetics rabbit anti-mouse IgA). After 5–7 days in an 8% CO_2, 37°C incubator, 1 ml of a sterile agarose–phosphate-buffered saline mix (same agarose concentration as in the 5 ml underlayer) containing 0.07–0.1 ml of protein A-absorbed guinea pig complement is added. Plaques appear within 1–2 hr and clones can be picked immediately or within 1–2 days.

If it is necessary to facilitate plaques, the size and clarity of the plaques vary with different batches of antiserum. We screen batches of commercial rabbit antisera and then purchase reasonable supplies of a good batch. We use commercial lyophilized guinea pig complement because in our hands rabbit complement has been less satisfactory. The protein A absorbs guinea pig antibodies from the complement, which may be cytotoxic for mouse cells, and prevents the killing of the myeloma or hybridoma cells. Titering the amount of complement to the lowest possible level is also important for maintaining myeloma and hybridoma viability.

We have found that the major technical problems in combining cloning in agarose with plaque formation are the inherent instability of antigen-coupled sheep red blood cells and difficulties in spreading the red cells evenly. The general properties and especially the stability of the sheep red cells vary from batch to batch and, when a single animal is used, from bleed to bleed. This is a greater problem when analyzing agarose clones since the red cells must remain intact for days, while in the standard Jerne plaque technique they need only remain intact for a few hours. While there are many ways to couple proteins to SRBC, the need for them to remain intact for 1 week or more limits the options. For example, antigens or haptens are efficiently and simply attached to SRBC by diazotization,[46,47] but this decreases the stability of the cells. A milder coupling reagent can be generated by converting the diazonium reagent to a substituted imidoester,[48] and red cells coupled to hapten with this reagent are stable enough to be used with agarose clones. However, the preparation of this reagent requires more work and reagents and is only useful if the antigen can be converted to a diazonium salt.

Chromium chloride has been used widely in immunology to couple antigens to red blood cells.[49-51] The procedure is simple and quite reproducible. Since it maintains the stability of the red cells, we have used it routinely to prepare antigen-coupled red cells for plaquing over agarose clones. Sterile SRBC are washed three times in sterile saline to remove phosphate ions that will inhibit the coupling reaction. The SRBC are resuspended so as to make a 10% solution and 7 μl of sterile (filtered) 0.5 M chromium chloride is added per 0.2 ml of SRBC. Then 10 μl of antigen (in our studies we use 20 mg/ml) of hapten-conjugated keyhole limpet hemocyanin, KLH) is added to the reaction, which then proceeds with occasional gentle mixing for 1.5–2.0 hr at room temperature. The coupled cells are then washed three times in double buffered saline (0.077 M NaCl, 0.08 M phosphate buffer, pH 7.3) The supernatant of the first wash may contain some hemoglobin, indicating that a few cells lysed, but the amount of lysis should be minimal. The coupled sterile red cells can be stored for as long as 3 weeks in double buffered saline or in serum-free medium. However, it is safer to prepare fresh cells every week.

As already mentioned, the efficiency of coupling and the stability of the cells vary somewhat from batch to batch of SRBC. However, the preparation of the chromium chloride itself has been reported to be the major variable in the procedure. We have used chromium chloride that is dissolved in distilled water and, as has been suggested in the literature, allowed to "age" at 4°C for at least 1 month. Some workers have found the coupling is improved if the chromium chloride is buffered, but we have not observed a difference. The relative concentrations of SRBC, antigen, and chromium chloride to obtain optimum coupling may vary with different antigens and must be determined empirically.

A major advantage of the chromium chloride method is its versatility. It can be used for protein antigens, for haptens that are coupled to the proteins prior to conjugation, and for preparing staph A protein or antibody-conjugated SRBC for use in the reverse plaque assay.[52,53] In the reverse plaque assays staph A protein or anti-immunoglobulin antibody is attached to the SRBC. The SRBC are then mixed with antibody-forming cells in either the Jerne (agar)[44] or Cunningham (liquid phase)[54] methods and the secreted immunoglobulin binds to the surrounding red cells. Facilitating anti-immunoglobulin and complement are added to lyse the sensitized red blood cells and form a plaque. The benefit of reverse plaque assays is that they do not require that the antibody secreted by the myeloma or hybridoma bind a particular antigen. In principle, mutants could be detected by using conventional antisera or monoclonals as either the facilitating or conjugated antibody. However, it should be noted that we and others that we have consulted have not yet been able to obtain reverse plaques over agarose clones.

The SRBC must be evenly dispersed in order to obtain clear macroscopic plaques. Care must be taken to see that the coupled SRBC are not nonspecifically aggregated, that the cells are evenly suspended before addition to agarose, and that the 1 ml containing the SRBC is spread evenly by gently rotating the dish before it is placed at 4°C. The clarity of the plaques also depends upon the density of SRBC. While low concentrations give larger plaques, their margins are less sharp and it is more difficult to distinguish plaque-forming and non-plaque-forming clones. If too high a density of SRBC is used, the red cells obscure clones that do not form plaques, making it difficult to identify non-plaque-forming mutant myelomas and hybridomas. We use a final concentration between 0.8 and 1.0%.

It is clear from all of the above that the plaque assays described are relatively delicate. In addition, in most of the situations described the mutant is detected as a clone that does not form a plaque. Just as with the immunoplate assay described in Section 4.1.1, this requires that each mutant must be individually recovered and characterized. However, once the reagents have been properly titered, the distinction between plaque-forming and non-plaque-forming clones is often easier than with the antigen or antibody overlay technique. Certainly, if one is looking for variants that form plaques against a background of non-plaque-formers, this is the preferable assay, since the plates can be scored by direct examination.

Mosmann and Baumal hae described a combination of the immunoplate and plaquing assays.[55] Myeloma cells are cloned in agarose as in the immunoplate assay (Section 3.2.1), except that SRBC are included with the myeloma cells. After 5 days, the clones and SRBC are overlayed with agarose containing a mixture of antibody reactive with the immunoglobulin secreted by the myeloma and antibody that will lyse the SRBC. One day later, an amount of complement is added that is just enough to lyse the SRBC in the presence of the amount of anti-SRBC present. The anti-immunoglobulin combines with the secreted immunoglobulin around those clones that are producing it. These antigen–antibody complexes fix complement in the local area around the clone, preventing the complement from combining with the antibody on the surface of SRBC. All of the SRBC on the plate are lysed except those that are close to the secreting myeloma cells, and the producing clones are therefore marked by a grossly visible red spot. Mutant clones are not surrounded by unlysed SRBC. Again, in most situations this is a negative assay. However, just as with other plaque assays, if one is looking for positive event or revertants, it could be very useful.

3.2.3. Replica Immunoabsorption

Replica plating has been a powerful tool in the isolation of bacterial mutants and could be equally useful for analyzing myeloma and hybridoma clones. However, since myelomas and hybridomas float off when they are grown on top of semisolid medium, it is not technically possible to use the standard procedure. Based on the ability of nitrocellulose filters to bind protein molecules, a replica immunoabsorption procedure has been developed.[56] Cells are cloned in soft agarose over feeder cells in the manner described previously. An extra layer of 1.2 ml of agarose medium is overlayed over the cell layer in order to protect the clones. At about the 100-cell stage a sterile nitrocellulose filter is applied over the clones. The secreted antibodies diffuse through the agarose and bind to the filter. After removing the filter, bound immunoglobulin can be detected by the binding of antigen or anti-immunoglobulin antibody-coated red blood cells or by the binding of radioactively labeled antigen or anti-immunoglobulin antibody. Since several filters can be incubated successively over the clones, several different parameters can be measured. For example, with one filter one could test for antibody production, while with another test for the loss of antigen binding or of a particular antigenic determinant. Although the method has been used primarily for detecting monoclonals with a given specificity, a scheme like the one just mentioned could be effective in screening for immunoglobulin mutants.

3.2.4. Fluorescence-Activated Cell Sorter

The fluorescence-activated cell sorter (FACS) can be used to isolate variants from cell lines that express surface immunoglobulin.[57–60] As a probe, one can use either flurochrome-conjugated antigen or antibody. The method works with conventional as well as with monoclonal reagents. As a further refinement, one can use an antigen such as dansyl chloride.[61] which changes its fluorescence when bound by surface immunoglobulin due to the hydrophobic environment of the antigen binding site. Since the more advanced sorters can sort according to two parameters simultaneously, it is possible to screen with two independent monoclonals, each tagged with a different fluorochrome. This could be particularly useful if, for instance, one were interested in selecting structural mutants and not ones that had lost the expression of surface immunoglobulin. One could use two fluoresceinated monoclonals that recognized independent antigenic determinants and set the FACS to isolate only those cells that reacted with one of the monoclonals but not with the other. Alternatively, if one did not have available the technology to do a double sort, a modification of the technique used by Rajewsky and colleagues to isolate cells with mutations in their H-2 (transplantation) antigens could be used.[60] They used two anti-H-2 monclonals that mutually inhibited each other's binding yet recognized independent determinants. They fluorescently labeled one of them, incubated cells with the two hybridomas with the unlabeled one in great excess, and sorted for cells that were fluorescent. Since the excess of unlabeled monoclonal prevents the staining of wild-type cells, only those variant cells that had lost the determinant seen by the unlabeled antibody but retained the determinant seen by the labeled monoclonal were fluorescent. This approach for the isolation of structural variants is particularly useful because it is a positive assay; it ignores nonproducing variants. With an appropriate pair of anti-immunoglobulin monoclonals, the method should be equally effective for isolating immunoglobulin structural mutants.

Technically, it should be noted that one run of the FACS is insufficient for isolating rare variants. Due to spillover, enrichment is only partial. Generally several cycles are required to generate a population that is enriched enough for cloning and random selection. In order to increase the signal-to-noise ratio and thereby improve the separation it is possible to covalently attach one's probe to highly fluorescent spheres rather than to a flurochrome.[62]

3.3. Selective Techniques

All of the techniques described above require screening many cells or clones to detect mutants. This has been possible because of the high frequency of structural mutants in myeloma and hybridoma cells. However, it is obvious that these approaches may limit the spectrum of mutants found. The cell sorter can be used to identify rare events, but because of the need to first enrich through a few cycles of sorting, it is more difficult to determine the exact frequency at which rare mutants arise. Selective techniques would clearly be very useful and are just beginning to be explored.

3.3.1. Complement-Mediated Cytotoxicity

Immunologists have for years used antibody-mediated, complement-dependent lysis to remove populations of cells from complex mixtures. It may appear surprising that this approach has not been used to select for structural mutants of immunoglobulins. In fact, Schrieber and his colleagues incubated an IgA-producing myeloma cell line (S107) with antibody against the variable region of the S107 immunoglobulin and complement and isolated resistant variants that were producing less antibody.[63] Monoclonal antibody and complement have been successfully used to select for point mutations in mouse transplantation antigens, suggesting the usefulness of this sort of selection.[64]

There have, however, been significant problems in applying this approach to selecting immunoglobulin mutants. First, the cells must not only be producing immunoglobulin but also must be synthesizing the membrane form of antibody, which inserts into the membrane as an integral membrane protein. Most cells that are secreting large amounts of immunoglobulin have little or none of the membrane form, which is primarily found in more undifferentiated antibody-producing cells. A second problem is that large amounts of secreted immunoglobulin tend to inhibit the attachment of anti-immunoglobulin to the small amounts of membrane Ig present. Cells can be washed free of secreted Ig and incubated in the cold with anti-Ig, but even this does not seem to be very effective. Cells can be evacuated of their intracellular pool of secreted Ig by first treating with the reversible inhibitor of protein synthesis cycloheximide. We have tried all of these approaches and so far have not been successful in greatly enriching for new kinds of mutants. We have found that, at least with the cell lines used, the surviving cells are initially resistant to killing and then in a few days return to sensitivity. This may be due to modulation of the expression of membrane Ig, but we have not proven this to be true. There is also a report that there are time-dependent variations in the expression of surface Ig after mutagenesis, suggesting that it is important to select at just the right time.[65]

3.3.2 Complement-Mediated Suicide

Kohler and Shulman[66] developed a suicide selection that is an elegant modification of complement-mediated killing. The surfaces of hybridoma cells secreting IgM antitrinitrophenol (TNP) (a small molecule or hapten that is commonly used by immunologists) are coated with TNP under conditions that do not kill the cells. The cells secrete antibodies that bind to the hapten, which is now an integral membrane protein. In the presence of complement this leads to their own self-destruction. This procedure enriches for cells that are either no longer secreting antibodies or are secreting structural variants that have altered binding of TNP and/or complement. The cycle can then be repeated with the surviving cells. Enrichment of 20- to 200-fold has been reported.

More recently, the complement suicide system has been used to obtain variants of an IgM-producing hybridoma against phosphocholine (PC) (another favorite hapten among immunologists).[67] Theoretically, this approach should work for any antigen that can be coupled to cell surfaces in a manner that maintains cell viability.

3.3.3. Toxin-Coupled Antibody

Conventional antibodies, and more recently hybridoma antibodies, have been coupled to cytotoxic agents such as α-amanitin and the A chains of diphtheria and ricin toxins in order to generate specific cytotoxic reagents.[68-70]

These conjugates have been shown to be effective in the *in vitro* killing of tumor cells and may have potential for therapy.[69,70] Anti-immunoglobulin conjugates with specificity for different parts of the immunoglobulin molecule exhibit selective killing.[68] Although to our knowledge this approach has not yet been successfully used for the isolation of structural or synthetic immunoglobulin mutants, the possibility is enticing. The potential problems are similar to those discussed for antibody-dependent, complement-mediated cytoxicity. The target cells may need to display surface immunoglobulin and not be secreting large amounts of immunoglobulin. The effectiveness of the selection could also depend upon how the conjugates of antibodies to toxins or drugs are processed and the lysosomal enzymes present in the particular cell line under study. Since only a few α chains of toxin are required to kill cells, this approach deserves to be explored thoroughly.

4. FREQUENCY AND PHENOTYPES OF MUTANTS

A wide variety of mutant mouse myeloma and hybridoma cells have been identified and characterized with respect to the immunoglobulins that they produce. As can be seen from Table II, most of the phenotypes that have been described in microorganisms also occur in cultured immunoglobulin-producing cells. However, this system differs from prokaryotic and other eukaryotic systems in the very high rate at which mutants arise. Many myeloma and hybridoma cell lines producing IgA and the different subclasses of IgG have been examined and all generate mutants spontaneously at rates between 1×10^{-3} and 4×10^{-4}/cell per generation.[3,4,31] Among these spontaneous mutants are ones with changes in immunoglobulin gene expression and in the amino acid sequence of the immunoglobulin polypeptide chains. These latter include major structural changes, such as deletions of whole domains or the expression of all or part of a new constant region (class switch), and point mutations in both the variable and constant regions of the heavy chain.

Table II
Variant Phenotypes in Mouse Myeloma and Hybridoma Cell Lines[a]

Synthesis variants
  Loss variants (H^-L^+, H^+L^-, H^-L^-)
  Quantitative variants (decreased or increased H and/or L synthesis)

Structural variants
  With major structural changes: deletions, subclass switch, long chains
  With minor structural changes: amino acid substitutions, changes in carbohydrates

[a]Reprinted with permission from *CRC Critical Reviews in Immunology*.[78]

As mentioned earlier, the frequency of mutants can be increased as much as 10- to 20-fold by mutagenesis with the agents described in Section 3.[3-5] In many experiments the frequency of mutants of all phenotypes was greater than 1% of the surviving cells. This extreme genetic instability is restricted to the immunoglobulin genes since myeloma cells resistant to bromodeoxyuridine, thioguanine, puromycin, and ouabain all arise at spontaneous frequencies of less than 10^{-6}. Revertants from thioguanine resistance also arise at similarly low frequencies.[71] It is, however, important to note that this comparison may not be valid since immunoglobulins are produced in large amounts by both myeloma and hybridoma cells, while the enzymes responsible for drug resistance represent a very small fraction of the protein synthesized by these cells and because the frequency of observed mutations will depend on the sensitivity of the screening system employed.

As noted in Section 2, a great deal is known about the structure and organization of immunoglobulin genes and the DNA rearrangements that occur during the differentiation of antibody-forming cells.[10] In addition, some recent studies have led most immunologists to believe that somatic mutations as well as gene rearrangements play important roles in the generation of antibody diversity.[13-16,72-77] Both the nature of some of the mutants that arise in cultured myeloma and hybridoma cells and the frequency with which they arise raise the possibility that they result from normal molecular events or are the reflection of the unusual aspects of immunoglobulin gene structure. This has led to the detailed characterization of the structural changes in the proteins and nucleic acids of a few mutants. We will review some of these studies because they illustrate how this somatic cell genetic system will ultimately be used to study the regulation of immunoglobulin gene expression, the plasticity of immunoglobulin and perhaps other animal cell genes, and structure–function relationships in antibody molecules. These studies also indicate that the phenotypic classification in Table II will have to be modified and that it will be possible to classify them according to their molecular defects. A more detailed review of the mutants that have been identified in myeloma and hybridoma cells has been presented by Morrison and Scharff.[78]

4.1. Frameshift Mutants

A number of spontaneous and mutagen-induced frameshift mutants have been identified. Among the spontaneous mutants originally identified by Milstein and his colleagues was one called IF3, which differed from the parental P3 IgG$_1$ immunoglobulin in its isoelectric point and in the size of its heavy chain.[31,32] Protein studies revealed that the C-terminal cyanogen bromide (CNBr) fragment of the parent had been replaced by a new fragment. The sequence of this fragment was identical to the parent up to residue 340, which is in the N-terminal part of the C_H3 domain (see Figure 1). Following residue 340 there was a sequence of 14 amino acids that were not present in the parent and then the protein terminated. The messenger RNA molecule was the same size as the parent as measured by sucrose gradient centrifugation, and the sequence of the relevant part of the messenger RNA suggested that two bases had been lost, leading to a frameshift and a premature UAA (ochre) termination at residue 355. The recent determination of the DNA sequence of the IgG_1 constant-region gene[79] is consistent with this mechanism.

The mutant M3.11 is a Melphalan-induced mutant of the MPC-11 IgG_{2b}-producing cell line, which lacks its entire C_H3 domain.[80] The C-terminal residue of the mutant C_H2 domain is asparagine, while that of the parent is lysine. Based on the sequence of the IgG_{2b} gene, it has been suggested that M3.11 also was the result of a -2 frameshift leading to a premature termination. This mutant was also interesting because only 60–70% of its heavy chains are glycosylated. The assembly, secretion, and serum half-life of the glycosylated and unglycosylated molecules are indistinguishable, thus suggesting that carbohydrate is not required for any of these processes, at least for this molecule.[81,82]

More than 14 additional short-chain mutants of the MPC-11 cell line have been identified and partially characterized.[78] The molecular weights of the H chains range between 35,000 and 50,000 Da, suggesting that mutations are occurring in many parts of the molecule. We have recently generated a large number of phenotypically similar mutants from an IgG_{2b}-producing hybridoma.[6] These also arose at a frequency of greater than 1% following mutagenesis.

Mutants of the S107 and W3082 IgA-producing cell lines with deletions of all or part of the C_H3 domain have also been identified.[83] Restriction analysis of the genes and Northern blots of the messenger RNAs suggest that these mutants are also the result of premature terminations, presumably resulting from either a frameshift or a point mutation. A mouse myeloma tumor producing a similar IgA mutant has also been studied.[84] These mutants form only HL half-molecules with abnormal disulfide bonds, suggesting that the interaction of C_H3 domains is important in forming H_2L_2 molecules. These mutants also lack the surface immunoglobulins found in the parent cells, confirming the importance of the C terminus in membrane attachment.

4.2. Point Mutants

A number of mutants have been identified that differ from the parental proteins by what appear to be point mutations. This type of mutation is especially interesting because single amino acid substitutions occur frequently in variable regions of heavy and light chains. It was therefore surprising that Milstein and his colleagues, using isoelectric focusing, identified two variants with point mutations in their constant regions while no variable-region mutants were recognized.[32] IF1 is another variant of P3, which, when analyzed at the protein level, was found to lack the C-terminal 83 residues of its heavy chain.[32,85] The messenger RNA that codes for this molecule cosediments on sucrose gradients with parental messenger but is translated into a short heavy chain in a cell-free system. The mutant is thought to have arisen through a single base change in the codon for Ser-358, which results in a termination codon. IF4, another variant of P3, appears to differ from the parent only at residue 415 of the heavy chain, where aspartic acid has been substituted for asparagine.[32] Analysis of the mRNA revealed that this was due to a base substitution and not the result of deamidation.

Spontaneous mutants with single amino acid substitutions in the heavy-chain variable region arise frequently in the S107 myeloma cell line.[35,42,43,86] which, as mentioned previously, secretes a phosphocholine (PC)-binding IgA antibody. Using antigen overlay (Section 4.1.1), and more recently plaquing methods (Section 4.1.2), clones have been isolated that have either decreased or lost their ability to bind phosphocholine-keyhole limpet hemocyanin. By SDS PAGE analysis, all the binding mutants produce normal size H and L chains and assemble the molecules into IgA polymers that are indistinguishable from those of the S107 parent. From one of the low-binding mutants, U_1, "revertants" can be obtained that have near wild-type binding. However, the "revertants" are not true revertants, in that they can all be shown to be structurally distinct from S107 by peptide mapping. The mutation rate for this system is high. A fluctuation analysis of the mutation from low to high antigen binding gave a mutation rate of approximately 2×10^{-4}/cell per generation.[86] Of the structural changes that have been identified, all are single or double amino acid substitutions in the H chain. U_4, a primary variant with just detectable binding, has a Glu to Ala interchange at residue 35 in the first hypervariable region.[43] X-ray diffraction studies suggest that the glutamic acid at residue 35 forms a hydrogen bond with the light chain, which is necessary to maintain the conformation of the antigen binding site, perhaps explaining how a single amino acid substitution can result in the complete loss of antigen binding. U_1, another primary variant, has an aspartic acid to alanine interchange in the fifth residue of the J segment (residue 101),[42] while a "revertant" from U_1, $S_3S_1{}^2$, has reverted back to aspartic acid at 101 but has an asparigine to threonine substitution at residue 83. Although localized point mutation is the simplest way to explain these changes, the complexity of a rearranging multigene family such as that of immunoglobulins raises the possibility of a more complex process, such as unequal crossing over. The genes from the variants are currently being cloned in order to better understand the mechanisms involved and to address the relationship between these mechanisms and the actual generation of antibody divesity *in vivo*. As already mentioned, recent studies comparing the sequence of germ-line genes and those expressed in antibody-producing myelomas and hybridomas suggest an important role for somatic mutation in the generation of diversity.[13-16,72-77]

4.3. Internal Deletion Mutants Associated with Changes in DNA or RNA

Another P3 variant, IF2, was found to have a shortened heavy chain.[32,85] Peptide fragment analysis showed that the C_H1 fragments were absent and that the hinge fragment was structurally altered. Sequencing of the new CNBr fragment revealed that IF3 possessed an internal deletion of 94 amino acids spanning residues 121–214. A new bond between Ser-120 and Val-215 was found. Comparison with the IgG_1 gene revealed that the entire C_H1 domain was missing.[87] *In vitro* synthesis with IF2 mRNA yields a deleted heavy chain. Sequencing of cDNA from IF2 mRNA demonstrated a deletion of the C_H1 codons.[88] Sucrose gradient sedimention shows that IF2 H-chain mRNA has a sedimentation coefficient of 16 S rather than the 17 S of wild-type message,[32] which is consistent with a deletion of approximately 300 bases. Restriction map analysis shows that the DNA deletion spans at least 5.5 kb, including the entire C_H1 domain as well as parts of the introns between V and C_H1 and between C_H1 and the hinge region.[89]

The mutant 10-1 is a deletion variant of MPC-11.[41] Unlike M311 (which was discussed earlier), its C_H2 and C_H3 domains (see Figure 1) are indistinguishable from that of MPC-11.[90] The deletion involves part of but not all of the C_H1 domain. Northern blot analysis indicates that 10-1 has a shortened H-chain MRNA as compared to MPC-11 (1.66 versus 1.85 kb).[91] However, restriction map analysis has not revealed any genomic DNA changes. Hence, the deletion appears to originate at the RNA level, perhaps due to a mutation in a splicing or other processing signal.

4.4. Class- and Subclass-Switch Mutants

As discussed in Section 2, the differentiation of normal antibody-forming cells is often associated with a switch from IgM to IgG or IgA production. At the gene level, this is accomplished by rearranging VDJ, which was 5' to the gene, to a site 3' to one of the other constant-region genes.[10] This rearrangement is associated with deletion of sequences 3' to VJD and 5' to the constant-region gene that is now being expressed. Subclones of myeloma and hybridoma cell lines have been identified that express a different constant region but the same variable region as the parental cell line.[78] It is not yet clear whether these are cells that have undergone further differentiation in culture using the normal mechanisms or have arisen through aberrant recombinations or rearrangements.

Some of the subclass switch variants arise at a very high frequency and have been identified using the immunoplate assay. For example, the MPC-11 cell line, which produces an IgG_{2b} immunoglobulin, generates IgG_{2a}-producing subclones at a frequency of 0.28%.[92] Some of these produce immunoglobulins with the MPC-11 variable region and probably the whole IgG_{2a} constant region,[93] while others produce hybrid heavy chains consisting of part of the IgG_{2b} constant region and part of the IgG_{2a} constant region.[94] The "recombination" in some hybrid molecules occurs within a domain. In addition, some of the MPC-11 mutants with internal or C-terminal deletions can generate secondary variants with normal sized chains by switching from IgG_{2b} to IgG_{2a} production.

In fact, Barbara Birshtein and Sherie Morrison and their colleagues have generated families of switch mutants, which are summarized in Figure 4.[78] Primary mutants with C-terminal deletions resulting in a 50,000-Da H chain acquired a normal sized H chain by switching to the γ_{2a} constant-region gene. The primary 10-1 mutant (see Section 4.3) with an internal deletion (47,000-Da H chain) generated secondary mutants either with normal size γ2a chain or mutants with still smaller H chains. These in turn converted to wild-type size or 47,000-Da γ_{2a} heavy chains. In the former case the rearrangement or recombination must have taken place 5' to the defect in 10-1, while the 47,000-Da γ2a molecules must have been generated by a change that occurred 3' to the defect, thereby retaining the mutant phenotype.

Rajewsky and his colleagues[57-59] and Herzenberg and his colleagues[61] have identified other class and subclass switches, using the fluorescent-activated cell sorter. Using the P3 cell line, they were able to identify rare sub-

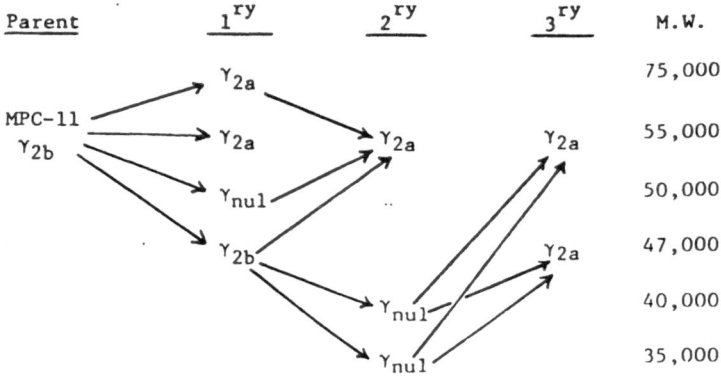

Figure 4. Genealogy of MPC-11 IgG_{2b} to IgG_{2a} subclass-switch mutants. (Reprinted with permission from *CRC Critical Reviews in Immunology*.[78])

clones that had switched from making IgG_1 to IgG_{2b}, IgG_{2a}, and IgA.[58] In general these subclones arose at spontaneous rates of 10^{-6}–10^{-7}/cell per generation. According to the deletion theory of subclass switches, revertants should not occur. However, reversion did occur at rates of 10^{-5}–10^{-6}/cell per generation. This latter finding plus the existence of hybrid molecules (from MPC-11 variants) suggests that at least some of the class and subclass switches may arise through unequal crossing over or mitotic recombination. Studies now in progress should define the molecular mechanisms involved.[95]

Hybridomas also undergo class switches.[59,96] One IgM-producing hybridoma switched from the expression of μ to δ (IgD) heavy chains but continued to express the parental variable region.[59] Another IgM-producing hybridoma generated an IgG_1-producing subclone, also still expressing the parental variable region.[96] Such class switches may be useful in tailor-making monoclonal antibodies for particular diagnostic or therapeutic tasks.[6]

5. DISCUSSION

Mouse myeloma and hybridoma cells provide an unusual somatic-cell genetic system. Mutants with a wide variety of phenotypes arise frequently. Because they secrete large amounts of the mutant gene product and form tumors in animals, it is possible to purify sufficient mutant protein to characterize their functional and structural changes. The extensive work on immunoglobulin gene structure and organization also makes it possible to determine the molecular mechanisms of mutation. On the other hand, the techniques currently available, while useful in identifying mutants, are cumbersome for studying rates of mutation. As has already been pointed out, selective or positive detection techniques are being developed that may facilitate such studies.

It is not clear whether the high spontaneous and mutagen-induced frequencies with which some mutants arise are related to the normal generation of antibody diversity or to the gene rearrangements that occur during the differentiation of normal antibody-forming cells. It seems likely that the instability of immunoglobulin genes at least reflects the unusual aspects of their structure that are involved in their evolution, expression, and diversity.

It is hoped that the continued isolation and molecular characterization of mutants will provide new and useful information on the mechanisms and enzymology of immunoglobulin gene rearrangement and expression. While somatic mutations in cultured cells similar to the abnormal gene rearrangement that occur *in vivo* have not yet been reported, such rearrangements are found in myeloma tumors and in the cultured cells derived from them. For example, the MPC-11 cell line produces intact H and L chains and a fragment of a κ light chain that contains a signal sequence and a constant region but no variable region.[97] The cytoplasmic messenger RNA also lacks variable-region sequences, but the nuclear precursor RNA contains them.[98] Analysis of the gene suggests that the V region underwent an aberrant rearrangement that brought it close to the C region but bypassed the J segment.[99] Since the J segment provides the 3′ splicing signal for the rearranged V region, this splice site is lost in this gene and the signal sequence is spliced directly to the C region. Other aberrancies appear to occur frequently in VJ rearrangements, leading to genes that are out of phase or contain in-phase deletions.[100,101] Such rearrangements also appear to occur in normal cells.[102] If somatic mutants with similar changes can be identified, it may be possible to learn more about the mechanisms responsible for their abnormalities and the frequency with which they occur.

A great deal has yet to be learned about the mechanisms responsible for gene expression in animal cells. One current popular approach is to change the sequence of genes in and around the origins of transcription using recombinant DNA technology and then to study the effects of these changes on the gene after it has been reintroduced into the cell. An alternative is to identify myeloma mutants with defects or changes in expression and then analyze the nature of the molecular changes responsible. As already noted, expression mutants arise frequently in cultured myeloma cells. Some of these nonproducing mutants still express messenger RNAs that are altered in their size or in the amount of messenger present.[103] Mutants have also been reported that produce increased amounts of immunoglobulin. For example, there is a mutant of the MOPC 315 cell line that produces approximately five times as much heavy chain and 10 times as much messenger as the parental cell.[104] This is associated with a change in the restriction map of the immunoglobulin gene. The detailed analysis of such mutants should provide insights into the regulation of expression of animal cell genes.

Finally, monoclonal antibodies have begun to play a major role in biology and medicine.[105] Mutant monoclonal antibodies can in some cases provide improved reagents that are tailor-made for certain diagnostic and therapeutic tasks.[6] The techniques developed to identify mutants of mouse myeloma cells are already being used for this purpose and promise to increase the usefulness of the hybridoma technology.

In conclusion, the isolation and characterization of mutants from cultured antibody-forming cells have already resulted in useful information. As the techniques for identifying such mutants improve, this somatic-cell genetic system will provide even more information on the molecular genetics of antibody production. The mechanisms responsible for the unusual instability of the immunoglobulin genes may or may not turn out to be of more general importance, but even if they are special, they will certainly lead to important insights about the mechanisms of gene stabilization and expression in animal cells.

ACKNOWLEDGMENTS. The authors wish to thank Ann Gorgoglione and Maria Sigismondo for their expert assistance in the preparation of this manuscript. One of the authors (DJZ) is a medical scientist trainee supported by NIHMS grant 5T32GM7288. The other author (MDS) received research support from the NIH (grants AI10702 and A15231), NSF (grant PCM77-25635), and ACS (grant NP-317).

REFERENCES

1. M. Potter, Immunoglobulin-producing tumors and myeloma proteins of mice, *Physiol. Rev.* *52*, 631–719 (1972).
2. E. A. Kabat, T. T. Wu, and H. Bilofsky, *Sequences of Immunoglobulin Chains*, Publication no. 80-2008, National Institutes of Health (1979).
3. R. Coffino and M. D. Scharff, Rate of somatic mutation in immunoglobulin production by mouse myeloma cells, *Proc. Natl. Acad. Sci. USA 68*, 219–223 (1971).
4. R. Baumal, B. K. Birshtein, P. Coffino, and M. D. Scharff, Mutations in immunoglobulin-producing mouse myeloma cells, *Science 182*, 164–166 (1973).
5. L. A. Wims and S. L. Morrison, ICR-191 and ethyl methanesulfonate induced mutagenesis at the immunoglobulin locus in the Y5606 cultured myeloma cell line, *Mutat. Res. 81*, 215–228 (1981).
6. D. E. Yelton, P. Thammana, C. Desaymard, S. B. Roberts, S.-P. Kwan, A. Giusti, D. J. Zack, R. R. Pollock, and M. D. Scharff, Monoclonal antibodies: The production of tailor made serological reagents, in: *From Gene to Protein: Translation into Biotechnology, The Four-teenth Miami Winter Symposium* (F. Ahmed, J. Shultz, E. E. Smith, and W. J. Whelan, eds.), Academic Press, New York (1982).
7. T. T. Wu and E. A. Kabat, An analysis of the variable regions of Bence–Jones proteins and myeloma light chains and their implications for antibody complementarity, *J. Exp. Med. 132*, 211–250 (1970).
8. D. Givol, The antibody combining site, *Int. Rev. Biochem. 23*, 71–125 (1979).
9. W. J. Dreyer and J. C. Bennett, the molecular basis of antibody formation. A paradox, *Proc. Natl. Acad. Sci. USA 54*, 864–869 (1965).
10. J. M. Adams, The organization and expression of immunoglobulin genes, *Immunol. Today 1*, 10–17 (1980).
11. C. Brack, M. Hirama, R. Lenhard-Schuller, and S. Tonegawa, A complete immunoglobulin gene is created by somatic recombination, *Cell 15*, 1–14 (1978).
12. P. Leder, E. E. Max, J. G. Seidman, S.-P. Kwan, M. Scharff, M. Nau, and B. Norman, Recombination events that activate, diversify, and delete immunoglobulin genes, *Cold Spring Harbor Sympl Quant. Biol. 45*, 859–865 (1981).
13. M. G. Weigert, I. M. Cesari, S. J. Yonkovich, and M. Cohn, Variability in the lambda light chain sequences of mouse antibody, *Nature 228*, 1045–1047 (1970).
14. S. Kim, M. Davis, E. Sinn, P. Patten, and L. Hood, Antibody diversity: Somatic hypermu-tation of rearranged V_H genes, *Cell 27*, 573–581 (1981).

15. D. Baltimore, Somatic mutation gains its place among the generators of diversity, *Cell 26*, 295–296 (1981).
16. M. Cohn, R. Langman, and W. Geckeler, Diversity 1980, *Prog. Immunol. 4*, 153–201 (1980).
17. P. Early, H. Huang, M. Davis, K. Calame, and L. Hood, An immunoglobulin heavy chain variable region gene is generated from three segments of DNA: V_H, D and J_H, *Cell 19*, 981–992 (1980).
18. E. E. Max, J. G. Seidman, and P. Leder, Sequences of five potential recombination sites encoded close to an immunoglobulin constant region gene, *Proc. Natl. Acad. Sci. USA 76*, 3450–3454 (1979).
19. H. Sakano, K. Huppi, G. Heinrich, and S. Tonegawa, Sequences at the somatic recombination sites of immunoglobulin light-chain genes, *Nature 280*, 288–294 (1979).
20. A. R. Lawton, P. W. Kincade, and M. D. Cooper, Sequential expression of germ line genes in development of immunoglobulin class diversity, *Fed. Proc. 34*, 33–39 (1975).
21. A. Shimizu, N. Takakashi, Y. Yamawaki-Kataoka, Y. Nishida, T. Kataoka, and T. Honjo, Ordering of mouse immunoglobulin heavy chain genes by molecular cloning, *Nature 289*, 149–153 (1981).
22. Y. Nishida, T. Kataoka, N. Ishida, S. Nakai, T. Kushimoto, I. Bottcher, and T. Honjo, Cloning of mouse immunoglobulin gene and its location within the heavy chain gene cluster, *Proc. Natl. Acad. Sci. USA 78*, 1581–1585 (1981).
23. K. W. Moore, J. Rogers, T. Hunkapiller, P. Early, C. Nottenburg, I. Weissman, H. Bazin, R. Wall, and L. E. Hood, Expression of IgD may use both DNA rearrangement and RNA splicing mechanisms, *Proc. Natl. Acad. Sci. USA 78*, 1800–1804 (1981).
24. R. Maki, W. Roeder, A. Traunecker, C. Sidman, M. Wabl, W. Raschke, and S. Tonegawa, The role of DNA rearrangement and alternative RNA processing in the expression of immunoglobulin delta genes, *Cell 24*, 353–365 (1981).
25. M. M. Davis, S. K. Kim, and L. E. Hood, DNA sequences mediating class switching in α-immunoglobulins, *Science 209*, 1360–1365 (1980).
26. H. Sakano, R. Maki, Y. Kurosawa, W. Roeder, and S. Tonegawa, Two types of somatic recombination are necessary for the generation of complete immunoglobulin heavy-chain genes, *Nature 286*, 676–683 (1980).
27. J.-L. Preud'homme, J. Buxbaum, and M. D. Scharff, Mutagenesis of mouse myeloma cells with Melphalan, *Nature 245*, 320–322 (1973).
28. B. W. Penman and W. G. Thilly, Concentration-dependent mutation of diploid human lymphoblasts by methytnitronitrosoguanidine: The importance of phenotypic lag, *Somatic Cell Genet. 2*, 325–330 (1976).
29. L. Jacobs and R. Demars, Quantification of chemical mutagenesis in diploid human fibroblasts: Induction of azaguanine-resistant mutants by N-methyl-N'-nitro-N-nitrosoguanidine, *Mutat. Res. 53*, 29–53 (1978).
30. U. Friedrich and P. Coffino, Mutagenesis in 549 mouse lymphoma cells: Induction of resistance to ouabain, 6-thioguanine and dibutycyl cyclic AMP, *Proc. Natl. Acad. Sci. USA 74*, 679–683 (1977).
31. R. G. H. Cotton, D. S. Secher, and C. Milstein, Somatic mutation and the origin of antibody diversity. Clonal variability of the immunoglobulin produced by MOPC 21 cells in culture, *Eur. J. Immunol. 3*, 135–140 (1973).
32. K. Adetugbo, C. Milstein, and D. S. Secher, Molecular analysis of spontaneous somatic mutants, *Nature 265*, 299–304 (1977).
33. P. Coffino, R. Laskov, and M. D. Scharff, Immunoglobulin production: Method for quantitatively detecting variant myeloma cells, *Science 167*, 186–188 (1970).

34. P. Coffino, R. Baumal, R. Laskov, and M. D. Scharff, Cloning of mouse myeloma cells and detection of rare variants, *J. Cell. Physiol. 79*, 429–400 (1972).
35. W. D. Cook and M. D. Scharff, Antigen-binding mutants of mouse myeloma cells, *Proc. Natl. Acad. Sci. USA 74*, 5687–5691 (1977).
36. R. J. Wang, Effect of room fluorescent light on the deterioration of tissue culture medium, *In Vitro 12*, 19–22 (1976).
37. B. K. Birshtein, J.-L. Preud'homme, and M. D. Scharff, Variants of mouse myeloma cells that produce short immunoglobulin heavy chains, *Proc. Natl. Acad. Sci. USA 71*, 3478–3482 (1974).
38. J.-L. Preud'homme, B. K. Birshtein, and M. D. Scharff, Variants of a mouse myeloma cell line that synthesize immunoglobulin heavy chains having an altered serotype, *Proc. Natl. Acad. Sci. USA 72*, 1427–1430 (1975).
39. S. Koskimies and B. K. Birshtein, Primary and secondary variants in immunoglobulin heavy chain production, *Nature 264*, 480–482 (1976).
40. T. Francus, B. Dharmgrongartama, R. Campbell, M. D. Scharff, and B. K. Birshtein, IgG$_{2a}$-producing variants of an IgG$_{2b}$-producing mouse myeloma cell line, *J. Exp. Med. 147*, 1535–1550 (1978).
41. S. L. Morrison, Murine heavy chain disease, *Eur. J. Immunol. 8*, 194–199 (1978).
42. W. D. Cook, S. Rudikoff, A. M. Giusti, and M. D. Scharff, Somatic mutation in a cultured mouse myeloma cell affects antigen binding, *Proc. Natl. Acad. Sci. USA 79*, 1240–1248 (1982).
43. S. Rudikoff, A. M. Giusti, W. D. Cook, and M. D. Scharff, A single amino acid substitution altering antigen binding specificity, *Proc. Natl. Acad. Sci USA 79*, 1979–1983 (1982).
44. N. K. Jerne and A. A. Nordin, Plaque formation in agar by single antibody-producing cells, *Science 140*, 405 (1963).
45. G. Kohler and C. Milstein, Continuous cultures of fused cells secreting antibody of predefined specificity, *Nature 256*, 495–497 (1975).
46. A. Nisonoff, Coupling of diazonium compounds to proteins, in: *Methods in Immunology and Immunochemistry* (C. A. Williams and M. W. Chase, eds.), Vol. 1, pp. 120–126, Academic Press, New York (1967).
47. B. Chesebro and H. Metzger, Affinity labeling of a phosphorylcholine binding mouse myeloma protein, *Biochem. 11*, 766–771 (1972).
48. P. C. Isakson, J. L. Honegger, and S. C. Kinsky, Preparation of stable erythrocyte target cells suitable for detection of the antibody response to the haptens azobenzenearsonate, azophenyltrimethylammonium and azophenylphosphorylcholine by plaque-forming cell assay, *J. Immunol. Methods 25*, 89–96 (1979).
49. E. R. Gold and H. H. Fudenberg, Chromic chloride: A coupling reagent for passive hemagglutination reactions, *J. Immunol. 99*, 859–866 (1967).
50. J. W. Goding, The chromic chloride method of coupling antigens to erythrocytes: Definition of some important parameters, *J. Immunol. Methods 10*, 61–66 (1976).
51. R. Kofler and G. Wick, Some methodologic aspects of the chromium chloride method for coupling antigen to erythrocytes, *J. Immunol. Methods 16*, 201–209 (1977).
52. G. A. Molinaro, E. Maron, and S. Dray, Antigen-secreting cells: Enumeration by means of hybrid-antibody coated erythrocytes in a reverse hemolytic plaque assay, *Proc. Natl. Acad. Sci. USA 71*, 1229–1233 (1974).
53. E. Gronowicz, A. Coutinho, and F. Melchers, A plaque assay for all cells secreting Ig of a given type or class, *Eur. J. Immunol. 6*, 588–590 (1976).
54. A. J. Cunningham and A. Szenberg, Further improvements in the plaque technique for detecting single antibody-forming cells, *Immunology 14*, 599–600 (1968).

55. T. Mosmann and R. Baumal, Macroscopic cloning assay using complement fixation to isolate secretion variants of myeloma cells, *J. Immunol. Methods 10*, 119–125 (1976).

56. J. Sharon, S. L. Morrison, and E. A. Kabat, Detection of specific hybridoma clones by replica immunoabsorption of their secreted antibodies, *Proc. Natl. Acad. Sci. USA 76*, 1420–1424 (1979).

57. B. Liesegang, A. Radbruch, and K. Rajewsky, Isolation of myeloma variants with predefined variant surface immunoglobulin by cell sorting, *Proc. Natl. Acad. Sci. USA 75*, 3901–3905 (1978).

58. A. Radbruch, B. Liesegang, and K. Rajewsky, Isolation of variants of mouse myeloma X63 that express changed immunoglobulin class, *Proc. Natl. Acad. Sci. USA 77*, 2909–2913 (1980).

59. M. S. Neuberger and K. Rajewsky, Switch from hapten-specific immunoglobulin M to immunoglobulin D secretion in a hybrid mouse cell line, *Proc. Natl. Acad. Sci. USA 78*, 1138–1142 (1981).

60. B. Holtkamp, M. Cramer, H. Lemke, and K. Rajewsky, Isolation of a cloned cell line expressing variant H-2K^k using fluorescence-activated cell sorting, *Nature 289*, 66–68 (1981).

61. J. L. Dangl, D. R. Parks, V. T. Oi, and L. A. Herzenberg, Rapid isolation of cloned isotype switch variants using fluorescence activated cell sorting, *J. Imm. Methods, 52*, 1–14 (1982).

62. D. R. Parks, V. M. Bryan, V. T. Oi, and L. A. Herzenberg, Antigen-specific identification and cloning of hybridomas with a fluorescence-activated cell sorter, *Proc. Natl. Acad. Sci. USA 76*, 1962–1966 (1979).

63. H. Schreiber and P. Leibson, Suppression of myeloma growth *in vitro* by anti-idiotypic antibodies: Inhibition of DNA synthesis and colony formation, *J. Natl. Cancer Inst. 60*, 225–233 (1978).

64. T. V. Rajan, H-2 Antigen variants in a cultured heterozygous mouse leukemia cell line, VII. Effect of selection with a hybridoma antibody, *Immunogenetics 10*, 423–431 (1980).

65. P. J. Leibson, H. Schreiber, M. R. Loken, S. Panem, and D. A. Rowley, Time-dependent resistance or susceptibility of tumor cells to cytotoxic antibody after exposure to a chemotherapeutic agent, *Proc. Natl. Acad. Sci USA 75*, 6202–6206 (1978).

66. G. Kohler and M. J. Shulman, Immunoglobulin M mutants, *Eur. J. Immunol. 10*, 467–476 (1980).

67. M. J. Shulman, C. Filkin, and C. Heusser, Mutations affecting the structure and function of immunoglobulin M, *Mol. and Cell. Biol. 2*, 1033–1043 (1982).

68. K. A. Krolick, C. Villemez, P. Isakson, J. W. Uhr, and E. S. Vitetta, Selective killing of normal or neoplastic B cells by antibodies coupled to the A chain of ricin, *Proc. Natl. Acad. Sci. USA 77*, 5419–5423 (1980).

69. D. G. Gilliband, Z. Steplewski, R. J. Collier, K. F. Mitchell, T. H. Chang, and H. Koprowski, Antibody-directed cytotoxic agents, Use of monoclonal antibody to direct the action of toxin A chains to colorectal carcinoma cells, *Proc. Natl. Acad. Sci. USA 77*, 4539–4543 (1980).

70. M.-T. B. Davis and J. F. Preston, A conjugate of α-amanitin and monoclonal immunoglobulin G to Thy 1.2 antigen is selectively toxic to T lymphoma cells, *Science 213*, 1385–1388 (1981).

71. D. H. Margulies, W. M. Kuehl, and M. D. Scharff, Somatic cell hybridization of mouse myeloma cells, *Cell 8*, 405–415 (1976).

72. P. J. Gearhart, N. D. Johnson, R. Douglas, and L. Hood, IgG antibodies to phosphorylcholine exhibit more diversity than their IgM counterparts, *Nature 219*, 29–34 (1981).

73. N. M. Gough and O. Bernard, Sequences of the joining region genes for immunoglobulin heavy chains and their role in generation of antibody diversity, *Proc. Natl. Acad. Sci. USA 78*, 509–513 (1981).

74. M. Pech, J. Hochtl, M. Schnell, and H. G. Zachau, Differences between germ-line and rearranged immunoglobulin V coding sequences suggest a localized mutation mechanism, *Nature 291,* 668–670 (1981).
75. E. Selsing and U. Storb, Somatic mutation of immunoglobulin light-chain variable-region genes. *Cell 25,* 47–58 (1981).
76. A. L. Bothewell, M. Paskind, M. Reth, T. Imanishi-Kari, K. Rajewsky, and D. Baltimore, Heavy chain variable region contribution to the NPb family of antibodies: Somatic mutation evident in a gamma 2a variable region, *Cell 24,* 625–637 (1981).
77. H. K. Gershenfeld, A. Tsukamoto, I. L. Weissman, and R. Joho, Somatic diversification is required to generate the V genes of MOPC 511 and MOPC 167 myeloma proteins, *Proc. Natl. Acad. Sci. USA 78,* 7674–7678 (1981).
78. S. L. Morrison and M. D. Scharff, Mutational events in mouse myeloma cells, *CRC Crit. Rev. Immunol. 3,* 1–22 (1981).
79. T. Honjo, M. Obata, Y. Yamawaki-Kataoka, T. Kataoka, T. Kawakamim, N. Takahashi, and Y. Mano, Cloning and complete nucleotide sequence of mouse immunoglobulin γ_1 chain gene, *Cell 18,* 559–568 (1979).
80. A. L. Kenter and B. K. Birshtein, Genetic mechanism accounting for precise immunoglobulin domain deletion in a variant of MPC 11 myeloma cells, *Science 206,* 1307–1309 (1979).
81. S. Weitzman and M. D. Scharff, Mouse myeloma mutants blocked in the assembly, glycosylation and secretion of immunoglobulin, *J. Mol. Biol. 102,* 237–252 (1976).
82. S. Weitzman, L. Palmer, and M. Grennon, Serum decay and placental transport of a mutant mouse myeloma immunoglobulin with defective polypeptide and oligosaccharide structure, *J. Immunol. 122,* 12–18 (1979).
83. D. J. Zack, S. L. Morrison, W. D. Cook, W. Dackowski, and M. D. Scharff, Somatically generated mouse myeloma variants synthesizing IgA half-molecules, *J. Exp. Med. 154,* 1554–1659 (1981).
84. E. A. Robinson and E. Appella, Amino acid sequence of a mouse myeloma immunoglobulin heavy chain (MOPC 47A) with a 100-residue deletion, *J. Biol. Chem. 254,* 11418–11430 (1979).
85. K. Adetugbo, Spontaneous somatic mutations, structural studies on mutant immunoglobulins, *J. Biol. Chem. 253,* 6076–6080 (1978).
86. W. Cook, C. Desaymard, A. Giusti, S.-P. Kwan, P. Thammana, D. Yelton, D. Zack, S. Rudikoff, and M. D. Scharff, Somatic mutations in the variable region of an antigen binding myeloma, in: *Immunoglobulin Idiotypes* (C. Janeway, E. E. Sercarz, and H. Wigzell, eds.), pp. 281–292, Academic Press, New York (1981).
87. H. Sakano, J. H. Rogers, K. Huppi, C. Brack, A. Traunecker, R. Maki, R. Wall, and S. Tonegawa, Domains and the hinge region of an immunoglobulin heavy chain are encoded in separate DNA segments, *Nature 277,* 627–633 (1979).
88. W. Dunnick, T. H. Rabbits, and C. Milstein, A mouse immunoglobulin heavy chain deletion mutant: Isolation of a cDNA clone and sequence analysis of the mRNA, *Nucl. Acids Res. 8,* 1475–1484 (1980).
89. W. Dunnick, T. H. Rabbits, and C. Milstein, An immunoglobulin deletion mutant with implications for the heavy-chain switch and RNA splicing, *Nature 286,* 669–675 (1980).
90. S. Morrison and B. Birshtein, personal communication.
91. R. J. Monk, S. L. Morrison, and C. Milcarek, Heavy-chain mutants derived from γ_{2b} mouse myeloma: Characterization of heavy-chain messenger ribonucleic acid, proteins, and secretion in deletion mutants and messenger ribonucleic acid in γ_{2a} mutant progeny, *Biochemistry 20,* 2330–2339 (1981).

92. W. D. Cook, B. Dharmgrongartama, and M. D. Scharff, Variable and constant region variants, in: *Cells of Immunoglobulin Synthesis* (B. Pernis and H. J. Vogel, eds.), pp. 99–112, Academic Press, New York (1979).

93. T. Francus and B. K. Birshtein, An IgG$_{2a}$-producing variant of an IgG$_{2b}$-producing mouse myeloma cell line. Structural studies on the Fc region of parent and variant heavy chains, *Biochemistry 17*, 4324–4331 (1978).

94. B. K. Birshtein, R. Campbell, and M. L. Greenberg, A $\gamma_{2b}\gamma_{2a}$ hybrid immunoglobulin heavy chain produced by a variant of the MPC-11 mouse myeloma cell line, *Biochemistry 19*, 1730–1737 (1980).

95. L. A. Eckhardt, S. A. Tilley, R. B. Lang, K. B. Marcu, and B. K. Birshtein, DNA rearrangements in MPC 11 immunoglobulin heavy chain class switch variants, *Proc. Natl. Acad. Sci. USA. 79*, 3006–3010 (1982).

96. P. Thammana and M. D. Scharff, Immunoglobulin heavy chain class switch from IgM to IgG in a hybridoma, *Europ. J. Imm. 13*, 614–619 (1983).

97. W. M. Kuehl and M. D. Scharff, Synthesis of a carboxyl-terminal (constant region) fragment of immunoglobulin light chain by a mouse myeloma cell line, *J. Mol. Biol. 89*, 409–421 (1974).

98. E. Choi, M. Kuehl, and R. Wall, RNA splicing generates a variant light chain from an aberrantly rearranged gene, *Nature 286*, 776–779 (1980).

99. J. G. Seidman and P. Leder, A mutant immunoglobulin light chain is formed by aberrant DNA- and RNA-splicing events, *Nature 286*, 779–783 (1980).

100. S.-P. Kwan, E. E. Max, J. G. Seidman, P. Leder, and M. D. Scharff, Two kappa immunoglobulin genes are expressed in the myeloma S107, *Cell 26*, 57–66 (1981).

101. O. Bernard, N. M. Gough, and J. M. Adams, Plasmacytomas with more than one immunoglobulin mRNA: Implications for allelic exclusion, *Proc. Natl. Acad. Sci. USA 78*, 5812–5816 (1981).

102. C. Coleclough, R. P. Perry, K. Karjalainen, and M. Weigert, Aberrant rearrangements contribute significantly to the allelic exclusion of immunoglobulin gene expression, *Nature 290*, 372–378 (1981).

103. M. Wallach, R. Ishay-Michaeli, David Givol, and Reuven Laskov, Immunoglobulin mRNA in myeloma mutants, *J. Imm. 128*, 684–690 (1982).

104. P. Ponte, M. Dean, V. H. Pepe, and G. Sonenshein, Regulation of heavy chain gene expression in mouse myeloma MOPC 315 cells, abstract, *From Gene to Protein: Translation into Biotechnology, The Fourteenth Miami Winter Symposium* (F. Ahmed, J. Shultz, E. E. Smith, and W. J. Whelan, eds.), Academic Press, New York, p. 86 (1982).

105. D. E. Yelton and M. D. Scharff, Monoclonal antibodies, a powerful new tool in biology and medicine, *Annu. Rev. Biochem. 50*, 657–680 (1981).

11

Detection of Chemically Induced Y-Chromosomal Nondisjunction in Human Spermatozoa

MARVIN S. LEGATOR AND ROBERT W. KAPP, JR.

1. INTRODUCTION

In the area of chemical mutagenesis certain procedures seem to gain considerable popularity even though their relevance to identifying human hazards is questionable or the genetic basis for the tests has yet to be established. Conversely, there are certain procedures where the potential for identifying genetic lesions in relevant systems is considerable, but their utilization is slow to develop. A procedure with great potential for identifying mutagens that induce cytogenetic changes in man is the detection of chemically induced increase in Y chromosomes in human sperm. This procedure, utilizing fluorochromes, may be one of the more important developments in recent years in the field of chemical mutagenesis. The amount of data, however, and presumably the number of investigators evaluating this technique are minimal. In this chapter, we will describe the studies that led to the development of this method, discuss the technique, and present data obtained using this procedure.

MARVIN S. LEGATOR • Division of Environmental Toxicology, Department of Preventive Medicine and Community Health, The University of Texas Medical Branch, Galveston, Texas 77550. ROBERT W. KAPP, JR. • East Laboratory, Bio/dynamics, Inc., East Millstone, New Jersey 08873.

2. BACKGROUND

The use of fluorescent dyes to study the organization of chromosomes was demonstrated by Caspersson and co-workers.[1-3] These investigators demonstrated that quinacrine-mustard enhances fluorescence at specific segments of plant chromosomes. This fluorescence results from preferential binding to certain regions of the chromosome, primarily in heterochromatic regions accessible to DNA bases. Barlow and Vosa,[4] using quinacrine, were able to detect Y chromosomes in mature spermatozoa. Human spermatozoa were smeared on slides, dried in air, washed in absolute ethanol for 5 min, and then stained for 20 min in 0.005% quinacrine. After slide preparation spermatozoa were viewed with fluorescent illumination. Chromatin in the heads of spermatozoa were found to fluoresce, with the basal third of the head presenting a denser fluorescent mass than the upper portion. The authors found that approximately 50% of the sperm stained showed a fluorescent body, which was called the "F" body, and concluded that this "F" body was a fluorescent site from the chromatin present in the distal segment of the long arm of the Y chromosome. These investigators believed that the "F" body represented the Y chromosome for the following reasons:

1. In mitotic and meiotic metaphase preparations, a segment of the Y chromosome fluoresces more strongly than any other chromosome.
2. In interphase nuclei of normal XY males, there is only one strongly fluorescent spot, while in nuclei from XYY males there are two such spots.
3. Nuclei of normal XX females exhibit no "F" bodies and in spermatozoa the frequency with which Y bodies are seen approaches that expected from a segregation of Y chromosome at meiosis.

Shortly after the initial study of Barlow and Vosa,[4] Sumner et al.[5] examined human sperm specimens stained with quinacrine hydrochloride and attempted to correlate fluorescence with DNA content using the feulgen reaction and optical density measurements. The authors found that a sperm with an "F" body contained significantly less DNA than the nonfluorescent sperm (-"F" body) and that this difference was equivalent to the calculated DNA difference between 23X and 23Y haploid chromosome compliments. Two "F" bodies were found in a little over 1% of the sperm examined and the sperm DNA content was found to be intermediate between the value determined for the X-bearing and Y-bearing sperm. From the studies of human sperm, the authors concluded that the double-fluorescent sperm have a 24 YY chromosome constitution. With the vast majority of doubly fluorescing sperm, the DNA content indicated that they were clearly not diploid, but disomic for the

Y chromosome. The authors concluded (1) that 24 YY sperm must result from nondisjunction of a Y chromosome at the second division of meiosis and therefore an equal number of 22 chromosome sperm deficient for a sex chromosome must also be present, and (2) second division nondisjunction does not involve the autosomes as frequently as the Y chromosomes, otherwise more than half of all sperm produced would be aneuploid. The authors cite evidence to indicate that there is a diminished efficiency of 24 YY sperm relative to normal sperm in achieving fertilization. The evidence for this is based on an approximate 15 times fewer cases of 47 XYY offspring than expected if YY sperm and 47 Y embryos were not at a disadvantage, and the lack of evidence of *in utero* loss of 47 XYY embryos, which indicates a loss of efficiency of YY sperm in achieving fertilization.

Sumner and Robinson[6] used an integrating microinterferometer to measure dry mass of sperm heads and since dry mass was found to be proportional to DNA content, dry mass could be used to measure DNA content. With this procedure the authors were able to confirm their earlier work indicating a difference in DNA content between spermatozoa showing an "F" body (Y-bearing) and spermatozoa with no such body (X-bearing). A difference of 2.13% was found between these two classes, which corresponded to the expected difference in DNA content between X- and Y-bearing sperm. The authors believed that this represented irrefutable evidence that human spermatozoa with one and no quinacrine-fluorescent spots represent Y- and X-bearing spermatozoa, respectively. The dry mass of spermatozoa with two spots proved to be significantly lower than that of X-bearing spermatozoa and as low as or lower than that of Y-bearing spermatozoa. Thus two "F" bodies could not be confirmed as being due to an extra Y. The authors suggest, however, that loss of material might occur during processing, producing an artificially low value for dry mass, and that present techniques may not be capable of resolving the error of the two "F" bodies in normal individuals. The background rate of this technique has, with amazing consistency, been reported to be approximately 1%. The 2.38% reported by these investigators may suggest that in an individual with XYY anomaly there is a selection against two "F"-bearing sperm but it still is significantly above the normal range. The following discussion of the work of Caspersson and Zech[3] would be consistent with this interpretation.

A key finding for the eventual development of the YFF procedure was made by Caspersson and Zech,[3] using fluorescent analysis with YFF individuals. Prior to this study, individuals with XYY anomaly had not been observed to produce XYY sons and therefore some geneticists concluded that there is a mechnism that eliminates the second Y from all spermatocytes. Thompson *et al.*[7] noted that all six sons of an XYY individual had normal XY chromosome compliment. They could find no conclusive evidence in either spermatogonial preparation or in first meiotic metaphases to indicate two Y chromosomes in an XYY individual. It was suggested that selection toward chromosomally normal spermatocytes occurs before meiosis in XYY males. Caspersson and Zech,[3] by the use of fluorescent staining, were able to show that, in fact, a sizable fraction of the spermatocytes from XYY individuals contained two Y's and suggested that, in theory at least, the individuals of XYY anomaly should be able to beget XYY sons, and indeed there have been such reported cases. This observation by Caspersson and Zech pertaining to spermatocytes of XYY individuals is extremely important for confirming that the "F" body is, indeed, the Y chromosome. This important observation seems to have been generally overlooked by individuals evaluating this procedure, and much discussion has transpired concerning the validity of the fluorescent staining for identifying the Y body. Although in the article by Caspersson and Zech, the exact percentage of extra fluorescent Y's in individuals with the XYY anomaly is not given, the specific statement indicates that a sizable fraction of the spermatocytes contain two Y's. A serious investigation has yet to be carried out to indicate the percentage of extra Y bodies in spermatocytes of XYY irdividuals.

3. AGENTS THAT INCREASE YFF BODIES IN HUMAN SPERM

The identification of "F" bodies in sperm by fluorescent dyes and the fact that the "F" bodies in all likelihood represent Y chromosomes suggested an important tool for identifying agents that induce chromosomal nondisjunction in human sperm. Kapp and coworkers[8-10] determined the effect of antineoplastic agents, fluoroscopy, X-rays, flagyl, and dibromochloropropane on increasing the frequency of double F bodies following treatment in selected individuals.

3.1. Methodology

The following procedure was used for determining the percentage of double "F" bodies after treatment.

1. Ejaculates were collected by masturbation into sterile, siliconized glass bottles, which were then brought to the laboratory for slide preparation.
2. Slides were prepared by placing one drop of semen upon a slide and then pressing another slide firmly against the first. The two slides were pulled apart to produce a uniform film and were then allowed to dry in a horizonal position for about 24 hr.

3. The dried semen slides were fixed in absolute methanol for 15 min and were then transferred to the following staining solution for 40 min: (a) 50 mg quinacrine dihydrochloride (Sigma Chemical Co., St. Louis), (b) 50 ml tap water, (c) 5 ml of ethanol. The slides were again drained for about 1 min and coverslipped in two drops of McIlvaine's buffer at pH 5.5 and left undisturbed in a horizontal position for 3 hr.

4. All slides were examined with fluorescent microscope using a 100× oil immersion objective, a darkfield condenser, and an HBO 200 high-pressure mercury vapor lamp as a light source. The exciter filter was a type BG-12, which peaked at 3655 Å with a secondary peak between 7000 and 8000 Å. The barrier filter absorbed frequencies below 4300 Å, whereby the primary fluorescence could be distinguished from the particular reaction for the specimen.

5. If the slides were scorable, up to 1000 spermatozoa were examined. If fewer than 400 spermatozoa were scored, the results were not used.

6. Each spermatozoan had to meet the following criteria in order to be considered for scoring: (a) normal size, (b) normal shape, (c) intact with complete membranes, (d) attached tail.

7. Once the scorability of each spermatozoan was established, the fluorescent body had to meet the following criteria in order to be scored: (a) it had to fall within the intact sperm head, (b) it had to lie in the focal plane of the sperm; (c) it had to form a distinct point of light rather than a large diffuse area of fluorescence, which usually characterizes overlapped chromatin.

The spermatozoa meeting the above criteria were scored into the following categories: (1) Spermatozoa with no fluorescent bodies, (2) spermatozoa with one fluorescent body (YF), (3) spermatozoa with two fluorescent bodies (YFF). Figure 1 illustrates the fluorescent bodies.

These categorized spermatozoa counts were taken from three representative areas of the slide surface. The number of sperm from each category (zero, one, and two "F" bodies) was expressed as a percent of the total number of spermatozoa examined.

3.2. Results to Date

Kapp and Jacobson[10] summarized the results of their study, which were presented as case studies, with the exception of the investigation of the industrial chemical dibromochloropropane. The consistency of this procedure is illustrated in Figure 2, where one individual was sampled 30 times in a 420-day period (mean of 1.3% sperm bearing double "F" bodies). In two other such control samples, a mean frequency of 1.2% and 1.3% YFF sperm was reported.

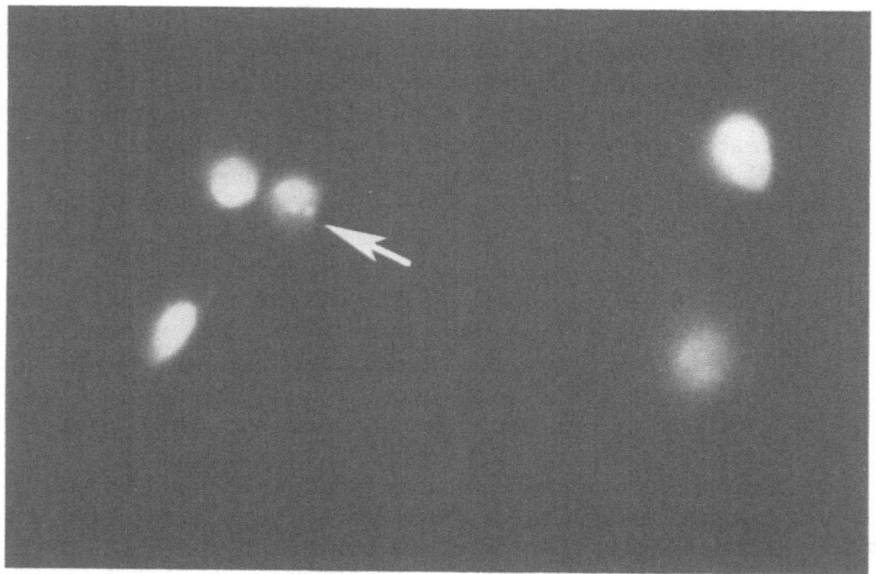

Figure 1. Photomicrograph of human spermatozoa stained with quinacrine dihydrochloride under fluorescent microscopy (1000×). The arrow denotes a fluorescent body. Since there are two such bodies in this sperm head, it is postulated that there are two Y chromosomes present. This implies that the Y chromosomes have failed to separate at anaphase II.

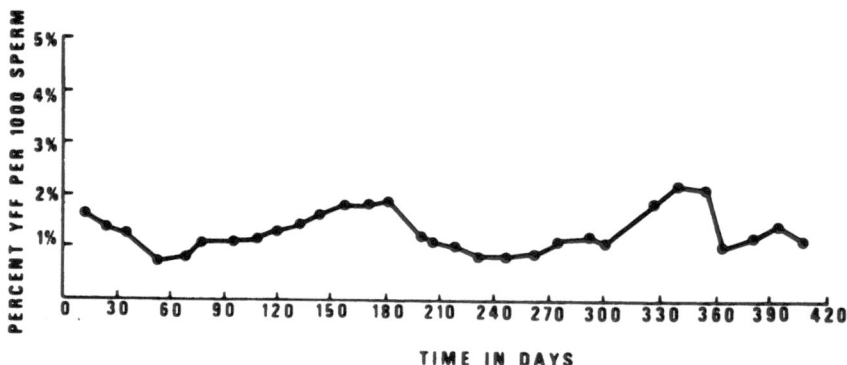

Figure 2. Control 1: Incidence of YFF sperm in 30 serial samples over 420 days from a 32-year-old white donor whose inseminations have resulted in over 100 successful pregnancies.

In this regard, it is interesting to note that in the work of Sumner *et al.*[5] the number of sperm with two Y bodies was reported as 1.26%. Indeed, investigations in the laboratory of one of the authors (MSL) as well as others that are using this technique seem to indicate that the normal background rate is fairly constant, where approximately 1% of the total sperm population exhibit double Y bodies. The results with various treatments are presented in Figures 3–6. Sequential studies of individuals exposed to adriamycin, occupational fluoroscopy, flagyl therapy plus diagnostic radiation, and X-ray therapy all indicate a marked increase in the YFF-bearing sperm varied with the treatment, but in most cases some decrease in number was seen in the 80th to 100th day following treatment.

Of considerable interest was the work carried out with nematocide, dibromochloropropane (DBCP), which is known to be an animal carcinogen and produce oligospermia and azoospermia in exposed workers. A single semen sample was collected from each of 30 individuals who had experienced occu-

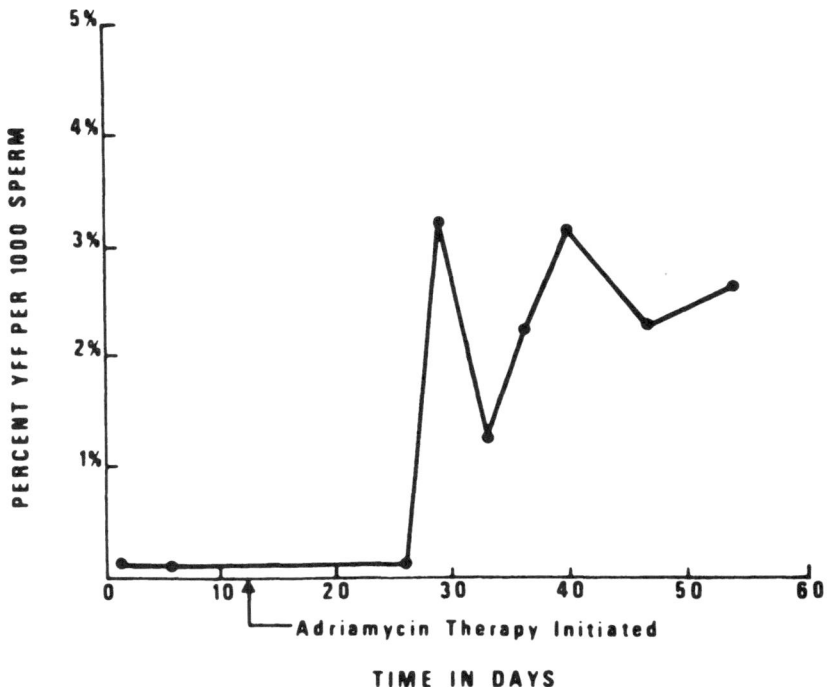

Figure 3. Exposed 2: Incidence of YFF sperm in nine serial samples over 55 days from a 22-year-old white donor who began treatment with adriamycin at the point of the arrow.

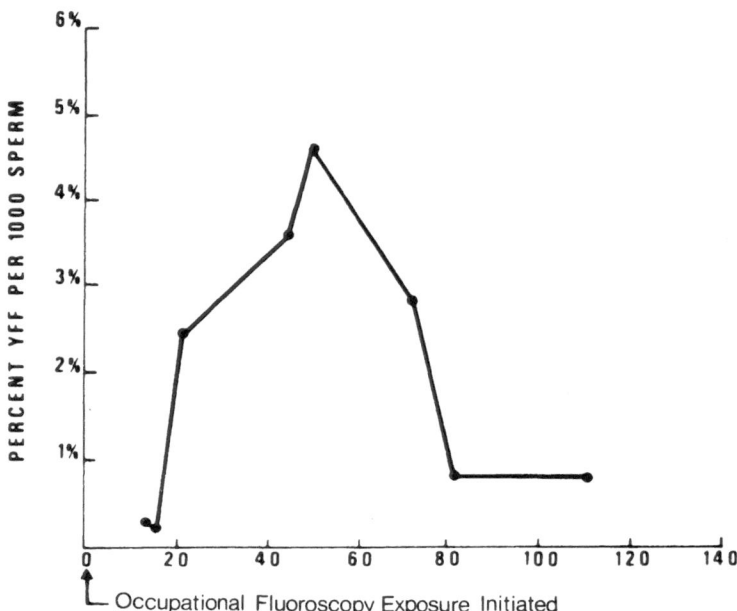

Figure 4. Exposed 3: Incidence of YFF sperm in eight serial samples over 110 days from a 28-year-old physician who began fluoroscopy residency at the point of the arrow.

pational exposure to DBCP. Of the 30 samples collected, 12 were azoospermic and were not analyzable by the YFF technique. The average age of the 18 workers examined was 33.8 years. The average length of worker exposure was 15.2 months (range 6–18 months).

Individual worker-exposure-level estimates were not available at the production plant; however, the exposure levels in the production area were estimated to be less than one part per million.[11] Table I displays data from the 18 men who had been exposed to DBCP and whose semen were analyzable (W-1 through W-18). It was found that the average YF frequency of these individuals was 41.8% (range 36.3–46.3), which is similar to that for the nonexposed individuals. Of interest is the fact that these DBCP-exposed workers showed a higher average YFF frequency (3.8%; range 2.0–5.3%) when compared to the initial sample from each of the three control individuals. Table II presents the distribution of individuals with normal (less than 2%) and abnormal (greater than 2%) incidence of YFF spermatozoa. As can be seen, all three of the initial samples of the nonexposed individuals fell within the normal range, while 16–18 DBCP-exposed workers fell outside the normal

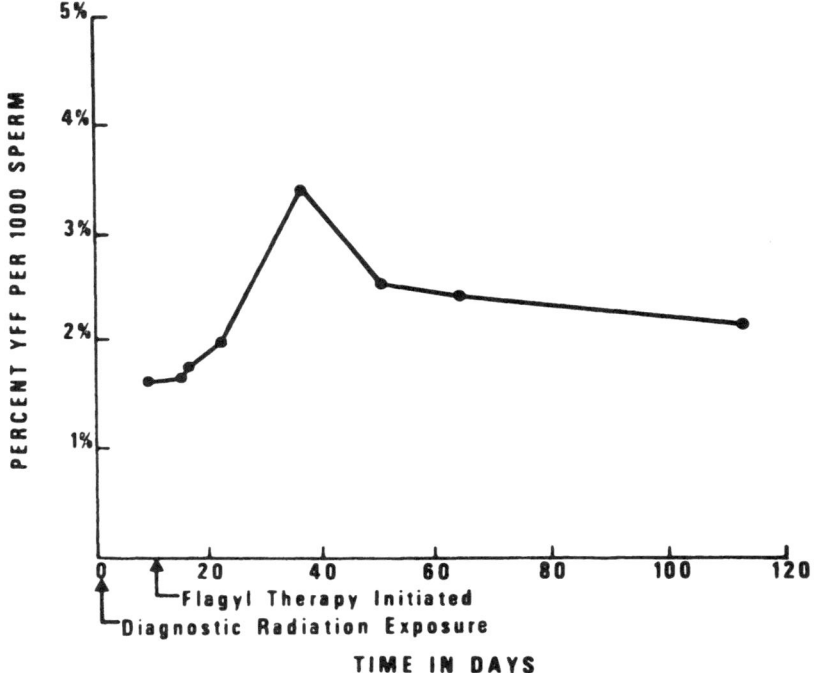

Figure 5. Exposed 4: Incidence of YFF sperm in eight serial samples over 118 days from a 32-year-old white research scientist who was exposed to diagnostic radiation 9 days before starting a 10-day regimen of flagyl.

range. The DBCP-exposed workers YFF values are statistically significantly elevated ($P < 0.01$) when compared to the nonexposed individuals as determined by χ^2 analysis with one degree of freedom.[8]

4. DISCUSSION

The preponderance of evidence would indicate that the brightly fluorescent "F" bodies represent the distal portion of the Y chromosomes. On the basis of dry mass measurements (dry mass being proportional to DNA content), Sumner and Robinson[6] stated that there is "irrefutable" evidence that human spermatozoa with one and no quinacrine-fluorescent spots represent Y- and X-bearing spermatozoa, respectively. This statement is bolstered by earlier work, where they as well as others have shown that with meiotic and mitotic

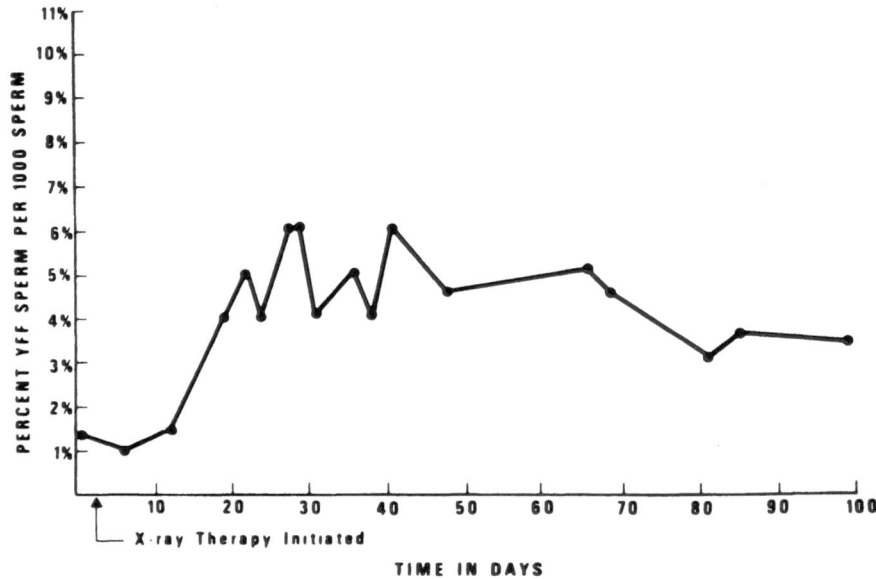

Figure 6. Exposed 5: Incidence of YFF sperm in 18 serial samples over 100 days from a 28-year-old white donor who was receiving X-ray therapy at the point of the arrow.

Table I
YF and YFF Frequencies in Semen Samples
from DBCP-Exposed Workmen

Case number	YF, %	YFF, %
16	44.5	3.3
17	41.3	2.8
18	42.3	5.0
19	40.0	4.5
20	41.5	3.8
21	46.3	3.8
22	42.5	2.0
23	40.3	2.8
24	37.3	4.0
25	41.3	4.3
26	36.3	2.0
27	40.5	5.0
28	43.3	5.3
29	39.0	3.5
30	43.0	4.0
31	46.0	4.0
32	39.5	4.5
33	44.8	4.0
Range	36.3–46.3	2–5.3
Mean	41.65 $\pm$ 2.76	3.81 $\pm$ 0.95

Table II
Distribution of Nonexposed and DBCP-Exposed Individuals as a
Function of the Percentage of YFF Sperm

Group	Number of individuals with YFF sperm	
	0–2%	2%
Nonexposed individuals	15	0
DBCP-exposed individuals	2	16

$\chi_1^2 = 22.5$; $P < 0.001$.

material from various sources the fluorescent spot could always be associated with the Y chromosome.

Several investigations have questioned the correlation between the "F" bodies and the Y chromosome. It has been suggested that the two "F" bodies may represent a single large "Y" chromosome with the two fluorescent spots.[6] In a study by Beatty,[12] 83% of Y chromosome were represented by "F" bodies and 79% of the haploid heads and 14.9% of the diploid heads were said to contain "adventitious" bodies that fluoresce like "F" bodies. It is difficult, however, to attribute a single "F" body as indicating a segment of a "Y" chromosome and question the origin of the second "F" body. The likelihood of the second "F" body not corresponding to the "Y" chromosome is further diminished when certain criteria are used for spermatozoa analysis, including: selection for normal size and shape, examining those sperm where the fluorescent body has to lie in the focal plane of the sperm, and requiring that the spots be distinct. It is difficult to perceive that "adventitious bodies" (bacteria or artifacts) would fall within the focal plane of the sperm head and fluoresce with the same intensity as a true "F" body. It is probable that contamination such as bacteria and debris would also be present at various sites within the preparation and with a frequency far greater than two discrete spots, which are the maximum usually observed in this procedure. Kapp and Jacobson[10] observed only 10/860,000 sperms analyzed (error rate less than 0.0012%) where more than two "F" bodies were found. "Adventitous" bodies if present would seem not to represent a major problem, and the criteria set forth for analysis minimize false readings.

From available evidence, primarily cytological, the most likely interpretation of data is that spermatozoa with two "F" bodies are indicative of a nondisjunctional event that occurred at the second meiotic division and represent YY sperm.

The most compelling evidence, however, for the nondisjunctional origin of the spermatozoa with two "F" bodies may be the studies carried out with agents that are known to cause genetic damage. Although the data base is limited, the case study approach carried out with this technique maximizes the inference of chemical causation. With adriamycin therapy, fluoroscopy, flagyl therapy plus diagnostic radiation, and X-ray therapy, in some cases individuals exhibiting near normal values before treatment showed a 300–600% increase in sperm with two "F" bodies after treatment, which was then followed by a gradual decrease of double "F" bodies in sperm.

The utility of this method is further illustrated with 18 workers exposed to the agricultural chemical dibromochloropropane. The marked increase of spermatozoa with two fluorescent bodies with this chemical is especially striking. This chemical is known to be carcinogenic, and to produce testicular atrophy, as well as oligospermia and azoospermia. The results of Kapp[9] indicate a genetic affect on individuals who were not rendered sterile by exposure to the chemical.

The fluorescent Y seems to be a unique property of humans and gorillas, and the lack of a suitable experimental animal model may, in part, be responsible for the slow development of this procedure. In human studies, the genetic importance of this technique, its noninvasive nature and relatively stable background rates, and the studies to date suggest that this is an excellent method for detecting mutagenic agents in high-risk populations. With the limited data base it is premature to forecast the eventual significance of this procedure; however, the profound potential of this procedure should mandate increased investigation.

REFERENCES

1. T. Caspersson, S. Farber, G. E. Foley, J. R. Kudynowski, E. J. Modest, E. Simonsson, U. Wagh, and L. Zech, Distinction between extra G-like chromosomes by quinacrine mustard fluorescence analysis, *Exp. Cell Res. 49*, 219–222 (1968).
2. T. Caspersson, S. Faber, G. E. Foley, J. R. Kudynowski, E. J. Modest, E. Simonsson, U. Wagh, and L. Zech, Chemical differentiation along metaphase chromosomes, *Exp. Cell. Res. 49*, 219 (1968).
3. T. Caspersson and L. Zech, Chromosome identification by fluorescence, in: *Medical Genetics* (V. A. McKusick and R. Claiborne, eds.), pp. 27–88, H. P. Publishing Co., New York (1973).
4. P. Barlow and D. G. Vosa, The Y chromosome in human spermatozoa, *Nature (London) 226*, 961–962 (1970).
5. A. T. Sumner, J. A. Robinson and J. J. Evans, Distinguishing between X, Y and YY-bearing human spermatozoa by fluorescence and DNA contact, *Nature New Biol. 22*, 231–233 (1971).
6. A. T. Sumner and J. A. Robinson, A difference in dry mass between the heads of X- and Y-bearing human spermatozoa, *J. Reprod. Fertil. 48*, 9–15 (1976).

7. H. Thompson, J. Mecylik, and F. Hecht, Reproduction and meiosis in XYY, *Lancet 2*, 831 (1967).

8. R. W. Kapp, Jr., D. J. Picciano, and C. C. Jacobson, Y Chromosomal nondisjunction in dibromochloropropane-exposed workmen, *Mutat. Res. 64*, 47–51 (1979).

9. R. W. Kapp, Jr. Detection of aneuploidy in human sperm, *Environ. Health Perspect. 31*, 27–31 (1979).

10. R. W. Kapp, Jr., and C. B. Jacobson, Analysis of human spermatozoa for Y chromosomes nondisjunction, *Teratog. Carcinog. Mutagen. 1*, 193–211 (1980).

11. OSHA, Occupational exposure to 1,2-dibromo-3-chloropropane. *Fed. Regist. 1977*, 45536–45549 (1977).

12. R. A. Beatty, F-Bodies as Y chromosome markers in mature human spermheads, *Cytogenet. Cell Genet. 18*, 33–49 (1977).

Index